THE MEXICAN TREASURY

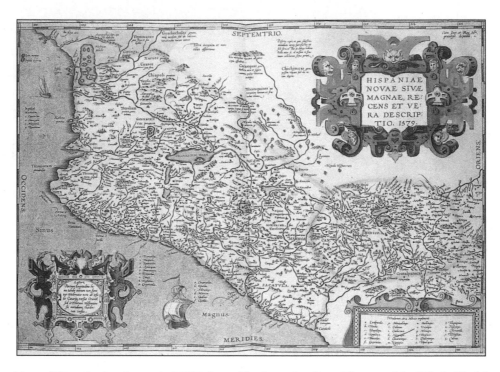

Map of New Spain, drawn in 1577, from Abraham Ortelius, *Theatre of the Whole World*, first English edition, edited and published by John Norton (London, 1606).

Courtesy of the British Library.

THE MEXICAN TREASURY

THE WRITINGS OF DR. FRANCISCO HERNÁNDEZ

SIMON VAREY

EDITOR

RAFAEL CHABRÁN

CYNTHIA L. CHAMBERLIN

SIMON VAREY

TRANSLATORS

STANFORD UNIVERSITY PRESS
Stanford, California

Stanford University Press
Stanford, California

© 2000 by the Board of Trustees of the
Leland Stanford Junior University

Printed in the United States of America

Library of Congress Cataloging-in-Publication Data

Hernández, Francisco, 1517–1587.
 The Mexican treasury : the writings of Dr. Francisco Hernández / edited by Simon
Varey ; translated by Rafael Chabrán, Cynthia L. Chamberlin, and Simon Varey.
  p. cm.
Includes index.
ISBN 0-8047-3963-3 (cloth : alk. paper)
 1. Natural history—Mexico—Pre-Linnean works. 2. Materia medica—Mexico—Early
works to 1800. I. Varey, Simon, 1951–   . II. Title.
QH107.H53 2000
508.72—dc21

                                                                            00-026519

Original printing 2000

Last figure indicates the year of this printing:

08 07 06 05 04 03 02 01 00

Typeset by Princeton Editorial Associates, Inc., Scottsdale, Arizona, in
9.75/16 Berkeley Old Style Medium.

CONTENTS

INTRODUCTION

The Hernández Texts • 3

RAFAEL CHABRÁN AND SIMON VAREY

The *Natural History of New Spain* • 26

JESÚS BUSTAMANTE

➷ THE TEXTS

MEXICO, 1571–1615

THE LOW COUNTRIES, 1630–1648

ILLUSTRATIONS

PREFACE AND ACKNOWLEDGMENTS

This volume contains a selection of English translations from the substantial corpus of writings by Francisco Hernández (1515–87), one of the foremost Spanish physicians of the sixteenth century, royal doctor, and, in the 1570s, chief medical officer in New Spain. King Philip II of Spain sent Hernández to the New World to research and describe the natural history of the region, assess the medicinal usefulness of the natural resources, and gather ethnographic materials for an anthropological history. When Hernández set out from Seville in 1570, he had already begun to translate Pliny's *Natural History* into Spanish and write a detailed commentary on it. By the time he returned to his homeland from New Spain in 1577, he had finished his edition of Pliny and written a vast *Natural History* of his own, together with an ethnographic volume that he called *Antiquities of New Spain,* a missionary poem, a practical index of medications used in New Spain, and several works (now lost) that had botanical and medical significance. The story of what happened to the manuscripts that Hernández left at his death is long, complex, and fascinating. The two introductory essays in this volume tell as much of that story as space permits.

In our texts, we offer a collection of writings representative not only of the varied accomplishments of Hernández but more particularly of the manner in which his work on Mexican natural history was disseminated, principally in the seventeenth and eighteenth centuries. Surprisingly, many of our selections have been unknown or unrecognized for more than two hundred years. Our texts constitute one of two volumes in which an international team of scholars explores the world of Francisco Hernández. Our companion volume, *Searching for the Secrets of Nature,* comprises a collection of essays interpreting the man and his achievements. The two volumes are intimately linked.

The task of translating the work of Francisco Hernández has taken us to many libraries, where we have incurred many debts. We are particularly grateful to the staffs of the British Library; the Wellcome Institute for the History of Medicine; the Universiteitsbibliotheek, Rijksuniversiteit Leiden; the Biblioteca Apostolica Vaticana and the Archivio Segreto Vaticano; the Facultad de Medicina at the Universität de Valencia; the Biblioteca Nacional, Madrid; the Ministerio de Hacienda, Madrid; the Archivo de Protocolos, Madrid; the Museo de Ciencias Naturales, Madrid; the Real

Academia Nacional de Medicina, Madrid; the library of the Palacio Real, Madrid; the Biblioteca Nícolas León, Antigua Facultad de Medicina, Mexico City; the Instituto de Biología, UNAM, Mexico City; the John Carter Brown Library, Providence, Rhode Island; the Henry E. Huntington Library, San Marino, California; the National Library of Medicine, Bethesda, Maryland; the William Andrews Clark Memorial Library, UCLA; and the Louise M. Darling Biomedical Library, UCLA.

Special thanks are due to José María López Piñero, who has supported and contributed to the whole of this project in countless, important ways. We have been beneficiaries of the generosity and learning of David McKitterick of Trinity College, Cambridge, and the late Fr. Leonard E. Boyle, O.P., prefect of the Biblioteca Apostolica Vaticana. Rachel Bindman has alerted us to several important sources in Italy. At the Clark Library we have been treated like royalty by Carol Sommer and Suzanne Tatian, and Teresa Johnson and Katharine Donahue have given us every assistance in the History Division of the Biomedical Library at UCLA.

The whole project has been completed under the aegis of the UCLA Center for Medieval and Renaissance Studies; as all the institutional affiliations and acknowledgments appear in full in our companion volume of essays, it seems nugatory to repeat them here. But it is both a duty and a pleasure to declare, loudly, that this volume was made not only possible but actual by major grants from the National Endowment for the Humanities and the Ahmanson Foundation. We are grateful to Hoechst, Marion, Roussel for a grant that has enabled us to include illustrations.

Last, we would like to thank David Hayes-Bautista and the Center for the Study of Latino Health and Culture, which he directs, for guidance and support, and Dora B. Weiner, who has served as director of what was known for a decade at UCLA as the Hernández Project.

ABBREVIATIONS

BN MS	Madrid, Biblioteca Nacional, MSS 22,436–22,439 (Hernández's drafts of the *Natural History of New Spain* and other writings)
Hac.	Madrid, Ministerio de Hacienda MSS 931–32 (Hernández's drafts of the *Natural History of New Spain* and other writings)
JCB MS	Providence, R.I., John Carter Brown Library, Codex Latin 5 (Nardo Antonio Recchi's selection of Hernández)
LMS	London, British Library, MS Sloane 1555 (Johannes de Laet's translation of Hernández)
M	Francisco Hernández, *Opera*, ed. Casimiro Gómez Ortega, 3 vols. (Madrid: Ibarra, 1790)
MB	Georg Marcgraf, *Historia rerum naturalium Brasiliae* (Leiden: Elsevier, 1648)
N	Juan Eusebio Nieremberg, *Historia naturae, maxime peregrine* (Antwerp: Moretus, 1635)
OC	Francisco Hernández, *Obras completas,* ed. Germán Somolinos d'Ardois et al., 7 vols. (Mexico City: UNAM, 1959–84)
QL	[Francisco Hernández], *Quatro libros: De la naturaleza, y virtudes de las plantas, y animales que estan recevidos en el uso de Medicina en la Nueva España . . .,* ed. Francisco Ximénez (Mexico City: Widow of Diego López Davalos,1615).
Somolinos	"Vida y obra de Francisco Hernández," *OC* 1:97–459
T	Francisco Hernández, *Rerum medicarum Novae Hispaniae thesaurus* (Rome: J. Mascardi, 1651).

A NOTE ON TEXTS AND TRANSLATIONS

Some hold translations not unlike to be
The wrong side of a Turkish tapestry

             —James Howell (1653)

As selections of the writings of Hernández passed through the presses in different languages and countries, his texts underwent the usual transformations and deformations. The resulting texts are sometimes corrupt, but on the whole they demonstrate a remarkable fidelity to the surviving manuscripts, even though many of the printed texts are not derived directly from those papers. In addition, early editors added their own comments and observations, weaving them, sometimes seamlessly, into Hernández's prose. Some of those editors simply paraphrased Hernández. We have not attempted to disengage Hernández from his editors: rather, we present the texts the same way they were presented in earlier times. If our text looks or sounds inconsistent, the reason is that it is a historical text that represents many more voices than Hernández's alone.

In the interests of clarity we have adopted a few other practices, occasionally at the expense of total textual integrity. We have broken up Hernández's typically endless Renaissance sentences, thus often ignoring the conjunctions that litter the pages of our source texts. Like many of his contemporaries, Hernández was also liberal with relative pronouns, so that the identity of the correct antecedent is often obscured: if so, we repeat the original substantive provided we can identify it. A similar kind of obscurity occurs because Hernández's earliest editor systematically moved sentences around without amending the surrounding text that was affected by this rearrangement. The surviving manuscripts usually (but not always) guide us in these cases, and we have consequently emended the text to restore an authorial intention, even if the intention was never carried into print. Finally, for variety's sake, we have sought synonyms for overworked all-purpose words, but we maintain characteristic phrases containing Hernández's synonymia (such as "well known and familiar") because they are nuances of rhetorical importance, especially to an author who was exposed early to Erasmian thought.

Names are left in the vernacular unless they have a familiar English form. Thus although we refer to Philip II (not Felipe II), we do not attempt to anglicize Martín Enríquez or, for that matter, Francisco Hernández. Spanish accents are retained in Spanish words and names. Because Náhuatl words are all stressed on the penultimate syllable, accents are unnecessary, but Spanish-speakers pronounce and accent them according to Spanish rules. We retain those Spanish accents on Náhuatl words as a courtesy to those who prefer them, and we trust that readers who can live without such accents will mentally delete them. We hope that this compromise is not too awkward.

The achievements of Hernández were immense and diverse. Nearly everything he wrote was composed in Latin—functional rather than elegant (though the language of his poems can be graceful), sometimes bafflingly obscure, occasionally ungrammatical, careless from time to time, and reduced here and there to a staccato sequence of sentence fragments that look much like unrevised notes. As Hernández's vocabulary in his descriptions of plants and their medicinal applications is usually straightforward, we employ expressions such as the slightly archaic "provokes sweat" rather than "sudorific," as renderings closer to his style. We endeavor in general to represent Hernández's style, which his earliest editors often preserved, but we see little purpose in re-creating his errors, so we silently correct his faulty grammar, insert nouns to prevent his participles from dangling, simplify his syntax, restore lost words, and delete accidental repetitions. We do not attempt to render or otherwise reproduce inconsistencies of punctuation or errors that can be confidently attributed to the press, such as turned letters (most commonly *u* for *n*, producing readings that could be plausible but make no sense in context, such as *unas* [ones] for *uvas* [grapes] in Spanish), two separate words printed together, one word split in two, and repeated letters. In the translations, brackets [ ] indicate additions to the text of fragments that we believe to have been in the source text originally but that are now lost or illegible. Bent brackets ⟨ ⟩ indicate the translators' conjectural additions to a text.

Náhuatl orthography was neither standardized nor consistent in the period represented by the texts in this volume. We have generally retained the old spellings of the texts themselves unless words are garbled beyond recognition, but we have used modern orthography in titles, headings, and index entries.

We envision this translation as a text that must be as clear and readable as is consistent with Hernández's Latin or Spanish and the various other languages and forms into which his writings were translated in the seventeenth and eighteenth centuries. As our purpose is not to produce a parallel text but an English text, we have glossed only glaring errors, inconsistencies, and obscurities in our source texts. We have sought to annotate sparingly and tactfully. The liberties we have taken with the text are conservative, for the writings of Hernández are far greater than the work of his translators, and we wish to keep matters that way.

CHRONOLOGY OF THE TEXTS OF FRANCISCO HERNÁNDEZ

1566–67   Hernández completes a large portion of his edition of Pliny, *Natural History.*

1570–77   While in New Spain, Hernández finishes his edition of Pliny, composes the *Antiquities of New Spain* and *Natural History of New Spain,* writes *The Christian Doctrine,* and completes a large number of lesser works.

1580   Philip II orders his physician, Nardo Antonio Recchi, to make a selection from Hernández's *Natural History of New Spain.* Hernández writes *An Epistle to Arias Montano.*

1587   Hernández dies in Madrid.

1590   In the second edition of *Historia natural y moral de las Indias* (Barcelona), José Acosta gives a short account of Hernández's expedition to New Spain and the resulting manuscripts.

1592   Fabio Colonna, *Phytobasanos* (Naples), mentions the description of *tlapatl* that had first appeared in the Hernández manuscripts and notes Recchi's work in progress.

1597   Jaime Honorato Pomar commissions a volume of paintings of plants and animals, some copied directly from Hernández's originals.

1598   A notarized copy of Hernández's *Index medicamentorum,* in Spanish, is made. The text is attributed to Gregorio López, with whose other work it is copied, and is acquired by Cardinal Riti.

1603   Federico Cesi, Duke of Aquasparta, founds the Accademia dei Lincei in Rome. Cesi acquires a manuscript copy of Recchi's selection of Hernández with the intention that it should be the new academy's leading publication.

1607   Juan Barrios, *Verdadera medicina, cirugía y astrología* (Mexico City) includes a different version, again in Spanish, of the *Index medicamentorum.*

1609   Barrios publishes a treatise on chocolate, in which he quotes Hernández and states that he owns a manuscript copy of Recchi's selection from the *Natural History.*

1614   Cesi proposes to Johannes Faber and Theodore Müller that they undertake a trip to Mexico to verify various aspects of the Recchi manuscript.

1615   Barrios's copy of Recchi's manuscript, translated into Spanish, is edited by Francisco Ximénez and published in Mexico City as the *Quatro libros.*

1616   Colonna's *Minus cognitarum stirpium* includes one chapter drawn in part from Recchi's manuscript.

1625–30   A director of the Dutch West India Company, Johannes de Laet, translates the text of the

Quatro libros back into Latin. He may have had a manuscript copy first, then the printed book. Selections from his own Latin appear, translated again, in Dutch in *Beschrijving van West-Indien* (Leiden: Elsevier, 1630).

1628   Faber publishes *Animalia mexicana descriptionibus scholiisque exposita,* his annotated edition of Hernández's descriptions of Mexican animals. The Accademia dei Lincei apparently produces a prospectus for Hernández, *Rerum medicarum Novae Hispaniae thesaurus,* which will finally be published in 1651.

1633   De Laet expands his description of the New World, incorporates more selections from his translation of Hernández, and puts his Dutch text into Latin as *Novus Orbis,* published by Elsevier in Leiden.

1635   The Jesuit scholar Juan Eusebio Nieremberg includes 160 chapters from the *Natural History* and a substantial portion of the *Antiquities* in his *Historia naturae,* published by Moretus in Antwerp.

1640   De Laet's Latin text of 1633 is translated into French and published, again by Elsevier, in Leiden.

1648   De Laet edits the works on Brazilian botany and medicine by Willem Piso, *De medicina Brasiliensi,* and Georg Marcgraf, *Historia rerum naturalium Brasiliae,* published together in one volume (Leiden: Elsevier). Marcgraf (d. 1643) cites thirty-three descriptions from Hernández, supplied by de Laet.

1651   After half a century of perseverance, the Accademia dei Lincei finally publishes the large folio edition of Hernández, *Rerum medicarum Novae Hispaniae thesaurus,* with learned commentaries by the academicians.

1658   Piso brings out a second edition of his 1648 work, with several plagiarisms and unwarranted claims of authorship. He now includes a few texts by Hernández, taken from Marcgraf or de Laet.

1659   An English physician, Robert Lovell, includes the therapeutic information about ninety-five Mexican plants, taken from the *Quatro libros* or the Rome edition of Hernández (who is not acknowledged), in *Pambotanologia,* published in Oxford. A second edition comes out in 1665.

1662   In *The Indian Nectar,* a treatise on chocolate, Henry Stubbe quotes from Hernández.

1685   John Chamberlayne cites Hernández as the principal authority on cacao in part of his

translation of one of three tracts, together published as *The Manner of Making of Coffee, Tea, and Chocolate.*

1686   The first volume of John Ray's immense *Historia plantarum* uses Hernández as one of its many authorities. Volume 2 (1688) contains an appendix devoted solely to Hernández, consisting of a summary of the contents of the Rome edition, preceded by a brief introductory essay.

1687–88   Hans Sloane conducts botanical and medical research in Jamaica.

c. 1689   Another Englishman, James Newton, writes an herbal, which draws on six Hernández texts from the Rome edition, Marcgraf, and de Laet. Edited by his son, the work is published posthumously in 1752.

1696   Abraham Munting, *Naauwkeurige Beschrijving der Aardgewassen,* devoted mainly to European plants, quotes briefly from the Rome edition and the *Quatro libros* in a few places. Sloane publishes an index of Jamaican plants, using Hernández as one of his many authorities.

c. 1690–1707   James Petiver, a London apothecary, annotates his copies of Nieremberg and Piso, with cross-references to Hernández.

1707   Sloane's *Natural History of Jamaica,* vol. 1, includes more than forty extracts from Hernández on Mexican plants.

1715   Petiver publishes a very short illustrated pamphlet in English that includes two descriptions of plants taken from Hernández.

1725   Sloane, *Natural History of Jamaica,* vol. 2, adds a few more selections from Hernández in English.

1752   James Newton's *Enchyridion* is published.

1766–72   Arnaud Vosmaer includes descriptions of the rattlesnake and bison, based on the Rome edition of Hernández and on Marcgraf and Nieremberg, in his book on exotic quadrupeds, birds, and snakes, *Natuurkundige Beschrijving eener uitmuntende verzameling van zeldzame gedierten, bestaande in Oost- en Westindische viervoetige dieren, vogelen en slangen.*

1790   The *Opera* of Hernández, vols. 1–3, edited by Casimiro Gómez Ortega, is printed by Joaquín Ibarra and published in Madrid.

1842   The first volume of the *Colección de documentos inéditos para la historia de España,* edited by Martín Fernández Navarrete, Miguel Salvá, and Pedro Sainz de Baranda, contains six letters from Hernández to King

Philip II and one to Juan de Ovando, president of the Council of the Indies.

1888   Two new editions of the *Quatro libros*: Antonio Peñafiel's is published in Mexico City, Nicolás León's in Morelia.

1926   Facsimile reprint of the manuscript of Hernández's *Antiquities* (Mexico City).

1933   Maximino Martínez publishes *Las plantas medicinales de México,* dedicated to the memory of Hernández and relying on him for descriptions of seventy-one plants still used for medicinal purposes in Mexico.

1942–45   The Instituto de Biología de México produces a Spanish translation of the Madrid edition of 1790.

1945   Joaquín García Pimentel produces a Spanish translation of the *Antiquities* (Mexico City).

1959–84   The *Obras completas* of Hernández appear in seven volumes, published by the Universidad Nacional Autónoma de México.

THE MEXICAN TREASURY

INTRODUCTION

THE HERNÁNDEZ TEXTS

RAFAEL CHABRÁN

SIMON VAREY

In a lifetime that began when Thomas More was drafting *Utopia* and ended as the king of Spain was fitting out the Invincible Armada, Francisco Hernández rose from relative obscurity to become one of the greatest physicians, historians, and naturalists in Spanish history. Nothing if not prolific, Hernández translated the thirty-seven books of Pliny's *Natural History* into Spanish and wrote long commentaries on them; he wrote a lengthy missionary poem on Christian doctrine, composed commentaries on Galen and Aristotle, and compiled a historical survey of New Spain. Best of all, he described at length the natural history of the Valley of Mexico. This last work, the *Natural History of New Spain,* occupied sixteen folio volumes (six of text, ten of paintings illustrating the plants and animals he had described). Like most of his other work, the *Natural History* was written in Latin, but Hernández himself began a Spanish translation of it and had some of it translated into Náhuatl as well. Hernández's most important work, the *Natural History* has never been published in its entirety in any language, not even in the *Obras completas,* and only a tiny fragment of it has appeared in English before. The texts we present in this volume are centered on the *Natural History,* supported by selections from the other works and various related documents, such as Hernández's will, two remarkable poems, his ethnographic "antiquities," the formal instructions from the king outlining what he was to do in Mexico, and Hernández's letters to the king in which he reported on his progress and invented excuses not to send his work back to Spain.

Hernández himself considered that, by producing his Spanish edition of Pliny and his own *Natural History,* he had completed two complementary natural histories that together covered the whole world. His Pliny is obviously an achievement of major importance, but it is far too large for us to represent in this volume, which concentrates on America rather than Europe. It may be small consolation, but the commentaries on Pliny do at least contain scattered autobiographical remarks, which afford us almost the only evidence we have of Hernández before his period of fame. For example, it is from the commentaries on Pliny that we learn that Hernández worked at Guadalupe "being doctor at that monastery and hospital" and that one of his

3

principal activities there was dissection, most famously of a chameleon.[1]

Hernández had begun work on Pliny by the 1560s, though he finished it in Mexico in the 1570s. He appears to have written little else before 1567, when he was promoted to the position of royal doctor. Three years later, he received the formal instructions outlining his duties on a scientific expedition to Spanish America that would change his life. The *Natural History* was the fruit—though not the only one—of Hernández's royally mandated expedition to New Spain, which began with his departure from Seville in September 1570 and ended with his weary return in May 1577. Concentrating on those years, our essay volume contains ample interpretation of Hernández's life and accomplishments. This, our text volume, contains a selection of the written accomplishments themselves. This introduction focuses on the dissemination of the text of the *Natural History* down to the end of the eighteenth century. In the manuscript volumes of the *Natural History*, Hernández wrote descriptions of more than 3,000 plants, 40 quadrupeds, 229 birds, 58 reptiles, 30 insects, 54 aquatic animals, and 35 minerals. The descriptions of plants, in particular, are framed by his desire to ascertain the medicinal usefulness of the natural life of New Spain. Hernández hired native artists to make paintings—not drawings—of many of the species that he described. Not every description was paired with a painting.

When Hernández returned to Spain in 1577, either he had two copies of his manuscripts with him, or he set about making a second copy. One copy, his corrected drafts, survives today, split between two repositories in Madrid, and is described in the next essay by Jesús Bustamante. A second copy, incorporating the corrections from those drafts, was presented to King Philip II. The king's copy was destroyed by the terrible fire that caused extensive damage to the Escorial in June 1671. Fortunately, about 1626 Andrés de los Reyes, the Escorial librarian, had drawn up an index of the manuscript volumes that were burned. He did so at the request of Cassiano dal Pozzo, the antiquarian and collector

who played an important role in the eventual publication of Hernández in Rome and whose papers are now dispersed all over Europe. This index found a permanent home at the School of Medicine at the University of Montpellier (MS H101). Philip's neglect had already ensured the eventual destruction of Hernández's sketches of plants by casually hanging them on the walls of his private apartments in the Escorial, and those that he did not "display" like that went up in smoke anyway. By the time of the fire, the Hernández manuscripts had already been partially copied, translated, and printed. The paintings, too, had been copied, but mostly as engravings in a fairly traditional European style. A few of them were copied as paintings, revealing their fascinating blend of Mexican and European perspectives. Today, some sixty paintings survive in the *Codex Pomar* in Valencia.[2]

No single edition of Hernández can be complete or comprehensive, although the seven modern volumes of the *Obras completas* appear to come close. One reason that they do not represent Hernández completely is that the text of the *Obras* takes no account of the fact that his works were selected, edited, borrowed, incorporated, and otherwise subjected to normal Renaissance practice. There can be no single, stable text. Even though three major editions of Hernández were published in 1615, 1651, and 1790, they are selections of his *Natural History*. These are the *Quatro libros* (Mexico City, 1615); the Rome edition, *Rerum medicarum Novae Hispaniae thesaurus* (Rome, 1651); and the Madrid edition, *Opera* (Madrid, 1790). Portions of Hernández's work appeared in different forms and different languages, in books of topography and travel as well as works on natural history and therapeutics. Some of those renderings of his texts remained in manuscript, but most were printed. In his discussion of the surviving manuscript drafts of the *Natural History* in Hernández's hand, Bustamante addresses the question of how Hernández arranged and rearranged his materials. To organize an edition of Hernández's *Natural History* the way the author finally envisaged it would be desirable, but it is not the way anyone has ever read it. It is not our purpose in this volume to re-create

1. Quotation from BN MS 2,864, bk. 8, chap. 27, fol. 197r; he says much the same at bk. 8, chap. 33, fol. 213v; on dissection, BN MS 2,865, bk. 11, introduction, fol. 188v.

2. Facsimile ed., with introduction by José María López Piñero (Valencia: Vicent García, 1990).

Hernández's final wishes. At the risk of doing his memory a disservice, our selections (and thus their translations) are designed to reflect the historical patterns of dissemination of the work of Hernández. Our intention in organizing the volume in this way is to present selections of texts that give modern readers a sense of which portions of Hernández's vast corpus entered scientific discourse and spread across two continents in the seventeenth and eighteenth centuries. In this introduction we attempt to discuss all the relevant texts that enabled subsequent generations to come to know the major achievement of Francisco Hernández.

Recchi's Selection:
John Carter Brown Library Codex Latin 5

In January 1580, Philip II asked one of his royal doctors, Nardo Antonio Recchi, to make a selection from the *Natural History* of Hernández. Recchi's selection is extremely important, because it was the basis for most of the dissemination of Hernández for two centuries. It makes sense to begin our discussion of the Hernández texts with an account of Recchi's selection. One copy of this selection, the manuscript at the John Carter Brown Library, Codex Latin 5, is a major document in the tangled and complex story of the Hernández manuscripts. Apparently in Recchi's hand for the most part (though there is clear evidence of another hand), it consists of 241 folios, occupied by a Latin text of Hernández. The volume belonged to Francisco Xavier, Cardinal de Zelada, whose bookplate is pasted on the front endpaper. The eighteenth-century binding is evidently Zelada's as well.

Recchi has long been accused of distorting Hernández or reducing him in some way that misrepresented him. José Mariano Beristáin was especially scornful of this "wretched compendium," which "truly reduced the noble work of Hernández to a mere manual of domestic medicine."[3] José M. López Piñero and José Pardo Tomás go a long way toward rehabilitating Recchi when they stress that what he made was a selection and, with relatively minor editorial adjustments, a selection that did not seriously mar the original text.[4] The first page of writing in the Brown manuscript confirms that Recchi did nothing more (although that was crucially important) than rearrange the material: "Four books on the materia medica of New Spain, collected according to the decree of Philip II, invincible king of Spain and the Indies, by the distinguished Doctor Francisco Hernández in the New World and arranged in order by Doctor Nardo Antonio Recchi, physician to the same monarch." The implication of this descriptive title is clear: Recchi arranged the material in order (*in ordinem digesta*), suggesting that what Hernández had delivered was disordered. In the English-speaking world, Recchi's work has sometimes been called a "digest," or more commonly a "compendium," and that has led quite unjustifiably to the mistaken notion that Recchi somehow abridged each chapter of Hernández.[5]

This surviving manuscript never went through a printing house, but other copies of it became the basis for the *Quatro libros* and the *Rerum medicarum Novae Hispaniae thesaurus*.[6] Although the text of Codex Latin 5 is valuable simply as a basis (if not the sole basis) of the final printed edition in Latin, this Recchi manuscript is important for another reason. The last few leaves of the manuscript

3. José Mariano Beristáin, *Biblioteca hispano americana septentrional,* 3 vols. (Mexico City, 1816–21), 3d ed. (Mexico City: Ediciones Fuente Cultural, 1947), pt. 3, pp. 18, 23. Beristáin was not alone in this opinion: the author of *Mercurio peruano,* no. 228 (March 10, 1793), considered that Recchi "has made useless all those objects of natural history, as is customary among people in the medical profession" (p. 169, in *Mercurio peruano de historia, literatura, y noticias públicas* 7 [January–April 1793]), while Gómez Ortega thought Recchi's selection was medically not very useful (M, 1, preface).

4. José M. López Piñero and José Pardo Tomás, *Nuevos materiales y noticias sobre la Historia de las Plantas de Nueva España, de Francisco Hernández* (Valencia: Instituto de Estudios Documentales e Históricos sobre la Ciencia, Universitàt de València, CSIC, 1994), 67.

5. Admittedly, digest seems to be the preferred term among booksellers rather than scholars. The term probably comes from a misunderstanding of the Latin. Nettie Lee Benson, "The Ill-Fated Works of Francisco Hernández," *Library Chronicle of the University of Texas* 5 (1953): 18–19 and passim, refers to Recchi's work consistently as a "compendium."

6. We discuss the issue of this manuscript and printing house practice in "Medical Natural History in the Renaissance: The Strange Case of Francisco Hernández," *Huntington Library Quarterly* 57 (1994): 134–35. A parallel text (Latin and Spanish) edition of this manuscript, albeit without its valuable indexes, has recently been published: *De materia medica Novae Hispaniae: El manuscrito de Recchi,* ed. Raquel Alvarez Peláez and Florentino Fernández González, 2 vols. (Madrid: Ediciones Doce Calles, 1998).

contain two indexes showing two different kinds of entries. These indicate that one list of Recchi's selections was drawn up first and that further selections were added at a later date, a few of them inserted between the lines in the first list but most of them added at the end. We know from Reyes's index that Hernández had arranged his material according to a Mexican system, but Recchi rearranged Hernández's chapters into customary European classifications. To do this, Recchi had to take chapters that were scattered all over the original manuscripts and bring them together according to the type of plants they described. His method, witnessed by his indexes, reveals that he took Hernández's texts at face value, wherever a herb is described, for instance, as sharp or bitter. Recchi's numbers in these additional index entries refer to the Escorial texts, as they are supposed to have done: but then that means that the *main* indexes in the Brown manuscript do not refer to the Escorial volumes at all, thus proving that Recchi had access to another copy of Hernández in manuscript.

Using the Montpellier (MS H101) and Brown manuscripts and the surviving drafts together, we can establish that the original Hernández texts, the one at the Escorial and probably also some other one that Recchi used, were continuously foliated across all the volumes, each volume containing roughly 200 to 250 folios, much like the drafts. Evidently there was some kind of subdivision, as the chapter numbers in Recchi's index indicate. The now lost Escorial copy no doubt contained virtually everything that was in the surviving drafts: the point was not that Hernández rewrote anything to suit the king's taste but that he rearranged the material. Although the Montpellier manuscript shows the order of the whole work when it entered the Escorial, it does not explain why that order was the one for which Hernández opted. López Piñero and Pardo propose, convincingly, that it was organized according to Nahua practice and that the order is thus mostly etymological.[7]

Recchi's manuscript selection of Hernández quickly became standard in the late sixteenth century, and the original Escorial text, whose integrity is at least witnessed by the Montpellier manuscript, was only partially restored by the belated Madrid edition's printing of texts apparently based on Hernández's corrected drafts.

The *Index medicamentorum*

A famous, strange looking text appears in one of Mexico's earliest and most important treatises on medicine, the *Verdadera medicina, cirugía, y astrología* by Juan Barrios, a large, long, and original work that has received nothing close to its due since it was published in Mexico City by Fernando Balli in 1607.[8] Only five copies of Barrios's work are known to exist, the best of which appears to be the one at the Facultad de Medicina at the University of Valencia, although many pages have been seriously damaged by worming, with occasional loss of text; the next best copy is that at the Wellcome Institute in London. The odd text that concerns us here is an eleven-folio section consisting of an index of diseases and the native Mexican plants that are used to cure them. Barrios attributes it to Dr. Francisco Hernández. When Barrios's book was published, none of Hernández's original work had yet appeared in print, and Hernández himself had been dead for two decades.

Although the text attached to Barrios's work has often been mentioned, described, and dismissed, it took until 1993 for anyone actually to recognize what it was. In their important study of Hernández manuscripts and printed works, López Piñero and Pardo note the dismissive comments by García Icazbalceta and Germán Somolinos d'Ardois before going on to point out that what Barrios printed was nothing more complex than a Spanish translation of a Latin index that would eventually be printed in its bare form as the index to the contents of Recchi's selection.

7. López Piñero and Pardo, *Nuevos materiales,* 43–58. There is further evidence of Hernández's willingness to adopt Nahua philosophy and to adapt his own preconceptions accordingly. See David A. Boruchoff, "The Conflict of Natural History and Moral Philosophy in *De antiquitatibus novae Hispaniae* of Francisco Hernández," *Revista canadiense de estudios hispanicos* 17 (1993): 241–58, and

Jesús Bustamante, "De la naturaleza y los naturales americanos en el siglo XVI: Algunas cuestiones críticas sobre la obra de Francisco Hernández," *Revista de Indias* 52, nos. 195–96 (1992): 297–328.

8. An English text of the whole of Barrios's book will appear in *Latino Medical Classics,* a series founded in 1997 by the Center for the Study of Latino Health and Culture at UCLA.

López Piñero and Pardo present a table that shows that the headings are identical, and they add a representative sample of texts to demonstrate that Barrios took his material from Recchi, with "minor variants of detail." Yet there is another, earlier text that is quite remarkably similar but has never been recognized for what it is. It is attached to *El Tesoro de Medicinas,* attributed to Gregorio López (1542–96).

A native of Madrid, López was known as a hermit who lived an ascetic existence throughout his thirty-three years of relative solitude in New Spain. He arrived in Veracruz in 1562, aged twenty, but for our purposes the most important period of his life was the decade from 1580 to 1589, which he spent at the hospital of Hoaxtépec, where Hernández is known to have worked in the 1570s. According to López's first biographer—or rather, hagiographer—Francisco Losa (1563?–1642), it was in the 1580s that López composed "a book of many medicinal remedies for various illnesses, drawn from personal experience and from his great knowledge of properties and natural virtues of plants."[9] This book was actually entitled *De la virtud de las Yerbas* and has long been thought to have been based somehow on the work of Hernández, with whom López is thus presumed to have had some contact in New Spain during Hernández's seven-year sojourn, as is entirely likely for a young man interested in medicine. Just as important, Hernández had been practicing in Guadalupe between 1558 and 1562, precisely when López is known to have visited the famous monastery on his way to Seville, prior to sailing for Mexico. Felipe Picatoste spoke truer words than anyone has ever realized when, in 1891, he described the manuscript of López in the Biblioteca Nacional, Madrid: "This book contains much that was undoubtedly taken from Hernández," and he thought it had been copied for Ximénez, who would edit Hernández in 1615.[10]

Introducing a reprint of the fourth edition of López's work, published as *Tesoro de Medicina* in 1727, Francisco Guerra notes two surviving manuscripts of this book: the one Picatoste described, which has 371 folios, 311 plus a section taken largely from Mesué, Oviedo, and Palacios; and one in the Archivio Segreto of the Vatican, which contains 204 folios, of which folios 173–204 contain a section on New World plants. The Vatican manuscript, a notarized copy made in the 1590s, became part of the Mexican/American collection assembled by Cardinal Riti.

The most interesting features of López's section on the medicinal plants of New Spain are that it was never printed until Guerra's transcript appeared in 1982 and that it is the work of Francisco Hernández, a point that has eluded scholars even though the evidence is clear. If the New World section was in López's hand and attached to other manuscripts that have not survived, why was it always omitted from the printed texts of López? We think it most likely that it was not written by López, nor necessarily even written down by him, but more probably added to blank leaves at the end of another manuscript. For convenience, we will call it López's index. His index and that of Recchi/Barrios are not identical, but collation of the two texts reveals that they had a common ancestor. Barrios translated Recchi, who is always supposed to have drawn up the index to his own arrangement of the Hernández materials that he selected for the *Thesaurus.* But the existence of López's index brings that supposition into question until we can establish whether or not López had access to Recchi, or Recchi to López.

The texts by López and Barrios both contain frequent spelling errors, but the errors are consistent. The texts sometimes agree in that they mention the same selection of plants, but just as frequently one text cites more than the other. There is no consistency in this matter: sometimes López has more material, sometimes Barrios. One brief example may suffice to demonstrate the kinship of the two texts:

[López, MS Riti 1716, fol. 174r]:
For headache from a cold cause, chapter 1
Place texaxapotla in the nostrils, and inhale its vapor that way, or a scant handful of leaves of the tzocuilpatli taken in water, or smoke it with the gum of copalliquahuithl, or with the bark or root of that tree, or the

---

9. The severely abridged English editions of Losa garble this passage. López has not been canonized, but he has been venerated. See Fernando Ocaranza, *Gregorio López, el hombre celestial* (Mexico City: Xochitl, 1944).

10. Felipe Picatoste y Rodríguez, *Apuntes para una biblioteca científica española del siglo XVI* (Madrid: Manuel Tello, 1891), 172.

yyauhtli, taken. Or, one dram of the roots of nauhteputz taken orally, or the resin of xochicocotzoquahuitl applied to the forehead and temples. Or, two drams of the root of izpatli taken. Or, the stones and fruit of the hoitzochitl dissolved in water and instilled in the nostrils, or, the leaves of the ecapatli crushed and applied.

[Barrios, Verdadera medicina, fol. 59r]

For headaches from cold.

Take the vapor or sniff the leaves of the texaxapotla, or the leaves of the tzocuilpatli, or the gum of the copalquahuitl, or smoke it with the root or branches, or take the yyauhtli, or take the weight of one real of the root of the nauhteputz, or the resin of the xuchiocotzoquahuitl, placed on the forehead or drink the weight of two reals of the root of Itzpatli, or the fruit of the huitzxuchitl, ground and put in the nostrils; or place on the head the mashed leaves of the ecapatli.

Evidence of these kinds occurs on every page: the wording has a common core but is always divergent, because López and Recchi/Barrios must have worked from different but closely related manuscripts. The confusing evidence means that López worked from a manuscript that almost certainly could not have been the basis of anything Recchi ever did. A third version of this index, in Spanish, came to light as this book was in production. It is part of Madrid, Universidad Complutense, Facultad de Medicina, MS 6.151 Her., fols. 390–509v. The main part of the text, fols. 75–383v, is a Spanish translation of Recchi's selection of Hernández. As we have not yet been able to study this manuscript in detail, we have not incorporated discussion of it in this introduction, although it has allowed us to refine some of our findings about other extant texts.

The index is a text in its own right, no mere guide to the contents of a book but a list of diseases and how to cure them with medicines made from Mexican plants. The index was probably already in existence in 1580 when Recchi was given the task of making his selection from Hernández. No one has ever known what Recchi's principles of selection

were. Because the Hernández manuscripts, following a Mexican arrangement, were confusing to Recchi, it would have been very simple for Recchi to have used this index—in some form—as a guide to what he ought to select.

The index appears to be related somehow to parts of book 10 of the *Florentine Codex,* where fray Bernadino de Sahagún presented a similar but much shorter sequence (sixty-nine headings, where Barrios and López have more than two hundred). His list "was examined" by eight Mexican doctors.[11] Sahagún's list of illnesses is not the same, nor are most of the plants the same as those quoted by Barrios, López, or the Complutense manuscript. It would be natural to conclude that his list and Hernández's were simply different texts, representing different ways of presenting comparable kinds of information, were it not for a teasing allusion in a letter from the viceroy to the king. Other parts of Sahagún's work influenced the second version of Hernández's *Antiquities* as late as 1577: Hernández drew on them and translated them. Georges Baudot quotes from the letter of Viceroy Enríquez to Philip II, April 22, 1577: "I believe that in Spain there are many versions of most of [Sahagún's work], although I do not know if all of it, and the protomédico took his part."[12] Baudot interprets this last clause to mean that the work of Hernández "was going to meet the same prohibitions" as the work of Sahagún, that is, that it would be censored. But could it be that "his part" is the part of the text that Hernández had contributed to Sahagún and that he, Hernández, has now taken it with him to Spain? Enríquez had written on March 30 to say that Hernández had left New Spain. Although the scant evidence is obviously inconclusive, this raises the extraordinary possibility that the parts on medicine in book 10 of the *Florentine Codex* might have been written by Francisco Hernández.

The *Quatro libros*

The first milestone after the publication of the *Index medicamentorum* by Barrios was a much more substantial text,

11. *The Florentine Codex: General History of the Things of New Spain,* trans. Arthur J. O. Anderson and Charles E. Dibble, pt. 11 (Santa Fe, N.M., and Salt Lake City, Utah: School of American Research and the Museum of New Mexico, 1961), bk. 10, chap. 28, pp. 139–63.

12. Georges Baudot, *Utopia and History in Mexico: The First Chroniclers of Mexican Civilization (1520–1569),* trans. Bernard R. Ortiz de Montellano and Thelma Ortiz de Montellano (Denver: University Press of Colorado, 1995), 502, quoting Archivo General de Indias, México, no. 69, dossier 4, fol. 2r.

based on a manuscript of Recchi's selection. The manuscript itself, unknown today, had been "signed" by Francisco Valles. We now know that it belonged, at least as late as 1609, to Barrios.[13] In 1615 fray Francisco Ximénez saw through the press Quatro libros. De la naturaleza, y virtudes de las plantas, y animales. The text of the Quatro libros is organized into four books, each subdivided into sections. The first three books are on aromatics, trees, plants, and fruits; herbs with a sharp taste; herbs that taste salty or sweet; and herbs that have a bitter taste or no taste at all; the fourth book deals with animals and minerals whose derivatives can be used as medicines. Two tables list illnesses and remedies (not based on the Index medicamentorum). Altogether the book contains 478 chapters translated into Spanish from Hernández's work, with some annotations and additions supplied by Ximénez. The stated purpose of this book was to be a handbook for use in places where there was no accessible pharmacy.

Until the appearance of the Complutense manuscript, it was not always clear where Hernández ended and Ximénez began, because although the editor was deferential to the author, he would occasionally add a note from his own experience without distinguishing it as such. Apart from a frontispiece portrayal of Saint Dominic, the book has no illustrations, so that identification of plants with confusingly similar names is sometimes impossible.[14] A lay hospital brother who arrived in New Spain in 1605, Ximénez worked at some time in the Hospital de la Santa Cruz, where he was in charge of the hospital's pharmacy. He apparently had received no formal medical training, but he did write a book, Memoria para la salud, now lost. His only tangible contribution to the history of medicine is thus his edition of Hernández.

The Huntington Library copy of the Quatro libros, which Henry Harrisse bought in Paris in 1871, is not only in exceptionally good condition for a handbook that was meant to be used frequently: it is also annotated. The ink has faded, but the barely legible annotations reveal that someone wrote in the margins, in Spanish, key words, mostly indicating parts of the body that are mentioned in the text. Clearly, the annotations were meant to serve as a quick finding aid for practical purposes, and so they confirm exactly what the book was intended to do.

We do not know the extent of the print run of the Quatro libros, but it was probably small—perhaps a few hundred copies—as most Mexican imprints of its time seem to have been. Copies of the Quatro libros have always been rare, especially in Europe, where, as we shall see, only one or two copies turned up in the seventeenth century. They were promptly put to good use.

THE LOW COUNTRIES, C. 1630–1648

Johannes de Laet's Translation of Hernández (British Library, MS Sloane 1555)

The bibliographical and textual history of Netherlandish editions of Hernández's work in New Spain has been subjected to distortion by omission, however unintentional. Hernández's great biographer Somolinos mentioned in a footnote a book that he had probably never been able to consult, and which he clearly had not read, because it is in Dutch: Nieuwe Wereldt, ofte Beschrijvinghe van West-Indien (Leiden, 1625), by Johannes de Laet.[15] Much less well known than any other text of Hernández is the manuscript behind this book, a Latin translation by de Laet from a

13. "His books were held in high esteem, and approved by Dr. Valles, and by the other royal doctors. By the king's order Dr. Nardo Antonio abbreviated them, and I have his original signed by Dr. Valles" (Barrios, Del chocolate [1609], reprinted in Antonio de León Pinelo, Question moral si el chocolate quebranta el ayuno eclesiastico [Madrid, 1636], fol. 117v).

14. The Nahua would commonly give the same name to several different plants or to plants that look alike or have the same properties but grow in different places. In an anticipation of the Bauhinian and Linnaean binomial systems, Hernández tried to get around this problem by adding place names, but without illustrations some plants are still unidentifiable.

15. The second edition, Beschrijvinghe van West-Indien (Leiden, 1630), was followed by a much expanded and revised Latin edition, Novus Orbis seu descriptionis Indiae occidentalis libri XVIII (Leiden, 1633), and a French translation with a few revisions and corrections of the Latin, L'histoire du Nouveau Monde, ou description des Indes occidentales (Leiden, 1640). Of course few people in the world read Dutch, and outside the Netherlands de Laet's Dutch work has never received more than passing attention. The clue that gives the game away, repeated over and over again, is that de Laet's title is so often misquoted, starting with Somolinos, as Beschrijvinghe van West-Indien door. "Door" is not a part of the title: it means "by."

Spanish manuscript by Hernández. As far as we know, nobody has ever described de Laet's manuscript or attempted to assess its significance.[16] In the 1620s and 1630s, this accomplished scholar and celebrated geographer—soon to prepare his own edition of Pliny—was translating Hernández back into Latin and into Dutch.[17] De Laet either acquired or had access to a manuscript of Hernández's Mexican work in Spanish, which he proceeded to translate into his own Latin. This became the basis for some translations into Dutch, which he put in the second edition of his book in 1630. We can be sure that Carolus Clusius, the foremost botanist of his time, would have used Hernández if he had been able to do so, but there is no sign of Hernández in any of Clusius's works, not even the posthumous *Histoire des drogues*.[18] De Laet's citations in 1630 thus constituted the first appearance of Hernández in the Netherlands and the first to have a significant readership anywhere in Europe.

A Calvinist who left his native Antwerp apparently for religious reasons, de Laet had been since 1621 a director of the Dutch West India Company, for whose employees' use he compiled his *Nieuwe Wereldt*.[19] The first two editions of de Laet's substantial book constitute a practical guide describing the plants, landscape, climate, customs, and miscellaneous observations of travelers to various parts of the Caribbean and Central and South America. These two editions of de Laet's book could not have reached a wide readership, simply because they were written in Dutch, but when the Latin edition appeared in 1633, it turned out to be a completely different, vastly improved and expanded text. The Latin or French editions were acquired by libraries and interested individuals all over Europe. All four editions of de Laet were published, as was everything else he wrote, by Elsevier in Leiden.

The first Dutch edition of de Laet includes some summary descriptions of the best-known Mexican plants quoted from José Acosta and Gabriel Alonso de Herrera. The medicinal properties of the *tunas* and the sheer versatility of the maguey persuaded de Laet that "New Spain is one of the best provinces of the New World and the most practicable to live in" ([1625 ed.], 5.1, p. 144). Cacao and corn turn up, in summary fashion, as do the armadillo and the crocodile, in the section devoted to Guatemala (bk. 7, caps. 1, 7), but in this 1625 edition there is no sign of Hernández at all. The first sign that de Laet had translated Hernández is *Beschrijvinghe van West-Indien* (Leiden, 1630), the second Dutch edition. Descriptions of twenty-seven plants taken from Hernández appear in this text, with those that are included in the sections on New Spain, Guatemala, and Michoacán being attributed directly to him. Acosta, Herrera, Nicolás Monardes, and others were now augmented by Hernández. Some of the descriptions of plants included in the books on other parts of the Spanish territories, including Peru, are unattributed and therefore harder to recognize, but in fact they are all Dutch translations of Hernández.

De Laet made further extensive use of his own translation, which he paraphrased, in the Latin edition, *Novus Orbis* (Leiden, 1633). Sixty-nine descriptions of plants taken from Hernández were incorporated in de Laet's printed Latin and French texts of 1633 and 1640. Descriptions of three of those plants were repeated in different sections of the book, and two that had been included in his 1630 Dutch were now omitted. In the 1633 Latin edition, de Laet included thirteen animals, eight of which had appeared in the 1630 Dutch, three minerals, and bezoar—the most common "stone" used in the European pharmacy.

De Laet's manuscript was eventually acquired by Hans Sloane, possibly as early as the decade of the 1680s, though the exact date of acquisition is unknown. Sloane started collecting manuscripts about 1680, and he certainly knew de Laet's work by the 1690s, but in print Sloane referred only to

---

16. There are a few passing allusions to this manuscript by P. J. P. Whitehead and M. Boeseman, *A Portrait of Dutch Seventeenth Century Brazil: Animals, Plants, and People by the Artists of Johan Maurits of Nassau* (Amsterdam: North-Holland Publishing Co., 1989). Their main focus is on Willem Piso and Georg Marcgraf and, where de Laet is concerned, his manuscript edition of Marcgraf (British Library, MS Sloane 1554).

17. De Laet's edition of Pliny was published in 3 volumes (Leiden, 1635). His other works include accounts of India and Persia.

18. Carolus Clusius, *Histoire des drogues, espiceries, et de certains medicamens simples, qui naissent e's Indes & en l'Amerique* (Lyon, 1619), a French edition of da Orta, Acosta, Alpino, and Monardes. See our commentary in "Hernández in the Netherlands and England," in *Searching for the Secrets of Nature*.

19. On de Laet leaving Antwerp, Johan Mensinga, biographical sketch of Abraham Munting, in Munting, *Naauwkeurige Beschrijving der Aardgewassen* (Utrecht, 1696), sig. [3]3 verso.

de Laet's printed texts, not to his manuscript.[20] Sloane's collections of books, manuscripts, specimens, herbaria, and miscellaneous objects formed the nucleus of the British Museum, which he enabled to be founded in 1753, and the manuscript has remained there ever since.[21]

The manuscript, British Library MS Sloane 1555, gives no explicit indication that Hernández is the original author; the title is "Plantarum Americanarum Descriptio," in nine books. MS Sloane 1555 is a small folio, of 98 leaves, all written in de Laet's neat, small hand.[22] The binding is contemporary. The first leaf of the manuscript has a list of the Mexican names of thirty plants, with the heading "D. Piso missa." We take the heading to mean that the descriptions, rather than the plants themselves, were sent to de Laet by his friend and colleague Willem Piso, chiefly because in the 1620s or 1630s, when de Laet made the translation, the young Piso had not yet gone to Brazil, where he would subsequently encounter some of these plants and send some of them back to Leiden.

Obviously, de Laet would have used a Latin text if he had had access to one, so we can be certain that he did not know Recchi's version as such—besides which, he never mentions Recchi by name in print or in manuscript. De Laet began his translation at some time between the two editions in Dutch, that is, between 1625 and 1630. By the time he produced his 1633 Latin edition, all that remained of Acosta's description of the maguey was a reference to his name. The way in which de Laet finally swept aside Acosta and Herrera and replaced them with the detailed descriptions of Hernández for the Latin edition suggests that as soon as de Laet discovered a text of Hernández in the late 1620s, he recognized its superiority and began to work it straight into the second Dutch edition of his own book; then between 1630 and 1633 he began to reshape his work. As

de Laet refined his work on the New World, his major innovations were chapters on the natural history of the region, and most of them were based extensively on Hernández. De Laet's subsequent Latin and French editions included many more selections, not only from Hernández but also from Monardes, Clusius, and López de Gomara.

De Laet's manuscript divides the Hernández materials into nine books, each one at first sight corresponding to the nine subdivisions that make up the four books of the *Quatro libros*. The first seven books of de Laet's manuscript describe plants. The eighth contains only three descriptions of animals, which are followed by three leaves that were left blank to make room for the rest of the animals, but that book was never completed. The ninth book contains the chapters on minerals. The organization of de Laet's material is, in places, the same as that of the *Quatro libros*, but he or his source text rearranged considerable portions, and he includes one chapter, on the *cempoalxóchitl* (3.69), that appears otherwise only in Nieremberg's 1635 text (which de Laet did not know until it was published), and chapters on the *tetocuilpatli* (3.38) and *tzocuilpatli* (4.2) that appear in print nowhere else at all.

By October 18, 1636, de Laet had seen copies of the *Quatro libros* and Nieremberg's *Historia naturae*, because he said so in a letter to Lucas Holste, and in a later letter he told Cassiano dal Pozzo that he had translated the work of Ximénez that was published in Mexico.[23] We know that one copy of the *Quatro libros* later in the century traveled from the Netherlands to London. As far as we know there is no copy of the *Quatro libros* in the Netherlands today, but one of the two copies in England, at Cambridge University Library, has a Dutch provenance and might have been the one that de Laet saw.[24] Yet de Laet's manuscript is not a straight translation of the *Quatro libros,* as we know not only

20. Sloane's earliest references to de Laet in print appear in his *Catalogus plantarum quae in insulae Jamaica sponte proveniunt* (London, 1696), which is, in effect, an index to his magnum opus, the *Natural History of Jamaica,* 2 vols. (London, 1707–25), which we discuss below.

21. Meaning the British Library, until 1997 housed in the British Museum but latterly not a part of it. The herbaria were transferred to the new Natural History Museum (then the British Museum [Natural History]) in 1880–81.

22. When he wrote in Latin, his handwriting was small and neat,

but his personal letters in Dutch are written in a different, florid style (compare, e.g., six letters in Latin to Claudius Salmasius, 1642–43, and one letter in Dutch to Arnoldus Buchelius, July 23, 1629, University Library, Leiden, MSS Pap. 7 and BPL 246).

23. Leiden, March 20, 1649; Université de Montpellier, Ecole de Médecine, MS H 268, fol. 80. Even as late as 1649 the Latin word *edita* is ambiguous, meaning either published or edited.

24. The Cambridge copy was acquired by John Moore at some time—probably late—in the seventeenth century. The other copy in England is at the British Library.

because his translations are often not especially close to Ximénez but also because he incorporates some texts that are not in the *Quatro libros* (but which are in the surviving manuscript drafts in Madrid), and he organizes some books in an entirely different order. The *Quatro libros* contains 478 chapters (424 plants, 27 animals, 26 minerals); de Laet's manuscript has 446 chapters (417 plants, 3 animals, and the same 26 minerals).

Translators and editors sometimes reorganize texts as they go along, but the ordering of de Laet's text, compared with the order shown by the Montpellier index, indicates that de Laet was not using a copy of Hernández's Spanish manuscript text from the Escorial—indeed, he could hardly have done so for practical and political reasons.[25] In *Novus Orbis* (1633; 5.23, p. 264) de Laet faithfully recorded an anecdote, which Ximénez embellished, that Hernández was on the point of losing his life after tasting the toxic leaves of the oleander. This anecdote appears nowhere else except the Complutense manuscript, so here, at least, is evidence that de Laet knew either the *Quatro libros* or the manuscript from which it was printed.[26] By no means were all the translations in de Laet's manuscript used in the Latin and French editions of his book, which contained more anyway than his Dutch editions, so that his is the most important single surviving manuscript because, along with Nieremberg's selections (discussed in the next section), de Laet's version is apparently an alternative arrangement and slightly different selection of Hernández, very close to the *Quatro libros*, certainly, but not identical to it.

Thus there were two divergent sets of texts in circulation in the early 1630s: the family of texts now represented by de Laet's manuscript and the *Quatro libros*, and the family represented by the Brown manuscript and the Rome edition of 1651. It seems certain that de Laet translated a Spanish translation of Recchi's selection, and in the

absence of other evidence, that is an assumption we are making. It is typical of this whole story that we introduce de Laet's manuscript in this section yet we conclude by discussing Recchi's. The evidence of de Laet's manuscript seems to mean that probably six discrete texts of Recchi existed:

1. the one that is now John Carter Brown Library Codex Latin 5
2. the manuscript, signed by Valles, owned by Barrios, and later used by Ximénez for the *Quatro libros*
3. one in Spanish that was used by de Laet
4. one that Recchi presented to the king
5. one that Recchi kept for himself, which passed into Cesi's hands and became the Rome edition
6. the Spanish text that became the Complutense manuscript

Juan Eusebio Nieremberg's *Historia naturae*

Working in Madrid with quite different manuscripts at the Imperial College, the Jesuit scholar Juan Eusebio Nieremberg incorporated 160 descriptions of plants, animals, and minerals from Hernández in his *Historia naturae, maxime peregrine*. This was another Low Countries venture, but, unlike de Laet's work, which was published in Leiden by Elsevier, Nieremberg's belonged to the now fading world of the Spanish Netherlands: his handsome book was published in that famous corner of Antwerp's Vrijdagmarkt by Balthasar Moretus at the Golden Compasses in 1635.[27] Nieremberg was certainly not the first to examine the Madrid manuscripts. Antonio de León Pinelo said in 1629 that he had seen three manuscript volumes of Hernández's work on the plants of New Spain, one on the animals, and one other on various subjects, including the Great Temple of Tenochtitlán. The drafts, he added, were in the Jesuits' college, and the corrected version in the author's hand, with illustrations,

25. De Laet's text does not resemble Hernández's translation, which exists in his hand but is very far from complete (BN MS 22,439).

26. This anecdote raises another pertinent question: from whom did Ximénez, who did not have any personal contact with Hernández in New Spain, learn about this incident?

27. Little scholarly and critical attention has been paid to this work. Commentaries on Nieremberg, such as Hughes Didier's *Vida y pensamiento de Juan E. Nieremberg,* translated by M. Navarro Car-

nicer (Madrid: Universidad Pontífica de Salamanca, 1976), concentrate solely on the spiritual writings. For discussion of Nieremberg, see Somolinos, 303–4. López Piñero and Pardo discuss the *Historia naturae* in *Nuevos materiales,* as do we in *Los manuscritos hernandinos y su difusión en los Países Bajos y Inglaterra* (Valencia: Instituto de Estudios Documentales e Históricos sobre la Ciencia, Universitàt de València, CSIC, forthcoming). The writings of Nieremberg (1595–1658) on aspects of natural magic and occult philosophy were important influences on Athanasius Kircher.

in the Escorial.[28] Nieremberg seems to have worked from both. Echoing Beristáin, Somolinos argues with some justice that Nieremberg's work is more important than the later Rome edition because it was taken directly from Hernández's manuscripts whereas the Rome edition had to rely solely on Recchi's selection. Nieremberg's selections include some chapters from the subsequently destroyed Escorial manuscripts, so that in about forty verifiable cases his texts of Hernández are unique.

Georg Marcgraf

Further extracts from Hernández in Latin, derived from de Laet's translation, appeared in a volume that contained two separate but closely related works that de Laet himself edited: Willem Piso's *De medicina Brasiliensi* and Georg Marcgraf's *Historia rerum naturalium Brasiliae,* printed by Elsevier and virtually always found today bound together in one volume, as they were issued (Leiden, 1648). Piso's work on Brazilian medicine makes no direct use of Hernández, but Marcgraf's companion work on Brazilian natural history incorporates thirty-three descriptions from the *Quatro libros* and de Laet.

Prince Johan Maurits employed Piso and Marcgraf to undertake their survey of the natural history of Brazil (1638–41). Piso (or Pies) was born in the early years of the seventeenth century, probably in Leiden, where he studied and practiced as a physician before settling in Amsterdam. Georg Marcgraf, from Liebstad in Meissen, far the more talented, was hired for the Brazil expedition in his threefold capacity as physician, scientist, and geographer. He was also an accomplished astronomer.

In 1643 Marcgraf was sent to Angola, where he died, and his encrypted notes from the Brazilian expedition were deciphered, then combined with Piso's work, by de Laet. The whole edited text was ready by 1646, but there was a delay in obtaining all the illustrations, and the work finally appeared in early 1648.[29] The resulting volume is a lavishly illustrated guide to the botany and zoology of northeastern Brazil, along with some commentary on meteorology, ethnology, and straightforward geography. The portions of the text that draw on Hernández are, as one would expect, annotations describing species common to Brazil and Mexico— twenty-seven plants and six animals. De Laet supplied all the annotations, which explains why he appears sometimes to intrude, speaking in his own voice and referring to his own work. The attributions are usually to Ximénez rather than Hernández.

These long-neglected Netherlandish translations show that, in one form or another, a relatively small but significant portion of Hernández's work was being made accessible about two decades before the belated appearance of the celebrated Italian edition of Recchi's version of his work, *Rerum medicarum Novae Hispaniae thesaurus.* In 1658, the Piso/Marcgraf volume on Brazil went into a second, much inferior edition, in which Piso introduced descriptions of the armadillo and the possum into his animal section, both derived from Hernández and Ximénez but taken without acknowledgment from Marcgraf. Many more allusions to Mexican plants appear in the 1658 edition under Piso's name, even though he had not been responsible for the botanical work. But by then Marcgraf and de Laet were both dead.

Hendrik and Abraham Munting

Two other Dutchmen, neither of them well known outside the Netherlands, both distantly connected with de Laet,

28. Antonio de León Pinelo, *Epitome de la biblioteca oriental i occidental, nautica i geografica* (Madrid, 1629). The drafts that he saw are those that we have mentioned above and that Bustamante describes below. They are now divided between the Biblioteca Nacional and the Ministerio de Hacienda. León Pinelo also made the extraordinary remark that the work of Hernández had been published in Frankfurt. His "authority" for this was Pietro Lasena, *Homeri Nepenthes seu de abolendo luctu liber* (Leiden, 1624), who does refer (81–82) to Hernández, but Lasena was describing Recchi's manuscript and the Lincei's intention to publish it. León Pinelo almost certainly saw the Lincei's edition listed in a catalog of the Frankfurt book fair (see Pierre Dupuy to Gerolamo Aleandro, Paris,

May 4, 1628, asking for a copy, even though he doubts that it was printed in Rome: books from the fair, he adds, do not reach Paris "because of the German wars" [*Il Carteggio Lincei,* Atti della Reale Accademia Nazionale dei Lincei, ser. 6, Memorie della classe di scienze morali, storiche, e filologiche 7 (Rome, 1938; reprint, Rome: Accademia Nazionale dei Lincei, 1996), 1165]). What is certain is that Johannes Faber's section on animals that was added to the *Rerum medicarum Novae Hispaniae thesaurus* has a title page dated 1628, but it was printed by Mascardi in Rome, not Frankfurt.

29. Information from Whitehead and Boeseman, *Portrait of Dutch Seventeenth Century Brazil.*

have a small role to play here. In 1642 Hendrick Munting (1583–1658) was appointed adjunct professor of botany and founded the second botanical garden in the Netherlands, at Groningen.[30] Marcgraf tells us that Munting cultivated *Canna indica* at Groningen, though where he obtained it originally no one knows.[31] Early in the seventeenth century Munting had been on what amounted to a ten-year grand tour of Europe, establishing a network of contacts and obtaining seeds and specimens to take back to the Netherlands. In London in 1604 he met his countryman Mathias L'Obel, the English king's botanist. Two years later, in Rome, Munting apparently stayed at the house of Johannes Faber and met a renowned expert on herbs and their medicinal preparations, Hendrik de Raaf. Munting made the journey to Naples specifically to meet Fabio Colonna, though his major career move there was to get himself appointed as personal physician to the prince of Gonzaga. Thus Munting established contact with two future commentators on Hernández, one of whom, Colonna, had already published his *Phytobasanos* (1592) with its mention of Recchi (but not Hernández) and his description of *tlápatl* (*Datura stramonium* L.).[32] Hendrik Munting may have established his collection of American plants as a result of this European tour. However he acquired them, Munting listed in his catalog about forty American plants that grew in his garden at Groningen, and because nearly all of them are listed in the contemporaneous catalog from Padua, one might guess that the one garden supplied the other with specimens or seeds.[33]

One of Munting's fourteen sons, Abraham (1626–83), would be, like his father, professor of botany at the University of Groningen, but he became even more distinguished. Abraham Munting's first book, the lavishly illustrated *Waare Oeffening der Planten* (Leeuwaarden, 1672) went quickly into a second edition the following year, and two more printings followed in 1682. In any of its early printings, Abraham Munting's work has a special linguistic and taxonomic

value because it is an important source of Dutch names for 65 trees, 64 shrubs, and 449 herbs, all of them European. Munting's most significant work is the posthumous, revised, and much expanded version of his first one, with the title changed to *Naauwkeurige Beschrijving der Aardgewassen* (Leiden and Utrecht, 1696). This is a massive, illustrated folio on medical botany, with an emphasis on the plants of the Netherlands and Germany.

The main text of Munting's posthumous and generally underrated work describes applications, methods of preparation, virtues, and, at the beginning of each chapter, the names of plants in five languages. For the medicinal virtues, Dioscorides, Galen, and Pliny are the main authorities, but Munting also uses Dodoens, Renodaeus, and Camerarius. The whole work seems as far removed from Hernández and Mexico as it could possibly be. Yet Hernández and Monardes appear occasionally, under "virtues." Munting gives references to Recchi and Hernández indifferently when he is citing the Rome edition and refers to Ximénez by name once or twice, suggesting that there was a copy of the *Quatro libros* in use in the Netherlands, probably in the late 1670s or early 1680s.

Franz Kiggelaer, "botanophile," made a Latin translation of Munting's work, which appeared as *Phytographia curiosa* in 1713 (reprint, 1727). Munting's connection with de Laet is explained in a prefatory biographical sketch by Johan Mensinga, who establishes that Hendrik Munting sent his son to Leiden to acquire the friendship of Adolf Vorstius (professor of botany) and de Laet. We know nothing more about the Muntings' connections, intellectual or personal, with either man. When de Laet died in 1653, Abraham Munting was still a young man of twenty-seven. We would guess that Munting the younger might have learned about Hernández, and in particular the *Quatro libros,* from contact with de Laet, especially when we see the sort of use that Munting made of the Mexican material.

---

30. The Muntings, father and son, are not especially well known even within the Netherlands: surprisingly, neither of them qualifies for a place in the *Nieuw Nederlandsch Biographisch Woordenboek,* the current dictionary of national biography.

31. MB 5.

32. See López Piñero and Pardo, *Nuevos materiales,* 78–79. Colonna said in 1592 that Recchi's work was in progress and in 1616 that the Lincei edition would "see the light."

33. Hendrik Munting, *Hortus, et universae materiae medicae Gazophylacium* (Groningen, 1646); Veslingius, *Catalogus plantarum horti gymnasi Patavini* (Padua, 1644).

ITALY, 1651

The Printing of the *Rerum medicarum Novae Hispaniae thesaurus*

Recchi selected texts from four manuscript volumes and organized his own selection of Hernández into four books, each one subdivided, in the arrangement familiar from the *Quatro libros*, an arrangement that the Rome edition of 1651 conceals even as it repeats, because it renumbers all the subdivisions as consecutive books. Chapters from the Brown manuscript are occasionally omitted from the Rome edition, the omissions usually occurring at the end of a book: such omissions may be editorial, but just as likely the result of a decision by a printer or compositor, because they always occur on the last leaf of a printer's sheet, where a new sheet would begin with the last two or three chapters. Even such a major and well-established printing house as Mascardi, like any other printer of the time, would not have had enough movable type in stock to set a long book such as this (950 folio pages) in less than about four months. To set all the type in one printing house, it would be necessary to set up two or three sheets at a time, each sheet representing, in this case, four printed pages. The staff would then print them, proofread them, correct them, and make the final print run, of perhaps five hundred copies.[34] The type would then be broken up, and the whole process would start again with the next set of sheets. For a large folio such as the Rome edition, it is most probable that the sheets were being printed by more than one printer elsewhere in Rome or in another city, simply to speed the process of producing the whole volume by having different parts of it set in type simultaneously. This would explain why each new "book" begins on a new sheet, because each printer's work could most conveniently be divided and assigned by book: Mascardi, or whoever oversaw the printing, would most likely split the manuscript where it was convenient, that is, between books

rather than between consecutive pages of continuous text. If a printer filled the sheet but had not quite reached the end of his portion of manuscript, he certainly would not begin another sheet if all the text left for him to set was not enough to fill the sheet. The text thus left over might be gathered together with any other bits of omitted text (from other printers) and printed as an appendix or as extra chapters. The omitted texts could just be left out altogether from the final printing.

Recchi himself certainly made not one but two copies of his selection, presenting one to the king and keeping the other. He personally may not have made any more copies, but others did. Yet it would be surprising to find one of Recchi's two personal copies being taken to Mexico and used by Ximénez. The copy that Recchi kept for himself is unlikely ever to have gone to Mexico, because it passed to his nephew Marco Antonio Petilio, who sold it to Prince Federico Cesi. Cesi wanted to publish an edition of this manuscript as the flagship publication of his new Accademia dei Lincei. He surely could not have known what he was letting himself in for, even though he had known about the work from Fabio Colonna. Colonna himself had had plans in the 1580s to publish an edition of Recchi's text, and he did eventually include one rather distant paraphrase of a few lines on the *cempoalxóchitl* (a marigold) in his *Minus cognitarum stirpium* (Rome, 1616). The ambitious Cesi even asked Theodore Müller to go to Mexico to "finish correcting a few things in the work of Recchi, . . . he left Rome on the 11th of April [1614]."[35]

Recchi's selection (however many copies there may be) was certainly the basis for the Lincei edition. One thing that does seem definite in this wilderness of uncertainties is that Recchi had a set of illustrations copied. The problem for Cesi was that Petilio had not sold him the illustrations. By 1611 Cesi had managed to lay his hands on a set of illustrations, however, because in May of that year he showed them

---

34. Among the stranger claims is one attributed to Claus Nissen, *Die Botanische Buchillustration: Ihre Geschichte und Bibliografie* 2nd ed. (Stuttgart: Hiersemann, 1966). According to a Christie's sale catalog (for June 24, 1992, p. 142), Nissen is supposed to have said that 2,000 copies were printed, that 1,000 destined for Spain were lost, and that surviving text sheets for 450 copies were finally reissued in 1649 and 1651. This seems to be a confused account of a

hypothesis proposed by Giuseppe Gabrielli, himself going on a plausible comment by Cassiano dal Pozzo, about 1,000 defective copies. For a convenient summary, see Somolinos, 411.

35. MS Vat. lat. 9681, fol. 1866. We are grateful to Rachel Bindman for alerting us to this information and providing us with a transcript of Cesi's letter.

to an admiring—and mildly frustrated—Galileo Galilei, the Accademia's newest recruit. Perhaps working from Recchi's copies of Hernández's originals, Cesi's group had by then apparently completed its own reproductions of the illustrations of five hundred Mexican plants. Galileo wrote to Piero Dini: "Then a few days ago, when, in the house of the illustrious and excellent Monsignore Prince Cesi, I saw the paintings of five hundred Indian plants, I had to affirm that either this is a fiction, denying that such plants exist in the world, or—if true, as it just might be—it is scourging and superfluous, as neither I nor any of those present knew their quality, virtue, or effects."[36] By 1613 the first woodcuts of these reproductions had been made, because Cesi was discussing sample illustrations done by Johann Gottfried: these were published in *Lynceorum Accademia mexicanarum plantarum imagines.* In 1619 Giorgio Nuvolo executed more woodcuts based on Recchi's copies, and these became the illustrations that would eventually be used in the Lincei's edition. In 1627 Matthäus Greuter engraved the first title page of the projected book, and a handsome, monumental design it is too. According to Francisco Guerra, Greuter changed the date on this title page from 1627 to 1628—easy enough in Roman numerals.[37]

The Lincei's book, which is often said to exist in five different states, was *Rerum medicarum Novae Hispaniae thesaurus,* beautifully printed and graced with a sumptuous engraved title page and a more sparely designed letterpress title page. Both title pages nicely suggest that the book is a monument to Hernández's industriousness, while they also announce its arrival in the new, public world of seventeenth-century printing. The first half of it (pp. 1–459) consists of ten books on Mexican plants, with woodcut illustrations; this section is followed by 375 pages on Mexican animals, 109 pages of commentary, an index, and a separate section

on animals. Cesi had enjoined Francesco Stelluti (1577–c. 1653) to oversee the work, in conjunction with Johannes Terrentius (Johann Schreck, c. 1580–1630), who was put in charge of the botanical section—the first half of the work.[38] Terrentius was aided by the Neapolitan scholar Fabio Colonna (1567/8–1650), who edited the plant section of Recchi's selection of Hernández.[39] The section on animals was assigned to Johannes Faber of Bamberg (Johann Schmidt, 1574–1629), and Cesi himself wrote a mighty, learned commentary on the classification of plants, separately published three centuries later as *Phytosophicarum tabularum ... prima pars* (Rome, 1904). The whole Rome edition is as valuable for the learned commentaries as it is for Recchi's version of Hernández's text.

The Lincei project was begun in earnest in 1610, but as two decades slipped by, Cesi seems to have intended to publish the whole book in 1628 (hence, supposedly, Greuter's alteration of the date on his title page). What happened next is uncertain. Guerra claims to have found evidence that ten copies with a 1628 title page might exist today—and so they may, and although some sheets survive with annotations in Cesi's hand (and he died in 1630), the book was not published in 1628.[40] These were tough times for the Lincei: three of the four commentators died by 1630, possibly just when they were again planning to issue this book, for a 1630 title page exists. No more is heard of the *Thesaurus* until 1648, when it might appear to have been published, with yet another new title page and a hastily updated dedication, necessary because its previous dedicatee, Cardinal Barberini, had been banished from Rome by Innocent X in 1644. The Lincei still had no more money for the project than before, and publication would have been impossible without the perseverance of Cesi's successor as the Accademia's president, Stelluti, who approached

36. *Il Carteggio Lincei,* 162.

37. Francisco Guerra, "La leyenda del Tesoro Messicano," *Atti dei convegni Lincei* 78 (1986): 312.

38. Stelluti was in charge of publication procedures as well as iconography. He obtained permission to publish from Pope Paul V as early as 1612. Terrentius worked on the project for only a very short time—probably one year or less—but he was evidently a fast worker. He had already finished his commentary by 1611, when he joined the Jesuits and left Rome on a mission to China, where he died.

39. Colonna—whom Linnaeus would later dub "the best of all botanists"—knew not only a great deal about botany but also enough Náhuatl to be able to correct the names of some plants. Incidentally, Colonna was the first to use the Greek *petalon* in the specialized sense of "petal." In his notes on Hernández, Colonna proposed the use of the term in its modern botanical sense, and in 1686 Ray endorsed this view by including the term this way in his own work.

40. Guerra, "Leyenda del Tesoro Messicano," 312. See n. 28, above, for the flawed claim that an edition was published in Frankfurt.

the Spanish ambassador in Rome for funds—and got them. Another title page is dated 1649, but the dedication to Philip IV is dated 1650. The book finally appeared with a newly dated title page in 1651.

We have seen the only complete copy with a 1628 title page in the United States, at the National Library of Medicine. The text in that and all differently dated copies that we have examined is identical in every respect, including such minutiae as broken letters, suggesting that the main body of the book was printed either repeatedly from the same type (impossible) or in a single set of sheets printed in 1628 that lay around somewhere for up to twenty-three years (not impossible but extremely unlikely for financial reasons), or in a single set of sheets printed in 1648 and used until the supply was exhausted in 1651.[41] This last hypothesis would mean that the dedications and title pages with the much earlier dates were printed in 1628 or 1630 in anticipation of a book that had not yet gone into production. The small, separately paginated section of Hernández devoted to Mexican animals and minerals, Johann Faber's *Animalia Mexicana descriptionibus scholiisque exposita,* is bound in at the end of most surviving copies of the *Rerum medicarum Novae Hispaniae thesaurus,* but it also exists as a separate entity with a 1628 title page. As a separate publication, it is extremely rare: the British Library and the Accademia Nazionale dei Lincei have copies, and another was offered recently at auction.[42] It is not even certain that this section was actually published in 1628. The most compelling evidence that there was no sign of the whole book in reality in 1628 or 1630 is that nobody in Europe seems to have seen it or even mentioned it. The best documentary evidence is the letter from de Laet to the Barberini librarian and fellow Netherlander Lucas Holste—also a member of the Lincei—dated October 18, 1636:

A book came into my hands that had been published in Mexico City, written in Spanish, about plants, animals, and minerals; its author was brother Francisco Ximénez, who took most of it from the books of Doctor Hernández, who had with great diligence described all of this at the order of the King of Spain, but because the author added no illustrations, his book is practically useless to us now. Several years ago we were expecting to see a compendium of this great work assembled by a very learned man, Nardo Antonio Recchi (as I gathered from Fabio Colonna), who had begun to compose it a long time ago. I saw a printed title page of this some years back; in conjunction with Elsevier last year we made inquiries in Rome about what hope there might be that this book exists; but I learned that the work had been interrupted or even discontinued because a similar book had been published by Nieremberg in the Low Countries. Yet his book, in my opinion, contains too little, and offers no illustrations apart from those that Clusius and others had already provided, which made me wonder why such a work would omit them. I am therefore asking you, distinguished sir, to explain how this matter stands, if you can find out the truth about it, and if this is how things are now, whether or not these are the true reasons, for I am missing the opportunity to add so many images; I have already received no few plants for the work of our American Company, and I took care to have them depicted from the living specimens.[43]

If de Laet's evidence was as exact as it looks, only a title page had been printed in 1628, and if so, it was probably used as a prospectus with two or three sample pages of text—not an uncommon practice. But this is the only suggestion that Nieremberg's work put a stop to the Lincei's.

Just as the *Quatro libros* generally did not reach Europe, so the *Thesaurus* did not reach Mexico. In Mexico, fray Agustín Vetancourt compiled his *Teatro mexicano* (Mexico City, 1698), which cites Barrios, Ximénez, and Farfán,

---

41. It seems that the Accademia itself was exhausted, too. It became moribund in 1651 and was never again a presence in Italian intellectual life until its revival in the early nineteenth century. Among the many studies of the Lincei, the most extensive and helpful is Giuseppe Gabrielli, *Contributi alla storia dell'Accademia dei Lincei,* 2 vols. (Rome: Accademia Nazionale dei Lincei, 1989). We have also benefited from Mario Biagioli, "Knowledge, Freedom, and Brotherly Love: Homosociality and the Accademia dei Lincei," *Configurations* 2 (1995): 139–66. As this book was in press, we also learned more about the Accademia from David Freedberg, to whom we are grateful.

42. Described in the Christie's catalog for Wednesday, June 24, 1992, p. 92.

43. A copy of de Laet's letter is preserved as Leiden, Universiteitsbibliotheek MS BPL 1830. We are grateful to the university library for permission to quote from this letter and for providing us with a photocopy of it. See also *Il Carteggio Linceo,* 1242–43. We have not yet found Holste's reply. A congratulatory verse by Holste to Faber appears in the *Thesaurus,* 839–40.

mentions Recchi, quotes from the *Quatro libros*, but makes no mention of the Lincei's edition either in the text or in the accompanying list of forty printed sources. Even if the Lincei project really was launched in 1628, no copies had reached the Netherlands either, and thus so few copies of the *Thesaurus* could have been in circulation then that de Laet's 1633 Latin edition, *Novus orbis seu descriptionis Indiae occidentalibus libri XVIII*, was truly the first printed work in Europe to make available substantial portions of Hernández's Mexican studies. But it was the Rome edition that became the standard text of Hernández, with the section on animals helping to generate the rival theories of Buffon and Clavijero in the late eighteenth century.[44]

ENGLAND, 1659–1752

Robert Lovell's *Pambotanologia*

In 1659 Robert Lovell produced a handbook entitled *Pambotanologia. Sive Enchiridion Botanicum. Or A Compleat Herball,* which contains an appendix listing close to two hundred therapeutics derived from plants in the East and West Indies. The West Indies section consists of ninety-five Mexican drugs. The texts of this portion of the appendix are Lovell's direct translations of appropriate and very short extracts taken from the *Quatro libros* and the *Rerum medicarum Novae Hispaniae thesaurus.* Lovell's abbreviated texts could come from either source, as they are all in both, but his language shows that in two cases he clearly used the Rome edition, in one he used Nieremberg, and the first three of his selections, *xochinacaztli, hoitzilóxitl,*

and *tlilxóchitl,* were translated from the *Quatro libros* rather than the Rome edition: again, this is evidence that the *Quatro libros* was available in England at mid-century. Nowhere is Hernández named as Lovell's source: indeed, only Richard Pulteney appears ever to have known that Hernández was Lovell's source or to have taken much notice of Lovell at all.[45]

The next substantial connection between Hernández and England comes by way of chocolate, in particular the lost treatise on chocolate by Juan Barrios. Even if Barrios's original treatise is lost, substantial enough extracts survive, yet they have been neglected until now. León Pinelo quoted Barrios at length in order to counter his argument about chocolate, and, in a parallel but unrelated treatment, a few short quotations in Spanish with English translations appeared in a learned work on chocolate, its medicinal applications, methods of preparation, and so forth by a Paracelsian sympathizer, Henry Stubbe. Stubbe's *The Indian Nectar* (London, 1662) was only the second treatise on chocolate in English ever to be printed; the first was a straightforward translation of a slim pamphlet by Antonio Colmenero de Ledesma, which Stubbe incorporated in his own work.[46] With a quixotic intertextual quirk, later versions of Colmenero would incorporate Stubbe. According to his preface, Stubbe was about to depart for Jamaica, where he expected to write an expanded and improved second edition of his work on chocolate, but instead he became a pamphleteer and controversialist who wrote about English religious politics.

Stubbe is responsible not only for providing extracts from Barrios.[47] He is also responsible for the first appear-

---

44. Discussed by Jaime Vilchis, "Globalizing the *Natural History,*" in *Searching for the Secrets of Nature.*

45. Lovell's book, said Pulteney, was "of so singular a complexion, as to merit notice in a work of this kind, were it only to regret the misapplication of talents, which demonstrate an extensive knowledge of books, a wonderful industry in the collection of his materials, and not less judgment in the arrangement. . . . At p. 482 begins an appendix on the drugs of the East and West Indies, extracted from the Arabians, and from HERNANDEZ" (*Historical and Biographical Sketches of the Progress of Botany in England, from its Origin to the Introduction of the Linnaean System.* 2 vols. [London, 1790], 1:181, 183). Educated at Christ Church, Oxford, Lovell is known to have practiced as a physician in Coventry, where he died in 1690, aged about sixty.

46. Stubbe (who signed his name thus) appears on the title page of *The Indian Nectar* as Stubbes. The standard study of Stubbe is James Jacob, *Henry Stubbe: Radical Protestantism and the Early Enlightenment* (Cambridge: Cambridge University Press, 1983). Harold J. Cook, "Physicians and the New Philosophy: Henry Stubbe and the Virtuosi-Physicians," in *The Medical Revolution of the Seventeenth Century,* ed. Roger French and Andrew Wear (Cambridge: Cambridge University Press, 1989), 246–71, is also useful. Colmenero, *Curioso tratado de la naturaleza y calidad del chocolate* (Madrid, 1631), translated into English as *A Curious Treatise of the Nature and Quality of Chocolate* by James Wadsworth (London, 1640; reprint, London, 1652).

47. A transcription of these extracts is reproduced by Simon Varey and Rafael Chabrán, "Mexican Medicine Comes to England," *Viator* 26 (1995): 352–53.

ance in English of comparable extracts on chocolate and the other medicinal ingredients included in Hernández's chapter on cacao. Stubbe had access by about the mid-seventeenth century to the Rome edition, but more surprisingly he had access also to "some citations" from a copy of the *Quatro libros*. Although it is valuable to see Hernández finding his way into English print, it is just as important that Stubbe used the voice of Hernández together with those of Juan de Cárdenas, Colmenero, and a Spanish doctor named Antonio de Robles Cornejo, who worked in Peru and later met Hernández in Madrid.[48] Stubbe apologizes to his readers "for representing so imperfectly the aforesaid *Indian* drinks; for the *Mexican Herbal* [i.e., *Rerum medicarum Novae Hispaniae thesaurus*] is so defective; . . . the *Spanish* is incomparably better, if I may judge thereof by some citations, I have seen."[49] All the same, Hernández emerges in context as one of several authorities, each of whom contributes his description, experience, assessment of the medicinal virtue, and discussion of the other ingredients that are added to cacao to make the compound medicine known as chocolate. In the Mexican pharmacy and in ordinary nonpharmaceutical chocolate drinks, the four principal additional ingredients, all valued for their medicinal effects as much as their flavor, were *achíotl* (more commonly known in England as anatto seed), corn, vanilla, and chili peppers.

By the 1670s the standard popular treatise on the three drinks together was a much reprinted, much translated pamphlet, attributed to Philippe Sylvestre Dufour and known in English as *The Manner of Making of Coffee, Tea, and Chocolate*. In the English edition of this little pamphlet (London, 1685) the section on chocolate was a new translation of Colmenero, by John Chamberlayne, who realized that Colmenero's account of chocolate was incomplete because it concentrated on the fruit of the cacao tree and its applications but omitted any mention of the tree itself and its cultivation. Because Colmenero had not described the

cacao plant (or rather, any of its four varieties that were commonly cultivated), Chamberlayne added a description and did the same for the plants that supplied the other principal ingredients.[50] Stubbe had provided the same information, but Chamberlayne did not take his texts describing these plants from Stubbe. Rather, Chamberlayne turned to the *Quatro libros* or the Rome edition, but it is hard to determine which, because Chamberlayne rendered his extracts in English without citing the Spanish or Latin and because his references to book and chapter are wild. Chamberlayne took further extracts of Hernández from the published Latin text of de Laet's *Novus Orbis* (1633), so that we have the transmission of a text from Hernández's original Latin to a Spanish translation to de Laet's Latin translation to Chamberlayne's translation of de Laet's Latin into English. It seems incredible that Chamberlayne is no further away from Hernández than he is. When Chamberlayne translated Colmenero, he was still only nineteen, embarking on a career of thoroughly miscellaneous writing.

Sir Hans Sloane and the *Natural History of Jamaica*

When the Duke of Albemarle was appointed governor of Jamaica in 1687, he took with him his personal physician, a twenty-seven-year-old Irishman named Hans Sloane. Sloane already had an established interest in medical botany and would have liked to have stayed in Jamaica longer than he did, but after eighteen months the duke died. The widowed duchess wanted to return to England at once and wanted Sloane to accompany her, so with all due gallantry he complied with her wishes. By the end of 1688, Sloane had laid the foundations for his only substantial printed work, *A Voyage to the Islands Madera, Barbados, Nieves, S. Christophers and Jamaica with the Natural History of the Herbs and Trees, Four-footed Beasts, Fishes, Birds, Insects, Reptiles, &c. of the last of those Islands*, in two large folio volumes, the whole known

---

48. Cárdenas had discussed cacao and chocolate, in three chapters of his *Primera parte de los problemas y secretos maravillosos de las Indias* (Mexico City, 1591). Robles Cornejo recorded his meeting with Hernández, in 1585, in an herbal approved for publication in 1617 but never published. The manuscript, which describes mostly Spanish plants but with some from New Spain, is Madrid, Real Jardín Botánico, Archivo, IV. 232 fol. 197.

49. Stubbe, *Indian Nectar,* 12.

50. In 1681 Giuseppe Donzelli incorporated the description of cacao from the Rome edition in his *Teatro farmaceutico.*

elliptically as the *Natural History of Jamaica*.[51] An important botanical, taxonomic, and medical work in its own right, Sloane's two lavish volumes contain exhaustive scholarly descriptions and exquisite engravings of more than four thousand plants native to Jamaica, many of them common to Mexico. Sloane drew on the work of most of the major writers and compilers we have mentioned in connection with Hernández, as well as virtually anyone else, dead or alive, who had anything significant, however brief or erroneous, to contribute to his subject.[52]

As Sloane painstakingly compiled the *Natural History of Jamaica*, this gifted linguist translated from the recognized Spanish sources and from Nieremberg, de Laet, Piso, and Marcgraf where relevant, and he incorporated forty-eight extracts from Hernández, together with comments on the accuracy or inaccuracy of the illustrations or the descriptions. Most writers before Sloane had shown respect for Hernández, to the point of accepting his descriptions uncritically, often because they knew of no systematic survey that would distinguish between species or between subspecies: with nothing to compare with his descriptions, Marcgraf, de Laet, and Nieremberg had taken Hernández as authoritative, and John Ray considered Hernández authoritative because he was the only one who had systematically described the Mexican material—even if some of his descriptions were defective.[53] It is clear that Ray and Sloane saw eye to eye about many things, including their judgments of Hernández. Although Sloane accepted Hernández's accuracy most of the time, he recognized confused identifications and descriptions in the Rome edition and the *Quatro libros* where others had seen no problems, and he noticed that the illustrations in the Rome edition did not always match their accompanying descriptions. If the Lincei scholars had come to similar conclusions, they kept their peace,

but only Sloane ever said anything about Hernández like this: "*Tlatlanquaye* and *Acapatli* of *Hernand.* and *Xim.* are so very confusedly Figured and Described, that I can make nothing of them, though I believe there are two sorts common to *New-Spain* and this Island, whereof this is one."[54] With such healthy and pragmatic skepticism, volume 1 (1707) and volume 2 (1725) of Sloane's *Natural History of Jamaica* made available, in English, significant portions of Hernández likely to interest English botanists, physicians, apothecaries, settlers, merchants, and consumers. Like the brief excerpts cited and translated by Stubbe, Sloane's more substantial translations have eluded the attention of Hernández scholars despite the renown of Sloane's work and its dissemination all over Europe.[55]

In the preface to volume 1 of *Jamaica* Sloane recounted some familiar parts of the story of Hernández and his expedition "to search after Natural Productions about Mexico; He design'd and describ'd many of the things he met with, at the Expence of 60000 Ducats; his Papers were put into the hands of Nardus Antonius Recchus, from whose Manuscripts they were by the Lyncei Publish'd at Rome, Anno 1649." Then, departing from any other commentators, Sloane noticed that the *Quatro libros* and the Lincei edition presented divergent texts, but he seems to have been the first to notice, or to care, that the real difference is not in what the two texts contain but in the order in which they are presented: "They were chang'd from their first order, as appears by the Spanish-Copy, Printed at Mexico; and 'tis pity that they were alter'd, and are so short and obscure."[56]

Sloane had also heard a rumor that the Hernández manuscripts deposited in the Escorial had survived the fire:

> Meeting with many of the Plants he describes in Jamaica, I had a great mind to be satisfied about them, and being

51. Each volume occupied Sloane for about eighteen years. Before either of them appeared in print, he put his manuscripts at the disposal of John Ray, whose *Historia plantarum* thus drew on Sloane's notes on Hernández, among others. Sloane also issued a most useful index, the *Catalogus plantarum quae in insula Jamaica sponte proveniunt* (London, 1696). These may be the only books to bear Sloane's name, but we should note his many contributions in the form of short papers read to the Royal Society and subsequently printed in the *Philosophical Transactions*, which he edited.

52. Sloane's encyclopedic approach is discussed in our as yet unpublished paper, "Try Deconstructing Sloane's *Natural History*

of Jamaica," read at a meeting of the South Central Society for Eighteenth-Century Studies, New Orleans, March 1996.

53. Ray, *Historia plantarum*, vol. 2, 2d ed. (1688), 1929–43.

54. Sloane, *Natural History of Jamaica*, 1:135.

55. Sloane's reputation among scholars today is not high, as witnessed by the tenor of several essays in *Sir Hans Sloane: Collector, Scientist, Antiquary*, ed. Arthur MacGregor (London: British Museum, 1995).

56. Sloane, *Natural History of Jamaica*, vol. 1, preface, n. pag.

told that the Original Draughts were in the King of Spain's Library, in the Escurial [sic] near Madrid, I wrote to Mr. Aglionby when he was Envoy from the late King William to the Court of Spain, to procure a Sight of that Work, and give me an Account of it. He was so obliging as to take the Pains to go thither, and was told that the Book was there, and that he should some time or other see it; which, tho' he endeavour'd several Times, yet he could never effect. Neither had other curious Travellers, better Fortune; for when they had heard of this Book, and (knowing of what importance it would be to see these Originals) did endeavour to procure a Sight of them, the Library-Keepers were so ignorant, to produce them, some other Book, no ways to the Purpose. Upon the whole matter, I am apt to think the Originals were carried to Rome, where the History was Publish'd, and that they remain'd there with Recchus his Nephew; where, If my Memory fail me not, Fabius Columna says he saw them, and that they are either to be found there, or at Naples, where Columna liv'd, that wrote Notes on them, or that they are lost.[57]

The allusion to Recchi's nephew is to Marco Petilio, who had sold the manuscript to Cesi. Curiously, Sloane equated Recchi's redaction with "the Originals" at the Escorial. Sloane went on to cite printed evidence in 1725 that he himself had been the factor that encouraged Joseph Pitton de Tournefort to send Charles Plumier to the West Indies to carry out his survey of native, medicinally useful plants.

> Dr. *Tournefort,* a Person of the greatest Curiosity in Things of this Nature, sent over to me from *Paris,* Dr. *Gundelscheimer,* to view what I had brought from *Jamaica.* ... This Gentleman, who was afterwards Physitian to the King of Prussia, and is since dead, carried back to Dr. *Tournefort* an Account of what I had brought from the *West-Indies,* and at the same Time a present, I made him amongst other Things, of Sixty very extraordinary Ferns, of which I had duplicates. This was the Occasion of Father *Plumier's* being sent to the *West-Indies,* as appears by [a] Passage in Labat.[58]

All of this is entirely plausible. What is apparently certain is that Tournefort had tried to find the Hernández manuscripts at the Escorial in 1688, even before Sloane's abortive attempt during Aglionby's first spell in Madrid, in 1692–93. In one of his prefaces Tournefort explains how he went in search of Hernández's descriptions of American plants: "There were some who supposed that this work was preserved in the rich royal library of the Escorial, near Madrid. But when I asked for the volumes of plants in the Hernández collections, several codices were shown to me but none dealt with plants from the Americas; they were all books of domestic plants, not exotics."[59] Other French writers cite Hernández, but less than their English counterparts.

The key to widespread European interest in Hernández was, of course, the appearance at last of the Rome edition. Once that edition of Hernández began to circulate, copies were acquired all over Europe. John Goodyer paid £1.14.0 for it in December 1652 (his copy is still at Magdalen College, Oxford); by March 24, 1670, the library of Nicolas Marchant contained two copies.[60] One came to Chatsworth, seat of the Dukes of Devonshire, and another was bought by the Royal Society, perhaps at Sloane's prompting; another went into the Huth collection (sold for £7 in June 1913), and in time copies appeared at Cambridge University Library, the Bodleian Library, and the library at Kew Gardens. Wolfenbüttel has a copy as well, as do the Bibliothèque Nationale in Paris, the Biblioteca Nacional in Madrid, and most other comprehensive libraries in Europe. The Rome edition was a major folio, an obvious purchase. Sir Thomas Browne bought a copy, which Sloane acquired when he bought Browne's entire library, and Browne cited it too, when he added a reference to the amphisbaena, or two-headed snake, to the 1672 edition of his eccentric *Pseudodoxia Epidemica.*[61] John Ray apparently did not have a personal copy of Hernández, but he certainly used the Rome editon in the 1680s, as did Tournefort in the 1690s, Charles Plumier in

57. Ibid. The reference is to Labat's "Journal of the Year 1697," 4:24.

58. Ibid.

59. Tournefort, *Institutiones rei herbariae* (Paris, 1700), "Isagoge," 44.

60. R. T. Gunther, *Early British Botanists and Their Gardens* (Oxford: Oxford University Press, 1922), 199. Paris, Bibliothèque du Muséum d'Histoire Naturelle, MS 447, "Catalogue des auteurs qui ont escrit des plantes depuis C[aspar] B[auhin]," fol. [2r], and "Catalogus librorum in Biblioteca Botanica, Dom: Nicolai Marchant," fol. 2r. The latter shows that Marchant had both editions of Piso/Marcgraf as well. Information from Alice Stroup, via Dora Weiner.

61. Bk. 3, chap. 15, in *Works,* ed. Geoffrey Keynes, 4 vols. (Chicago: University of Chicago Press, 1964), 2:207.

the 1700s, Pierre Pomet in the 1710s, and Jean Baptiste Labat in the 1720s. The last two of these authors were familiar with the *Quatro libros* as well, though both tended to summarize four or five authors at once, so their source texts are seldom clear.

Sloane had already begun to amass the largest single collection of medical and botanical materials that perhaps any individual has ever attempted to create. When it came to the American plants, he was familiar with all the writings that mattered, including the *Quatro libros,* perhaps from the bishop of Ely's collection, which was available to scholars in London. When John Moore became bishop of Ely in 1707, his library was already famous in Britain and the subject of jealous speculation about his methods of acquiring books. When the collection was bought by King George I and given to Cambridge University, in 1714, it did contain a copy of the *Quatro libros,* which had been in Dutch hands at some time before Moore obtained it. Moore had such an interest in medicine that some have thought him a physician.[62] At any rate, Sloane may have read this copy or possibly acquired his own by then. The present British Library copy may have been Sloane's, but his information about it in the *Natural History of Jamaica* seems to depend more on de Laet than on any copy Sloane may have had in front of him:

> However, it went with the Manuscript, from which that at Rome was publish'd; there was a Copy printed at Mexico in Spanish, in the Year 1615. Francisco Ximenes, one who attended the Sick of the Hospital in that City, publish'd it then, with Emendations, Notes, and the Additional Observations he had made of several Simples he had found in Espaniola, or Sto. Domingo, and other Islands of the West-Indies. John de Laet mentions this Book in Latin, and from him Vander Linden, in his Book de Scriptis Medicis has, I suppose, taken its Title, but I

verily believe it was never printed in any other Language than Spanish. John de Laet takes many things out of him, and puts them very often in a wrong Place, as additional to the Observations of Marcgrave in Brasile, in the Edition of that Author, publish'd by him in 1648. But that Fault may be easily pardon'd, in one who was no more than a Collector and Editor of Books wherein he did not pretend to any great Knowlege [*sic*].[63]

This was easily the most comprehensive account yet of the Hernández manuscripts. Subsequent searches still have not turned up "the originals" in Rome (where Spanish scholars looked in 1783) or in Naples. Who knows whether the Escorial librarians in the 1690s were misinformed, as Sloane's account makes them seem, or incompetent, as appears from Tournefort?

Sloane also mentions Piso and Marcgraf and their work on Brazil, adding that it was a pity Marcgraf died before he had finished working up the papers, because de Laet "tho' a learned man, yet was ignorant of *Natural History*" and Piso, "tho' a Practical Physician, yet had no great Knowledge of Natural things," leading to a less reliable edition than "one could wish," and he cared little for Piso's 1658 edition. But Sloane's purpose was to get at the truth, not condemn shoddy scholarship.

James Newton's *Enchyridion*

Tradition has it that in or around the year 1689 James Newton, an English physician and "a diligent and skilful botanist," compiled the only work he ever wrote, and one he left unfinished when he died in 1718.[64] Newton's work remained unpublished until 1752, when it was issued as *The Complete Herbal,* which contains, as an appendix, *Enchyridion Universale Plantarum: or, An Universal and Complete*

---

62. Moore's library was available to scholars, at Ely House (now demolished) in Holborn, London, but presumably it was housed there only after Moore was appointed to the see of Ely in 1707. We are indebted for much of this information to David McKitterick.
63. Sloane, *Natural History of Jamaica,* vol. 1, pref. n. pag. Sloane's allusion to van der Linden is puzzling, because in the first edition of *De scriptis medicis* van der Linden cites the Rome edition under its normal title and in the normal contemporary way: as *Nova plantarum* (Rome, 1651) under Hernández, and *Plantarum, animalium &c.* (1648) under Recchi. Sloane referred to Mercklin's edition of

van der Linden (1686), in which the Rome edition again appears twice, but each time with the date 1649.
64. The compliment is from Pulteney, *Sketches,* 1:234. The dating of Newton's work to 1689 originated with Johannes Dryander, who compiled the *Catalogus Bibliothecae historio-naturalis Josephi Banks,* 5 vols. (London, 1796–1800). Dryander noted (vol. 3 [1797], 37) that Newton referred to Ray's 1688 volume of the *Historia plantarum,* but not to anything published later and so assumed that that was about the date of composition.

History of Plants, with their Icons, in a Manual.[65] Newton was one of many people who had assisted Ray, probably with specific information, as Ray graciously acknowledged in the preface to his own *Historia plantarum.*[66] Nevertheless, Newton lapsed into obscurity even in his own lifetime.

The *Enchyridion,* Newton's section on apple trees (including one type of tomato), includes seven Mexican species whose descriptions Newton adopted from either the Rome edition, Nieremberg, or Ximénez by way of de Laet. The seven are *huitztomatzin, amacóztic, ahoacaquáhuitl, texotli* (Nieremberg), *tzopilotlzontecomatl,* which he called *tzopilotl* (Ximénez and de Laet), *tetlatia* (Nieremberg, Recchi), and *illamatzapotli* (Recchi). Newton questioned Recchi's identification of the *tzopilotlzontecomatl* and took only a small portion of his text from Recchi. The rest of Newton's text could have come from Ximénez, but if he used de Laet, as he says, Newton must have had access to de Laet's manuscript, because this plant was not included in any published edition of de Laet's book on the New World.[67]

James Petiver

James Petiver was a botanist, entomologist, and apothecary. Petiver's role in English work with connections to Hernández occurs mostly in his capacity as apothecary, because he was always looking for new ingredients to incorporate in his medications, and as a result of these interests he owned a formidable library, which might have included de Laet's manuscript translation of Hernández.[68] Petiver's life seems to have been a natural history of compulsive annotation: book after book contains cross-references in his small, neat hand. Of particular interest to us are his annotations to Nieremberg (in a copy now at UCLA's Clark Library) and to the 1658 Piso/Marcgraf (at the British Library, with most of his other books). The Clark copy of Nieremberg's book was sold as a duplicate by the British Museum in 1769, probably because its annotations would have been considered disfiguring at the time (two other copies, both clean and acquired, we think, in the eighteenth century, remain in the British Library today). Petiver's annotations in these volumes show an interest almost exclusively in Hernández, and in particular they provide cross-references to the Rome edition. Petiver also corrected some of the spellings of the Náhuatl names of plants in the chapter headings. The annotations to Nieremberg, probably made in the mid- to late 1690s, with references to Sloane added in or after 1707, mark the information he wanted or needed to help him make salable drugs.[69]

Petiver was the author of several works, including one very rare publication, *Hortus Peruvianus Medicinalis: or, The South-Sea Herbal* (London, 1715), which consists of three double columns of commentary keyed to five plates depicting a variety of plants from the Americas—not just from Peru, despite the implication of the title. Petiver's main sources are Louis Feuillet, who is named in the long subtitle as discoverer of most of these plants, then Pomet, Lémery, Ray, and Hernández. Curiously, Petiver gives no bibliographical information, so that any reader using this slim pamphlet would be expected to know who all these authorities were.

SPAIN, 1790

The Madrid Edition

Barely a decade after the expulsion of the Jesuits from Spain in 1767, Juan Bautista Muñoz, "cosmographer of the Indies," was working through manuscripts in the library at the Imperial College in Madrid, preparing his *Historia del Nuevo Mundo.* He came across the rough drafts of Hernández's work

---

65. The *Complete Herbal* was reprinted in London in 1798, 1802 (the "6th edition") and 1805. The *Enchyridion* was not included in these reprints.

66. Ray, *Historia plantarum,* vol. 1, n. pag., sig. A3vf.

67. And although the plant appears in Lovell, Newton cites much more than Lovell does.

68. His library included that rarity Colonna's *Phytobasanos* (1592), Hendrick Munting's 1646 catalog, Abraham Munting (1672), de

Laet in Dutch (1625), Thomas Trapham on Jamaica (1679), Monardes, and the Rome edition of Hernández (British Library, MS Sloane 3367, fols. 8r, 11v, 16r, 35v, 36r). For the possibility that Sloane acquired the de Laet manuscript from Petiver, see Whitehead and Boeseman, *Portrait of Dutch Seventeenth Century Brazil.*

69. British Library, MSS Sloane 2295, 2311–12, 2338, 2340, 2344, 2346, 2350, 2363–64, 2366, 2941 are Petiver's notebooks, crammed with remedies and his notes on a variety of diseases.

on Mexican materia medica, as well as the manuscript of Hernández's poem addressed to his friend and mentor Benito Arias Montano. Recognizing these documents for what they were, and realizing that they had been "lost" for 150 years, Muñoz alerted the noted physician and botanist Casimiro Gómez Ortega, who copied the manuscripts in 1786.[70] Those copies are now in the Museo de Ciencias Naturales in Madrid. Gómez Ortega at once prepared a new edition of Hernández's works based on these manuscripts: the *Opera* (Madrid, 1790), always known as the Madrid edition. In his preface Gómez Ortega wrote about the discovery of the Hernández manuscripts: the documents were found "not without divine design"; the discovery itself was a "most auspicious event." He added that the documents, which were written and corrected in Hernández's own hand, had been unearthed from their semirotten state by the labors of Muñoz as they "were disintegrating on the library shelves, and were doing constant battle with cockroaches and worms."[71]

The task of printing and publishing the Hernández manuscripts was given to Joaquín Ibarra (1725–85), the "royal printer" who was "recognized as the outstanding Spanish printer of modern times."[72] But Ibarra did not live to see Hernández's work in print, and the job was taken over by his widow. Coinciding with the high point of the Crown's support for science in the eighteenth century, the finished product was another handsome tribute to Hernández, in quarto on fine paper, albeit without any illustrations. Somolinos calls the Madrid edition the most personal or authentic of the Hernández editions. Even this edition was never completed; three volumes were published in 1790, but the projected fourth and fifth never materialized.[73] With more than three thousand descriptions of plants and the medicines derived from them, the Madrid edition put something like Hernández's original text on Mexican materia medica in print, in Spain, at last.

The story of the dissemination of Hernández texts does not end with the Madrid edition, as our chronology of his works indicates, but we do not have the space to chart the publication of letters to the king in 1842, or the translation of the Madrid edition into Spanish a century later, or the modern edition in Spanish, the *Obras completas*. Some works remained in manuscript until the appearance of the *Obras completas* and attracted no attention. These include *The Christian Doctrine, A Book of Stoic Problems, A Book of Stoic Questions,* and other, lesser pieces. We can now begin to see the relationships between the manuscripts and the many printed texts that included parts of Hernández's work on the natural history of New Spain. We conclude this essay with a stemma—which we believe is the first ever devoted to Hernández—that shows these relationships and demonstrates how widespread the dissemination of the work of Hernández on Mexican natural history really was and continues to be.[74]

70. Gómez Ortega (1741–1810) was director and professor of the Real Jardín Botánico, as well as court physician and royal pharmacist to Charles III. As Somolinos indicates (331), we do not know the exact date of Muñoz's discovery, but it must have been between 1775 and 1783. The papers are discussed in the next essay, by Jesús Bustamante, and the whole enterprise is discussed by Leoncio López-Ocón, "The Circulation of the Work of Hernández in Nineteenth-Century Spain," in *Searching for the Secrets of Nature.*

71. M 1:iv.

72. Diana Thomas, "The Book Trade in Ibarra's Madrid," *Library,* 6th ser., 5 (1983): 335. Somolinos said much the same (345). Copies of José Nicolás de Azara's letter to the Marqués de Sonora, Rome, July 20, 1785, and Gómez Ortega's letter to Sonora, Madrid, September 20, 1785, countering some of Azara's scholarly conclusions about Hernández, reveal the intellectual justification for a new edition in the 1780s. The purpose of the letters was to win Sonora's approval for funding (Madrid, Biblioteca Nacional, MS 22727, folletos 47–48). Official correspondence concerning the division of tasks, subsidies, and publication is now at the John Carter Brown Library.

73. Somolinos, 396. Volumes 1–3 contain, as planned, Hernández's poem to Arias Montano, which was thus published for the first time, and the bulk of the botanical studies. Volume 4 was to have contained sections on minerals and animals as well as some other aspects of natural history, and Gómez Ortega's commentaries; volume 5 was to have consisted of miscellanies and commentaries.

74. Pending our detailed study of the Complutense MS, we have omitted it from this diagram.

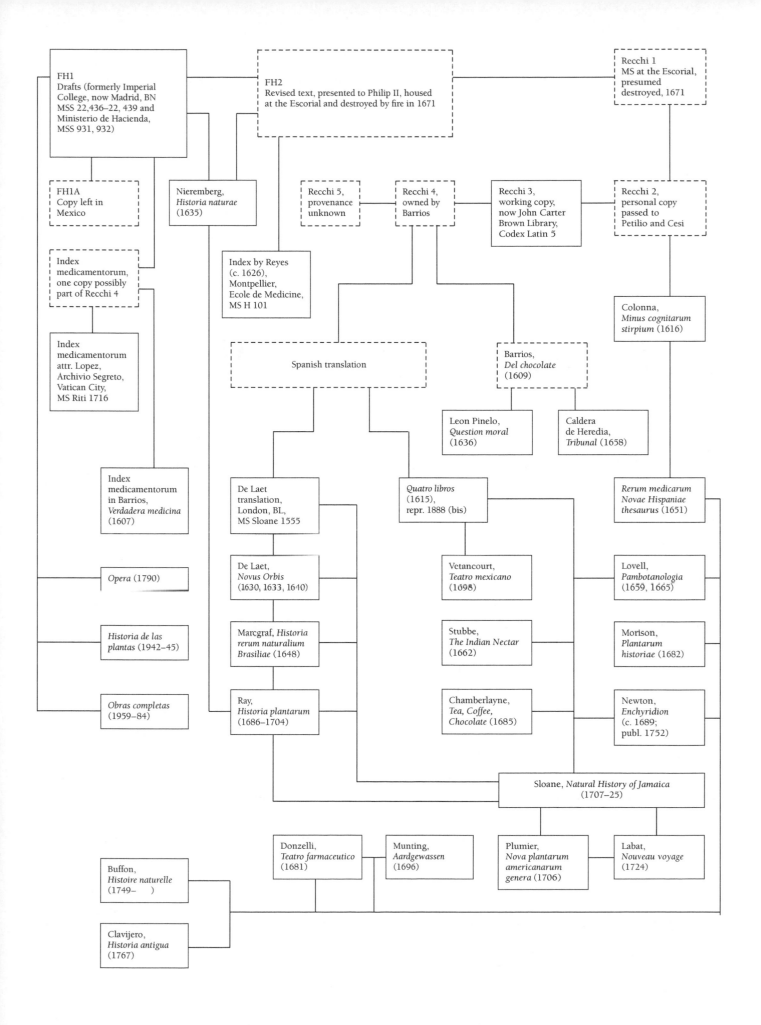

THE *NATURAL HISTORY OF NEW SPAIN*

JESÚS BUSTAMANTE

In the framework of the historiography of early modern Spain and its scientific achievements, Francisco Hernández's work on natural history has played a very special role, at least since the eighteenth century.[1] Spanish scholars could make long lists of more or less "brilliant" works by Iberian authors, but, for a vindication-oriented historiography, it was essential to find, in addition, some published work that could be considered an unambiguous contribution to the history of science. And that was the role assigned to the work of Hernández, because in contrast to so many works preserved in manuscript whose diffusion was dubious, the work of Philip II's *protomédico* seemed to be just what the scholars were looking for: a work whose manuscript had not survived but whose place and dissemination in the scientific world could not be doubted, since it had become known only through "European" (non-Spanish) editions and citations.

Toward the end of the eighteenth century the canonization of Hernández as the father of Spanish science led to the so-called rediscovery of his original manuscripts and to a truncated edition (Madrid, 1790), which contained only the *History of Plants*.[2] But throughout the nineteenth century, as "the question of Spanish science" received renewed and very polemical attention, back came the convenience of an acritical adoption of the texts edited in the two previous centuries. Preoccupied with the weighty question of the work's place and dissemination, rather than its originality or the significance of Hernández's whole project, both in itself and in the context of its time, scholars preferred to proceed—incredible as it seems—as if all traces of the original manuscripts of Hernández had been lost or destroyed.

In our own time we have inherited this tendency, which was even in a sense adopted by Germán Somolinos and the

---

1. This essay is derived from a larger research project (PB97-1125) financed by the DGES, Dirección General de Educación y Cultura, Spain.

2. See Fermín del Pino, "América y el desarrollo de la ciencia española en siglo XVIII: Tradición, innovación y representaciones

a propósito de Francisco Hernández," *La América Española en la época de las Luces: Tradición-innovación-representaciones* (Madrid: Ediciones de Cultura Hispánica, 1988), 121–43.

rest of the editorial board of the *Obras completas* of Hernández. In this edition, which most certainly is not complete as
the title claims, the *Natural History of New Spain* is simply a
translation of the Madrid edition of 1790 (consisting of no
more than the *History of Plants*), complemented by the one
book on animals that was tacked on at the end of the Rome
edition of Hernández (1651).[3] Nonetheless, the editors
undeniably knew of the existence of some manuscripts that
would have been more useful to them in reestablishing the
text of Hernández as he might have written it. As for the section on animals, textually the most difficult and problematic,
they knew that the Museum of Natural Sciences in Madrid
held two manuscripts comprising the copy of the original
text of Hernández on zoology that Casimiro Gómez Ortega
had had made in 1786 but that was not included in his
1790 edition.[4] As for the plants, they also knew about MS
932 in the library of the general archive of the Ministerio
de Hacienda in Madrid, which is nothing less than the second volume of the original manuscript of Hernández, yet
they scarcely used it. They did give a good deal of attention
to MS 931 in the same collection, which corresponds to volume 5 of the Hernández original and which was published
just about in its entirety in volume 6 of the *Obras completas*.[5]
I do not mean all this to be a facile criticism of an edition I
consider admirable, very useful, and full of value. I intend

only to call attention to limitations and assumptions that
we would do well to overcome.

The manuscripts of the *Natural History* of Hernández
were not irretrievably lost or destroyed; in fact, one might
well ask if they have ever been truly lost (even by the members of the editorial board of the *Obras completas*). Their
"disappearance," in my view, is due more to the critical position of those scholars, to what they were looking for, where
they were looking for it, and what they expected to find.
Such attitudes have certainly affected the study of Hernández, together with numerous other classic Spanish authors.

In the light of new perspectives and new research, the
original surviving manuscript of Hernández's work on
natural history has become conspicuous again: it has re-
appeared in its complete form—just as happened at the end
of the eighteenth century. And it is no accident that I am
neither the first nor the only one to "discover" the four volumes that complement the two that have remained all this
time at the Ministerio de Hacienda. At the very least, others
who have similarly discovered them include María del Car-
men Sánchez Téllez, Francisco Guerra, and José Luis
Valverde (when they were still in private hands) as well as
José María López Piñero and José Pardo Tomás.[6]

The purpose of this essay is to call attention to the
importance of the work of Hernández in itself, as an

3. Significant works that are omitted from the *Obras completas*
range from the description of the Great Temple of Mexico City (a
Latin translation of an original by fray Bernadino de Sahagún) to a
longer work of great intellectual scope, apparently not known to
the editors. I refer to the translation of the complete works of Saint
Dionysius the Areopagite. This is the first complete Spanish version
of this mystic, whose writings were very important during the
Renaissance as the primary Christian justification of Neoplatonism,
as the source of a major theory of names and knowledge, and as
one of the most accomplished accounts of the Great Chain of Being.
The work survives in a folio volume of one hundred leaves that
was prepared for the press but never printed: BN MS 10,813. See
Eulogio Pacho, "Versiones castellanas del Pseudo Dionisio Areo-
pagita," *Revista española de teología* 30 (1970): 245–64. For Renaissance views on Dionysius, see, among others, Frances A. Yates,
Giordano Bruno and the Hermetic Tradition (Chicago: University of
Chicago Press, 1964), 117–29.

4. Both manuscripts were described in detail by Somolinos,
1:428–29. They were first noticed by Agustín Jesús Barreiro, "Los
trabajos inéditos del Dr. Francisco Hernández sobre la gea y la fauna
mejicanas," *Revista de la Asociación Española para el Progreso de las
Ciencias* (1929): 161–75. José Tudela de la Orden mentioned them
and their location in *Los manuscritos de América en las bibliotecas
de España* (Madrid: Ediciones de Cultura Hispánica, 1954), 306; see

also María de los Angeles Calatayud, *Catálogo de las expediciones y
viajes científicos españoles a América y Filipinas (siglos XVIII y XIX):
Fondos del Archivo del Museo Nacional de Ciencias Naturales*
(Madrid: CSIC, 1984), 23.

5. Somolinos, 394, 396, 399, 424, 426–31; these manuscripts were
first described by Tudela, *Manuscritos de América*, 259–67.

6. Sánchez Téllez et al. were given access to volume 4 only (containing animals, minerals, and the indexes), and they mention the
owner only by his initials, C[arlos] I[báñez] M[uñoz]. See their
*La doctrina farmacéutica del Renacimiento en la obra de Francisco
Hernández, c. 1515–1587* (Granada: University of Granada, 1979),
15, 20–22. López Piñero and Pardo mention the manuscripts in
passing in *Nuevos materiales y noticias sobre la Historia de las Plantas de Nueva España de Francisco Hernández* (Valencia: Instituto de
Estudios Documentales e Históricos sobre la Ciencia, University of
Valencia, CSIC, 1994), 28–29, 39. The manuscripts were eventually donated to the Biblioteca Nacional on March 31, 1987, and the
donation was publicized in the library's regular newsletter. They
were first described by Julián Paz, *Catálogo de manuscritos de
América existentes en la Biblioteca Nacional,* 2d ed., revised by
Clotilde Olaran and Mercedes Jalón (Madrid: Ministerio de Cul-
tura/Biblioteca Nacional, 1992), 147. See also *Nuevos ingresos de
manuscritos en la Biblioteca Nacional (MSS. 22431–22608)* (Madrid:
Ministerio de Cultura/Biblioteca Nacional, 1994), 12–13.

intellectual and scientific microcosm, mediating between the Old and New Worlds but also steering its own path among different European traditions. This special quality arises in large part from both the failure of the complete, finished work and its success in the sense of its partial dissemination and adaptation by different scientific traditions over the course of four centuries.

For a study of this kind, the original manuscripts are exceptionally valuable, so let us move first to as detailed a description as space permits, together with some further materials that I consider important and a few preliminary conclusions about the ways in which Philip II's proto-médico conceived and constructed his *Natural History of New Spain*.

The Surviving Original Manuscripts of the *Natural History of New Spain* and Their Evolution

The surviving original manuscripts of the *Natural History* (that is, descriptions of the plants, animals, and minerals of New Spain, with their table, or index) form the main part of a collection of five folio volumes of manuscript, rebound now in six parts, which also contain other works and shorter pieces written by Hernández during his expedition to New Spain. This collection of manuscripts was always the personal property of Hernández and remained in his hands until his death in 1587. The papers then passed to his son, Juan Fernández, who had been his father's closest collaborator on the expedition in New Spain, was the acknowledged author of the "table" or index to the *Natural History,* and inherited all of his father's books.[7]

At an unknown date but prior to 1629, the manuscripts came into the Imperial College of the Society of Jesus in Madrid, where they remained "lost" until their "discovery" in the 1780s. Notwithstanding this, Antonio de León Pinelo, in his *Epitome* (1629), not only mentioned these manuscripts and their location but also described their distribution across five volumes.[8] Juan Eusebio Nieremberg, Jesuit and professor of physiology at the Imperial College itself, used these manuscripts for his own work and included extracts and complete chapters in his *Historia naturae, maxime peregrine.*[9]

Although Nicolás Antonio was familiar with León Pinelo's work, he surprisingly omitted these manuscripts altogether from his extremely important *Bibliotheca Hispana Nova* (1672). Antonio was the first to focus on the publishing history of Hernández and the first to give precedence to the manuscript drawn up by Recchi.[10] However, Andrés González Barcia's enlarged edition of León Pinelo's *Epitome* (1737) reemphasized the existence of the manuscripts and repeated their exact description and location.[11] The information did not go unnoticed, because in a letter dated June 24, 1753, Peter Löfling wrote to Linnaeus that according to the marquis of Grimaldi, "part of the manuscripts of Hernández must be in the library at the Escorial, and the rest in the Imperial College in Madrid, or at any rate some of it should be recoverable."[12] And in 1762 Joseph Quer declared that "many volumes of [Hernández] papers still survive in manuscript."[13]

In 1779 Juan Bautista Muñoz was commissioned to produce his *History of the New World*. Interested as he was in the description of the Great Temple in Mexico City, in that same year or the next, he "discovered" the manuscripts of Hernández exactly where everybody had been saying all along that they were to be found: at the Imperial College in Madrid. This "most auspicious event" began the process of editing, in 1785, which culminated in the edition of

---

7. See letter of March 24, 1576, and Hernández's will, below.

8. *Epitome de la biblioteca oriental i occidental, nautica i geografica* (Madrid, 1629), 127–28.

9. Nieremberg's many citations from Hernández are extensive and almost always explicit. He also says, "The autographs of this author are in my possession." Juan Eusebio Nieremberg, *Historia naturae, maxime peregrine* (Antwerp, 1635).

10. See the edition printed by Ibarra, *Bibliotheca hispana nova* (Madrid, 1783), 1:432.

11. Facsimile ed. (Barcelona: Ediciones de la Universidad, 1982), col. 858.

12. For correspondence between Linnaeus and Löfling, see *Memorias de la Real Sociedad Española de Historia Natural* 5 (1907): 11–134, this quotation at 96.

13. Joseph Quer, *Flora española o Historia de las plantas que se crian en España* (Madrid, 1762), dedication, n. p.

1790.[14] Yet since that date, not a single scholar has shown any direct interest in the manuscripts themselves, so they have been forgotten and "lost" again until their present "rediscovery," rebound in six volumes and split between two repositories.[15]

As far as I am aware, the manuscripts were dispersed during the very process of Gómez Ortega's editing them, but they were brought together again, probably at the Ministerio de Hacienda, and only then—for unknown reasons—split up once more the way they are now. Two volumes remained in the Ministerio, where they are today (MSS 931, 932), while the other three (rebound in four) remained in the possession of Carlos Ibáñez Muñoz until he donated them to the Biblioteca Nacional in 1987 (MSS 22,436–22,439).

The Surviving Manuscripts: Description

The five manuscript volumes of old—described by León Pinelo in 1629 and Gómez Ortega in 1790—constitute six folio volumes today. Five of them are bound in marbled leather of the eighteenth century (I should say after 1780), and the other binding is a good modern imitation. The spines are decorated with gilt bands and red and green labels indicating the author and contents, in abbreviated form. The labels on the first four volumes (i.e., the *Natural History*) also give the number of the volume. As a general rule these manuscripts, which are in a fairly good state of conservation, can be said to have been originally a fair copy on which Hernández then worked, making numerous corrections, additions, deletions, and rearrangements.[16]

The *History of the Plants of New Spain* occupies the first three volumes (i.e., BN MS 22,436; Ministerio de Hacienda,

MS 932; BN MS 22,437), which are foliated in two ways. Modern foliation starts at folio 1 in volumes 1 and 3, but there is also Hernández's own continuous foliation through all three volumes (designed to make the indexes easier to compile). The fourth volume (BN MS 22,438) contains all the books on animals and minerals, along with a second section containing the full botanical and zoological indexes compiled by Hernández's son. The fifth volume (Ministerio de Hacienda, MS 931), well known for years, comprises treatises on several diverse subjects (the antiquities of New Spain, geography, religion, philosophy, and so on) and is thus the most heterogeneous in every sense, even to the point of containing fair copies of one work but drafts or notes of another. The sixth and last volume (BN MS 22,439), the smallest and the only one in a modern binding, owes its origin to the desire on the part of one of its owners to separate physically the Spanish translation of the *History of Plants*, which in the old collation of the manuscripts was bound in at the end of the first volume. These manuscripts are described in detail in the appendix, below.

The *Natural History of New Spain* and the Surviving Manuscripts: The Organic Development of the Work

Contained among the more than thirteen hundred manuscript leaves in the six surviving volumes of manuscripts is the only known complete version of the *Natural History of New Spain*.[17] Contrary to custom, which repeats a statement of León Pinelo, these manuscripts are not drafts in the sense of being preparatory to a final version but rather are the final version, precisely the one on which the author worked harder and longer. The corrections, additions, and deletions,

14. The basic study of the rediscovery and this edition is Somolinos, 329–53, but it can be supplemented by Enrique Beltrán, "Una polémica sobre Francisco Hernández y su obra en 1785," *Anales de la Sociedad Mexicana de Historia de la Ciencia y de la Tecnología* 5 (1979): 59–73, and del Pino, "América y el desarrollo."

15. The history of this new "loss" is most significant, but as I am here only summarizing scattered information, I will not go into detail.

16. The volumes at the Biblioteca Nacional have been restored, but those at the Ministerio de Hacienda have not, even though the bindings are more worn and the paper is damp stained and shows

signs of mildew and even damage from mice (to which Gómez Ortega alluded in 1790).

17. The other works, which I will not discuss here, can be found in *OC*, vol. 6. I have discussed the specific problem of the *Antiquities* in "De la naturaleza y los naturales americanos en el siglo XVI: Algunas cuestiones críticas sobre la obra de Francisco Hernández," *Revista de Indias* 52, nos. 195–96 (1992): 297–328, and the relationship between Hernández and the work of Sahagún in *Fray Bernardino de Sahagún: Una revisión crítica de los manuscritos y de su proceso de composición* (Mexico City: UNAM, 1990), 353–65.

which make the manuscripts so messy and give them the appearance of a draft, in fact contribute much of value to any study of the work today, because they allow us to reconstruct the successive phases of development through which the work and Hernández's conceptions passed.

One must remember that, given the scope of the enterprise, Hernández constructed his *Natural History* through successive approaches, which did not affect the whole of the work's contents at the same time. Thus the successive phases of production meant continual, cumulative improvement of the manuscript, while simultaneously leaving traces, incongruities, and inconsistencies that together constitute a kind of subtextual archaeological stratigraphy. The resulting lack of homogeneity provides very useful material for study but also hinders a simplified exposition of the same.

This manuscript of the *Natural History,* broadly speaking, began as a fair copy of an earlier, revised manuscript that is now lost. In the process of transmission, many features of the original manuscript were absorbed imperceptibly in the new fair copy. This is especially obvious in the ordering of the material and, above all, in the numbering of the chapters, particularly in the botanical section but in the animal section as well, in which the numbering (not the contents) is full of inconsistencies, errors, gaps, and systemic repetitions. In fact, it is impossible to calculate exactly how many chapters each book contains, especially in the botanical portion of the work. All of this arises because a disorganized or reorganized original was copied in a new order. In any case, these inconsistencies reveal what must be an early alteration of the criteria for classification used by Hernández.

The resulting copy is a substantial manuscript that divides the *History of Plants* into twenty books with four appendixes (to books 3, 7, 8, and 9) and arranges the description of animals and minerals into six separate books. A further characteristic feature of this copy is that in the left margin of each chapter (plants and animals alike) Hernández added one or more numbers referring to the illustration

(or illustrations) corresponding to whatever is described in the text. Such references are very important because, unlike the chapters, which are ordered and reordered again and again, the illustrations are numbered pretty much in the order in which they were made (the numbers never needing to be altered), and so they enable us to use this numbering as a chronological guide to the process of collecting the botanical and zoological material.[18]

I should add that the structure of twenty books plus four appendixes seems to be a transformation from the original arrangement in the earlier, lost manuscript of one continuous sequence of twenty-four books. The surviving manuscript certainly contains too little evidence (or at least I have not found any) to prove that this sequence of twenty-four books ever existed.[19] However, Hernández alludes twice to this arrangement: first in a letter to Philip II on March 31, 1574, and the second time in a letter to Juan de Ovando on September 1 of the same year. If I am right in thinking that the twenty-four-book structure was unique to the lost manuscript, that letter to the king should indicate the date when the original manuscript in twenty-four books was completed and the decision taken to copy it. The letter to Ovando, in its turn, would signal the very moment at which the surviving manuscript was being copied.[20]

In any event, Hernández was dissatisfied with this new fair copy (that is, the surviving one) and began to correct it. This was the beginning of a lengthy series of phases of textual improvement whose rough chronology and precise limits demand a minutely detailed critical study. Let me mention here only the major phases, which are fairly clear and affect the complete or nearly complete work and which introduce new elements to the external appearance of the manuscript.

Hernández began to revise the text proper of his work, and, at the same time that he was correcting transcription errors, he was modifying his prose style, varying his phrasing, and, wherever possible, improving or enlarging the descriptions or the therapeutic applications. The earliest of

18. See Hernández's letter to the king, March 24, 1576, below.

19. By contrast, there are clear signs of a much older arrangement in four large books, subsequently divided into twenty books plus the four appendixes we have now.

20. Letter to the king, March 31, 1574.

these deletions, interlineations, and texts scribbled in the margins appear in the fair copy.

The doctor also intended to order the chapters in numerical sequence, especially in the botanical section. However, this task was left unfinished, not just because it was a complicated job but also because it was premature. The textual revision reveals that several chapters were wholly inadequate, dubious, or inappropriate—generally just a few brief notes with a generic description: to put these chapters right depended on obtaining new and accurate information. Yet there are other cases in which there was too much information, so that a chapter had to be split into two or more new chapters, or a whole series of chapters had to be moved to other places and so have their place in the classification system changed. Thus arose a type of correction in the chapter sequence that, so far from clarifying it, made it even more distorted and incoherent. Furthermore, this also entailed the drastic measure of cutting whole leaves that were then placed elsewhere in the manuscript, at least if such cutting did not affect any other chapters that were not to be moved; otherwise, with only an occasional exception, the cuts do not affect the foliation, which must have been done afterward.

Yet the problems do not stop here. The revision turned up repetitions. In a few cases the repetitions were simple: one plant is described in two different places (suggesting an initial doubt about classification or that the same plant may have had more than one name in Náhuatl, or both). In such cases Hernández chose the fuller description and the more etymologically appropriate native name (which would describe more of the plant's properties). Only then would the redundant chapter be crossed out and the word *superfluit* ("it is unnecessary") be added in the margin, again introducing unexpected variables in the sequence of chapters.

However, there are other, much less obvious cases of repetition. These occurred in those cases in which Hernández reckoned that several plants with different names might be one and the same but harbored a lingering doubt that they were the same species, that they were closely related

varieties, or that they were different plants with deceptively similar appearances. In these cases Hernández usually wrote in the margin *ya se vido* ("seen already"), which seems totally cryptic to us now, because the reader today almost never knows where such plants have been "seen" above. On other occasions, however, Hernández left more explicit notes in the margins, such as that he had sought more information about the plant, or that it should be compared with some other, or simply that it seemed to be the same as one that appeared somewhere else. It is notable that in not one of these doubtful cases was the chapter in question deleted, but instead it remained in abeyance while new information was being obtained or while he decided what to do with it.

The internal problems with the new manuscript still do not stop, even here. The textual revision also revealed gaps. The new copy did not bring together all the available botanical material; there were old drafts (from the early phase of the work during his sojourn in the surroundings of Mexico City) as well as new material (collected on his travels in New Spain, especially Michoacán and Pánuco) that contained information that was not incorporated in the main work. Hernández decided to incorporate them in the fair copy, but as he did not have enough space to insert them in their proper places, he put them all together in an additional book, whose internal arrangement followed that of the work as a whole, and placed it after the other botanical books. This extra text became book 21, with marginal references to the illustrations witnessing the corresponding source and chronology.

Having come this far, Hernández felt obliged to have a new fair copy of the work made, which was to be sent with some haste to Philip II. This was the origin of the manuscript, now lost, that was eventually placed in the Escorial and that, according to the evidence of Hernández's letters, was finished by March 20, 1575.[21] The surviving evidence of the Escorial manuscript, such as the version prepared by Nardo Antonio Recchi and—above all—the exact copy made by Cassiano dal Pozzo of the books on animals and minerals (used for the appendix to the Rome edition of

---

21. To the king, March 20, 1575, below. He said almost exactly the same thing to Ovando in an undated letter (see José Toribio Medina, *Biblioteca hispanoamericana (1493–1810)* [Santiago de Chile: The author, 1900], 2.288).

1651), confirms that the manuscript version made for the king did incorporate all the corrections and textual additions that Hernández had made in his own manuscript up to that moment.

At the very time that this new fair copy was being made, it became obvious that the sheer size of the work and the complexity of its internal organization (made manifest in the chaos of the chapter numbering, especially in the botanical books) had made the *Natural History* an unwieldy compilation. To make the work usable, it was essential to prepare a reference tool, an alphabetical index of the names of plants and animals contained in it that would indicate where they were treated in the text and which illustration or illustrations corresponded to them. This was the purpose of the "table," which Hernández's son completed while the copy was being made and while the doctor himself was concentrating on the second phase of his tasks on the expedition: experiments in hospitals that would test the medicinal properties of the plants he had described (this was the beginning of another series of works and manuscripts).

The compilation of the index meant having to foliate all the books on plants cumulatively, and the separate books on animals and minerals. The resulting index for two distinct sets of texts was not one table that combined them both but two: one for plants and one for animals. In the surviving manuscript these indexes have many interesting characteristics. The first and longer one, for the plants, is written in a neat hand in one column centered on the page, and the second, in a more cursive hand, is arranged in two columns per page, but the amount of information and its organization are identical in both indexes. The native name of the plant or animal determines its place in strict alphabetical order. To the right of that, like a textual complement (not always present) is a Latin equivalent, called "etymology" by Hernández. Then come the numbers that turn the table into an index: folio numbers for the text to the right, for the illustrations to the left.[22] The most telling feature of these tables is that both numbers, written at the same time as the names, refer to the copy for the king (the lost Escorial manuscript), as the sole surviving copy of the Escorial index proves without leaving the slightest room for doubt.[23] Only later—and in a much more cursive hand—was a second foliation added to the right, corresponding to the manuscript I have been describing; and to the left a second set of numbers for the illustrations corresponded, for the most part, to the sketches (*esquizos*) that Hernández kept with him, at least until he drew up his will in 1578.[24] This second numbering of the illustrations was added also to the general text of the surviving manuscript, in the left-hand margin next to the relevant chapter, where the new numbering is obviously different from the numbers written there in the first place.

This table, which brings together the index of the Escorial manuscript and that of the surviving manuscript, permits a unique critical comparison of the contents of the two manuscripts. Although such an analysis would be too long and intricate a task to undertake here, we can at least propose with some confidence that in the copy prepared for the king there was a serious effort to order the chapters in sequence and put them physically in the right places. However, everything suggests that many of the problems were left unresolved. In fact, book 21 was kept the way it was, an additional section tacked on after the rest of the botanical books.[25]

---

22. The structure of the table is described by Hernández in a letter to the king, March 24, 1576, below.

23. For an edition of that copy of the index (now at the University of Montpellier), see López Piñero and Pardo, *Nuevos materiales*.

24. A clear example of the connection between this second numeration and the esquizos is the last entry in the table of animals (MS 22,438, fol. 218). The entry is a last-minute addition, the "other maçacoatl": after indicating the folio number where the description can be found, Hernández wrote, "There is no sketch of this." References to the sketches or "little drawings" made on the spot in Mexico are scattered all over the manuscripts and in Hernández's letters, e.g., to the king, March 24, 1576, below, in which he makes it clear that he is sending the king finished illustrations, not the sketches. We know from his will that he still had the sketches in his possession, because he specifically bequeathed them to Philip. Although we do not know the exact date, the sketches did eventually pass into Philip II's hands, who, "for fear that, being unbound, these papers could easily be lost," ordered several people—among them fray Juan de San Gerónimo—to cut them and paste them onto sheets of linen, thus creating mannerist landscapes that were then hung on the walls of his apartments at the Escorial. There are numerous references and descriptions of them: I have used the *Colección de Documentos Inéditos para la Historia de España* 7 (1845): 6.

25. See letter to the king, March 24, 1576, below.

Hernández sent Philip II his copy in March 1576. The doctor, however, continued to work on his personal copy throughout that year and, actually, into the next. He completed another revision of the text, amending the style, making further additions and deletions, and improving some of the descriptions. Redundant chapters were now deleted, as were inadequate ones and the chapters that described plants that existed in Europe. However, the vast majority of doubtful cases were retained, even when—according to the marginal annotations—the plant had been identified as another, already described.

As in the previous revision, new materials were introduced. The additions that appear at the end of many of the books (frequently without any chapter numbers), and especially the additions gathered together as appendixes to books 3, 7, 8, and 11, all belong to this period. This was also when the complementary books on animals and minerals were compiled and added in the form of an appendix at the end of volume 3, exactly where the botanical descriptions end. In this concrete case it is not a question only of new materials but also of much more detailed and exact versions of chapters that existed earlier and could now be deleted or canceled in the form in which they appeared in the manuscript sent to the king.

Finally, it was in this period—still in Mexico but preparing to return to Spain—that Hernández wrote some personal notes in which he indicates how he means to continue and finish the *Natural History*; he lists the things he has to do before his departure from Mexico and on his arrival in Madrid, the books he has to get back, debts to settle, and business to finish. Several of these notes date in all probability from February or March 1577.[26]

Hernández's Project: The Internal Structure of the Botanical Work and the Keys to Its Organization

One property of the original manuscripts, with all their limitations, deletions, additions, and inconsistencies, is that they present the work of Hernández almost like a living thing, or at least as an enterprise subject to a continuous process of growth, maturation, and gradual change, which, however, never delivers a definitive end product. This is the process that I have sought to describe in a basic way. But as the manuscripts contain, in addition, some of the fundamental keys that Hernández used to organize his project on natural history, I turn to this issue now, albeit briefly and with reference only to the most complex portion of his work, the botanical.[27]

Francisco Hernández traveled to New Spain charged with the task of creating a natural history of the new territories or, more exactly, with the objective of compiling a "Pliny of the New World." That is to say, his obligation was to write down as much information as he could gather from local sources on the natural and medicinal things in America, consulting for this purpose "all the doctors, medicine men, herbalists, Indians, and other persons with knowledge in such matters."[28] The main object of his expedition was therefore to gather and make known the cumulative experience of local practitioners; thus a second purpose was neglected, reduced to the status of a merely desirable complement, the original medical experiments that Hernández could undertake: "You shall experience and test at first hand all the abovementioned if you can, but otherwise, you are to obtain information from the said persons."[29]

26. In the Madrid edition (1790), Gómez Ortega did a good job of editing the *History of Plants*. He aimed to publish the text as Hernández had left it in its final revision, so he omitted all the notes, comments, marginal references, erased and suppressed texts, and so on. The only really important variants are his division of book 21 into four (his books 21–24); his omission of virtually all the plants from the Philippines and East Indies (which were intended to form a separate essay); and his renumbering and rearrangement of the sequence of chapters in each book.

27. For a more detailed argument on this topic, see Jesús Bustamante, "Francisco Hernández, Plinio del Nuevo Mundo: Tradición clásica, teoría nominal y sistema terminológico indígena en una obra renacentista," in *Entre dos mundos: Fronteras culturales y agentes mediadores,* ed. B. Ares and S. Gruzinski (Seville: Escuela de Estudios Hispanoamericanos, 1997), 243–68.

28. "Instructions," below.

29. Ibid. On the question of the scientific expedition, see Jesús Bustamante, "La empresa natural de Felipe II y la primera expedición científica en suelo americano: La creación del modelo expedicionario renacentista," in *Felipe II (1527–1598): Europa y la monarquía católica,* ed. J. Martínez Millán (Madrid: Parteluz, 1998), 4:39–59.

This distinction is very important for an understanding of the written results of the expedition. The abundant information that could be gathered from local practitioners, mostly native doctors, was assembled in that peculiar modern Pliny that is the *Natural History of New Spain.* As for the original experiments on simple and compound medicines, they were written down to form several medical treatises outside—and complementary to—the *Natural History,* strictly speaking, and its structure. In fact, these experiments were intended as an academic and collective task that could only be undertaken systematically from December 1574 onward, when the *Natural History* was practically complete in terms of the materials it was to cover.

Despite the above, the *Natural History of New Spain* is not a straightforward compendium of ethnobotanical and ethnozoological descriptions, for two reasons; in the first place, as Hernández himself states, it includes experiences passed on to him by native inhabitants, as well as some of his own. Second, and more important, Hernández subjected all this information—both his own and the native inhabitants'—to the "medical rules" of European scholarship. That is, Hernández was not some neutral compiler but one who treated his information and his informants with a critical eye, discussing with them, comparing data, weighing—and selecting—evidence, and, especially, applying a rigorous method to the collection and description of his material.[30] The "new Pliny" is thus a compilation conducted according to a system, and its material was deeply and seriously mediated by its compiler.

For this task Hernández made good use of his solid training as a medical doctor and a surgeon, which combined eclectically several traditions of the learned Europe of the time (he was unsure whether to call himself *medico primario* or *protoiatro*). But Hernández certainly did not approach the nature of the New World from a direct, ingenuous European viewpoint. On the contrary, as a result of the royal instructions he was given and the concrete objective of his expedition, his approach to American nature was by the cultural

tradition of the native doctors, especially through those "experiences they have had for hundreds of years," which Hernández came precisely to collect.[31] All these factors have repercussions for the structure of the *Natural History,* a strange combination of cultural traditions that brought together European and native classification systems.

Annotations in the original manuscripts and the headings of the botanical books, omitted in the Madrid edition in the eighteenth century, confirm without a doubt that Hernández adopted as his organizing principle the traditional system of alphabetical order. But at the same time the key terms he opted to alphabetize were taken from the native languages, in particular Náhuatl, and so this criterion actually became a major source of problems.

For a start, Hernández felt obliged to establish fixed spellings for Náhuatl words at a time when there was no consistency.[32] Thus he systematically transcribed as *hoa* what was usually written as *ua, oa,* or *hua* (=/wa/); and he normalized *qua* as *cua* (=/kwa/), as appears from the very beginning of his work.

However, in the second place, the phonology of the native languages—especially Náhuatl—introduced a striking distortion in his alphabetical scheme. Entries for letters such as *c* and *t* (which actually conceal different phonemes) created disproportionately large categories, whereas for other letters, which Náhuatl lacks or does not use as initial letters, there were hardly any entries, or even none at all.[33] In this way, in the *History of Plants* it turned out to be impossible to establish an exact correspondence between "letter" and "book," and Hernández even found it necessary to reduce to appendixes some letters that he had considered originally to occupy books of their own. The distribution of letters and books is as follows:

Letter	Book	Notes
A	1–3	Originally one book, later split into three. *Bk 1
B	Appendix	Originally "appendix to book 1," later corrected to "appendix to book 3." Con-

---

30. See letter to the king, March 31, 1573, below, and Benítez Miura, "El Dr. Francisco Hernández: 1514–1578 (Cartas Inéditas)," *Anuario de estudios americanos* 7 (1950): 400.

31. To the king, March 31, 1573, below.

32. On this subject see E. Díaz Rubio and Jesús Bustamante, "La alfabetización de la lengua náhuatl," *Historiographia linguistica* 9 (1984): 189–211.

33. Such is the case with *b, d, f, g, l, r, s, v* [*u*], and *z*.

tains plants of the Philippines and East Indies beginning with *B*, to which others (including Mexican plants) beginning with *A* were added later.

C	4–7	Probably one book that was later split into four. *Bk 2
D	Appendix	Four plants from the Philippines and East Indies beginning with *D*. One Mexican plant beginning with *C* was added later.
E	8	
F & G	Appendix	Six plants of eastern origin beginning with *F* or *G*.
H	9	
Y	10–11	
L	Appendix	Originally "appendix to Book 3," corrected subsequently to "Appendix to Book 11." Philippine plants beginning with *L*; others beginning with *Y* (some Mexican) added later. Books 8 to 11 (letters *E* to *L*) probably made up a single book that was later split into four books with two appendixes. *Bk. 3
M	12	
N	13	
O	14	
P	15	
Q	16	
T	17–19	
X	20	There is no evidence to prove this, but books 12 to 20 (*M* to *X*) were probably one book (*Bk. 4). This hypothetical book 4 with letters *M* to *X* would have the same length as *book 2, containing the letter *C* only. On the early organization in four books, see note 19.

As I mentioned above, Hernández added a book 21, with its own alphabetical sequence from *A* to *X*, to the original alphabetical organization of twenty books.[34] In this second sequence, which brings together quite old materials from the expedition, Hernández used different, and in fact less advanced, orthographic criteria.[35]

In any case, book 21 was provisional and intended to be absorbed in the rest of the work. What Hernández meant to

do with his work, to start from the form in which his original manuscripts have survived, is outlined in some important notes written in MS 22,436, fols. 236v–237r. The first reads: "Merge major and minor alphabets." "Major alphabet" was Hernández's term for his twenty-book sequence; "minor alphabet" was book 21. His intention was to put them both together in a single sequence.

All of this raises another, intriguing issue in the organization of the *History of Plants:* if it was arranged alphabetically, why did it need an alphabetical index of the names of the plants? The answer is to be found in the analysis of the work itself, as well as in the second of Hernández's above-mentioned annotations: "And then put together [the genera] those of the same kind by name and virtue, although following the alphabetical order, using the table." The meaning of this annotation is further complemented and clarified by a third note: "Put together the ones that are the same or nearly so, and drop the superfluous ones."

The alphabetical sequence that Hernández used in his books is not just an alphabetical sequence of popular names of plants (the latter being the function of the index), as indicated by the index. The purpose of the alphabetical order of the books is to arrange the "genera" of the plants. To achieve this Hernández operated as follows: first, all the plants of the same kind (*congeneres*) were assembled in one group; second, a common name (in Náhuatl) was assigned to that group as a genus name; and third, Hernández used these genera names to establish the alphabetical order of the books.

For the definition of these groups, as the annotations cited above confirm, Hernández used a double criterion: the "virtue" of the plant, following a European model, and the Náhuatl name, with which he adapted himself unconsciously to a Mesoamerican classification system. In fact, although the European system was always there as a corrective, Hernández adopted the indigenous system to such an extent that he systematically applied Náhuatl terminology for all the botanical genera, even when there were traditional terms for them in Latin, backed by classical authority.

---

34. Gómez Ortega's arbitrary splitting of book 21 broke up a single alphabetical sequence into book 21 (*A* to *C*), 22 (*D* to *O*), 23 (*P* to *R*), and 24 (*S* to *X*).

35. He created entries, for example, under the letters *s* and *v* (or *u*). The latter are almost always written as *hu*.

Hernández ran into serious difficulties when he tried to combine both criteria and was frequently caught up in the native classification system or misled by the Náhuatl terminology. In these cases he created groups that made no sense from a European point of view.

For a clearer explanation of the above, I now present some examples. For this purpose I have chosen book 4, since it contains a long sequence of chapters that pose no problems either in order or in numbering and can thus be followed in any of the available editions. Although the letter corresponding to book 4 is *C*, the chapters from 16 to 20 deal with a series of plants, none of which begins with that letter: *Nux indica, bahey, sacsac, quauhcoyolli,* and *iczotl.* The reason that they appear where they do is that in Náhuatl they are all assembled under the genus name *coyolli.* And also, from the European viewpoint, there are no doubts as to integrating a single unit known by the Latin name of *palma.* But the method used by Hernández forces him to add to this group three other plants (chaps. 21–23), which, although not *palmae* by "virtue," bear the term *coyolli* in their popular native names: *quauhcoyolli chietlae, ycpac tecoyolli,* and *ycpac coyolli.* The advantages and drawbacks of the system are obvious.

It must be pointed out, though, that in many cases the double classification—by virtue and by name—is quite consistent. For example, in that same book 4, chapters 28 to 39 constitute a genus classified by the term *camohtli,* or more precisely by an alleged root *cam-* (which Hernández identified in all the names), its "virtue" lying in the fact that each plant is associated with the presence of a tubercle. Also, chapters 41 to 63 constitute a well-defined group, whose classifying term is *copalli,* translated by Hernández as "gum genus." In this case the "virtue" that defines the group is the principle of trees emitting "gum," "resin," or "amber" (forming in effect a sequence of subgenera).

At the same time there are other cases in which the classification is totally untenable from European scientific criteria. In book 4, chapters 64 to 68 constitute a genus defined by the Náhuatl word *chichioal-,* meaning "milk-bearing," or "teat." In this case Hernández was using a purely popular ethnobotanical term that refers to plants that give off milky sap, to plants that have the property of promoting the production of milk in women, or to plants whose leaves, fruit, or flowers look like a teat. Although none of these has any virtue in common, Hernández came to accept this group as just another genus.

The reason for this is that, like other naturalists of the period, Hernández hung on to an etymological dream that he thought he saw fulfilled in the Náhuatl language. As he himself said, "It is a wonder that among such rude and barbarous people, one hardly encounters a word that is not related to its significance and etymology, but rather almost all of them were adapted to things with such apt skill and wisdom that hearing the name alone is enough to indicate the natural properties that can be known or investigated."[36]

What Hernández in fact did was to apply, as part of his own natural philosophy, a theory of names inspired by Saint Dionysius the Areopagite (whom he translated). This theory was very similar to the one applied by Arias Montano in his own *Natural History,* although Montano—more conventionally—identified Hebrew as the etymological language.[37]

The double system of classification, together with the energy of the Náhuatl botanical culture that shines through his work, caused Hernández the most headaches. For one thing this particular combination made it almost impossible ever to perfect the organization. For another, it rendered Hernández's work almost unintelligible to European scholars, who promptly adapted it to their own exclusive scientific traditions. Paradoxically enough, it is the presence of all these problems and contradictions that makes the work of Hernández so worthy and interesting from the viewpoint of today's researchers.

---

36. *Antiquities* 2.20, below.

37. Benito Arias Montano, *Naturae Historia, prima in magni operis corpore pars* (Antwerp, 1601). This work was published by Jan Moretus.

APPENDIX

Volume 1: Biblioteca Nacional, MS 22,436

The manuscript contains 237 folios, to which in modern times 65 blank leaves have been added (to replace the Spanish translation of the History of Plants when it was removed to make the present volume 6). Hernández foliated his manuscript in the top right-hand corner of each recto, omitting folio 27. Modern foliation has been added in the lower right-hand corner of each recto, which corrects Hernández's erroneous omission. I follow the modern foliation here.

Without prologue or preface, the work begins on folio 1 with the title of book 1: "De historia plantarum nouae hispaniae Liber primus, francisco hernando medico atque historico philippi secundi Regis hispaniarum et indiarum , et totius noui orbis medico primario authore [The first book of the history of the plants of New Spain, by Francisco Hernández, doctor and historian to Philip II, King of Spain and the Indies, and principal doctor of all the New World]." This title, with minor variations, is repeated at the beginning of each book, but the whole work has no single title.[38] I omit here any mention of the actual contents and of the very problematic question of the chapters, which is treated separately later. The manuscript is made up as follows:

```
fols. 1–45    . . . . . .book 1
 fol. 46   . . . . . . . .blank
fols. 47–100   . . . .book 2
fols. 101–62   . . . .book 3
fols. 163–71   . . . .appendix to book 3
fols. 172–233   . . .book 4
fols. 234–35   . . . .blank
fols. 236–37   . . . .originally blank; subsequently 236v and
                      237r were completely covered with
                      personal notes by Hernández about his
                      project in general, the recompense he
                      expected from the king, and so on.
```

Hernández numbered the leaves from 1 to 235 (or 1 to 234, since he neglected to number folio 27), leaving the three last leaves (235–37) unnumbered.

Volume 2: Ministerio de Hacienda, MS 932

Clearly a continuation of the manuscript I have just described, this one contains 274 leaves without any modern pagination or foliation. It maintains, however, the foliation that Hernández gave it, again in the top right-hand corner of each recto, continuing where he left off in the previous volume. Thus this volume begins at folio 236. I follow this, the only foliation, here. The volume is made up as follows:

```
fols. 236–85   . . . .book 5
fols. 286–353   . . .book 6
fols. 354–80   . . . .book 7
fols. 381–82   . . . .blank
fols. 382v–383v  .appendix to book 7
fols. 384–98   . . . .book 8
 fol. 399 . . . . . . . .blank
fols. 400–401   . . .appendix to book 8
fols. 402–7   . . . . .blank
fols. 408–35   . . . .book 9
fols. 435v–438v  .blank
fols. 439–76   . . . .book 10
fols. 477–500   . . .book 11
fols. 501–4   . . . . .appendix to book 11
fols. 505–7   . . . . .blank
```

There are three more blank, unnumbered leaves.

Volume 3: Biblioteca Nacional, MS 22,437

This manuscript, which again is a continuation of the one previously described, has 308 leaves, once more with two sets of foliation, the recent numbering restricted to this volume alone (1–308), Hernández's own foliation continuing from the previous volume and including a few irregularities, especially at the end. I follow the modern numbering here, but I give Hernández's numbering in parentheses. The manuscript is made up as follows:

```
fols. 1–31 (508–38) . . . . . . . . .book 12
fols. 31v–32v (538v–539v) . . . .blank
fols. 33–48 (540–55) . . . . . . . .book 13
```

---

38. Variants in the titles of the books—except, of course, the book number—are basically stylistic, but because they are systematic and common to other of his works, they help to establish the relative chronology of the manuscripts. There are two main variants, one earlier and one later than the form quoted here. The earlier is what Hernández used in the first clean copy of his work. In this manuscript it appears only in book 21, where he uses *et* for *atque* and *protoiatro* for *primario*. The other is the final version used in this manuscript only in the titles of books 18 to 20, where he uses *ac* in place of *et* or *atque* and restores *primario*.

fols. 49–59 (556–66) . . . . .book 14

fols. 60–62 (567–69) . . . . .blank

fols. 63–88 (570–95) . . . . .book 15

fols. 88v–91v (595v–598v) . . . .blank

fols. 92–112 (599–619) . . . . . .book 16

fols. 112v–113v (619v–620v) . .blank

fols. 114–44 (621–51) . . . . . . .book 17

fols. 145–77 (652–84) . . . . . . .book 18

fols. 178–80 (685–87) . . . . . . .blank

fols. 181–202 (688–709) . . . . . .book 19

fols. 203–15 (710–22) . . . . . . .book 20

fols. 216–18 (723–25) . . . . . . .blank

fols. 219–93 (726–802) . . . . . .book 21

> The whole of book 21, which concludes the *History of Plants,* is a compilation of botanical materials organized from *A* to *Z* (Hernández called it a "minor alphabet") that gives rise to numerous leaves that have remained blank between the different classifying letters.
>
> It is important to note that Hernández did not number folios 253–55, which are three inserted quarto leaves, containing a fair copy of several notes on questions of natural history and on the expedition to New Spain. These same notes are duplicated in foul papers, on folios 252r–v and 256r–v (folios 764–65 in Hernández's numbering), which were originally blank.

fols. 294–308 (807–19) . .Books of animals and minerals.

> This section treats only new chapters or new redactions that enlarge or correct those in the main body of that series of books that actually appear in the following volume. As with the previous case, its division into books means that a few blank leaves were inserted. It should be noted that Hernández's foliation is very irregular here, since he omitted folios 803–6, and three leaves are numbered 817.

Volume 4: Biblioteca Nacional, MS 22,438

This manuscript contains 219 leaves with modern numbering. In this volume Hernández foliated only the text of the books on animals and minerals (fols. 1–121), that is, the part that he needed to compile the table, or index. I follow the modern foliation; I have occasionally added, in parentheses, the numbering of Hernández, which shows irregularities and changes of criteria. The manuscript is made up as follows:

fol. 1 . . . . .Prologue and dedication to Philip II

fols. 1v–2v . . . . .blank

fols. 3–20 . . . . .On the history of quadrupeds (fols. 1–17; he repeated 16)

fols. 21–73 (18–70) . . . . .On the history of birds

fols. 74–89 (71–86) . . . . .On the history of reptiles

fols. 90–95 . . . . .On the history of insects (fols. 91–96; Hernández neglected to number fols. 87–90)

fols. 96–110 (97–111) . . .On the history of water creatures

fols. 111–20 (112–21) . . .On the history of minerals

fols. 121–210 . . . . .Table, or index of the names of plants

> It is important to note that folio 172 is an inserted leaf, taken from a draft of the index and containing various verse compositions, no doubt considered as potential introductions to the eventual printed publication of the *Natural History.* One of them is "in praise of the author hexasticon," followed by one "by Juan Hernández on the portrait of his father," and finally, "an epigram to the archbishop of Mexico." I should say that all three verses were composed and in the hand of Juan Fernández or Hernández, son of the doctor, and author of the table where the verses are inserted.

fols. 211–19 . . . . .Table or index of the names of animals.

> This second table is in a different hand and is not organized the same way as the previous index. The index of animals in this volume occupies folios 211–18. On folio 218v, between trial swirls of the pen and odd phrases Hernández wrote a list of personal jottings about books he had lent to various friends in Mexico City. Folio 219 basically contains the index of animals appended to volume 3.

Volume 5: Ministerio de Hacienda, MS 931

This volume has no number on the spine, and the only indication there of the contents refers to the first essay in the volume, by which it is generally known. The manuscript contains 234 leaves of text, with modern numbering. The volume comprises a miscellany whose different parts Hernández numbered individually. I follow the modern numbering with that of Hernández given in parentheses.

The manuscript is made up as follows:

Volume 6: Biblioteca Nacional, MS 22,439

The only volume in a modern binding. The spine lacks a volume number and gives the contents as merely "Manuscripts." The volume contains 56 leaves of text with old foliation (1–56), followed by six blank, unnumbered leaves. As mentioned above, this volume came into being when an earlier owner decided that the Spanish translation of the *History of Plants* should have a volume to itself and so disbound it from the first volume. The volume is made up as follows:

Note: The translation of book 1 is complete, that of book 2 only the first fifteen chapters.

THE TEXTS

MEXICO, 1571–1615

THE INSTRUCTIONS
AND LETTERS TO THE KING

The formal instructions outlining Hernández's responsibilities in New Spain were signed by Philip II in early January 1570. Hernández set out from Seville in the late summer of 1570 and arrived in Veracruz in the spring of 1571. From Mexico he wrote regularly to Philip, reporting on the progress of his scientific research, always promising to send his work, but never sending it until 1576. Hernández's reluctance to part with his writings was linked with his repeated requests for permission to prolong his stay in Mexico. After 1575, fearing for the integrity of his work, Hernández began to plead for his return to Spain. Although the letters are framed by the required formal courtesies, the tone of Hernández's language is remarkably personal at times.

Sources: The instructions are preserved in Archivo General de la Nación, México, Reales cédulas (Dup.) 47, 262, and printed in José Toribio Medina, *Biblioteca hispano-americana* (1493–1810) (Santiago de Chile: The Author, 1900), 2:293–94. Some of the letters were also printed by Medina from copies in the Archivo de Indias. In all, seventeen letters of Hernández have been printed, fourteen to the king and three to Juan de Ovando. One letter to the king and five to Ovando appear in *Documentos inéditos para la historia de España,* vol. 1 (Madrid: Viuda de Calero, 1842); Medina included all but the first two to the king (*Biblioteca,* 2:273–97), but his extract of the letter from Viceroy Enríquez is telling in that it omits the part showing that Hernández's ethnographic work would be censored. José Luís Benítez Miura published five letters in *Anuario de estudios americanos* 7 (1950): 367–409. Benítez Miura is the sole printed source for two letters, and Medina for another four; otherwise all the letters have been printed in at least two places. Transcriptions vary. We have translated the printed texts.

The Instructions of Philip II
to Dr. Francisco Hernández

January 11, 1570

The King.—It is hereby ordered that you, Doctor Francisco Hernández, our physician, shall hold and occupy the office of our chief medical officer of the Indies, islands, and lands of the Ocean Sea,[1] to which office we have appointed you, and for all other matters relevant to the history of the natural things that you shall find in those parts, the following shall apply:

First, that with the first fleet to leave these realms for New Spain you shall embark and shall go first to that land and to no other of the said Indies because we are informed that more plants, herbs, and medicinal seeds are to be found there than elsewhere.

Item, you shall consult, wheresoever you go, all the doctors, medicine men, herbalists, Indians, and other persons with knowledge in such matters, if it seems to you that they have understanding and knowledge, and thus you shall gather information generally about herbs, trees, and medicinal plants in whichever province you are at the time.[2]

Further, you are to find out how the above-mentioned things are applied, what their uses are in practice, their powers, and in what quantities the said medicines are given, as well as the places in which they grow and their manner of cultivation, and whether their habitat be dry or moist, or if they grow among other trees and plants, and if they occur in different varieties, and you shall write down descriptions thereof.

Item, you shall experience and test at first hand all the above-mentioned if you can, but otherwise, you are to obtain information from the said persons, and once you are satisfied that you have an accurate account, you shall describe their nature, virtue, and temperament.

You shall cause to be sent here all the medicines or herbs and such like that you may see in those parts, provided that they are noteworthy in your judgment, and do not already grow in these realms.

As far as concerns the history that you shall compose, as we have understood that you have agreed to do it, we shall leave it to you and entrust it to your good judgment and learning.

Item, when you have concluded what you have undertaken to do in New Spain, you shall go from there and travel to the provinces of Peru, where you shall continue to investigate the above-mentioned matters entrusted to you.

Furthermore, you shall take notice that although the title of chief medical officer of all the Indies is given to you, you shall be obliged to reside in one of the pueblos in which the Court and Chancery are located, which you shall have chosen, and to carry out the duties of your office in the area around that pueblo, no further than five leagues from it, such that you neither encroach upon nor make use of the jurisdiction, nor make any calls beyond those five leagues, although you may examine and grant a license to persons in the said provinces who come before you of their own free will for this purpose to your seat and place of residence, notwithstanding that they may be from beyond those five leagues.

Further, you may not by virtue of your office examine, disturb, or prevent any person who holds a license from exercising it.

Since we have appointed Doctor Sánchez de Renedo our chief medical officer of the provinces of Peru and the mainland, we command that throughout the time during which you shall reside in those provinces by our mandate he shall not exercise his office in the district of the Court where you reside; it shall be understood that he may exercise it in the districts and under the jurisdiction of the other Courts in which you do not reside, in the said provinces of Peru and the mainland, subject to the title and instructions that we have given.

The rights that you shall have to conduct examinations and licenses must be subject to the regulation of the president and judges of the royal Court established in the said pueblo, in consideration of the quality of the land;[3] the said president and judges shall send to our Council of the Indies

---

1. Periphrasis for "America."
2. Hernández was instructed to collect information as much as samples, as his descriptions of plants often demonstrate. It was neither necessary nor possible for him to examine and test every medicinal plant, animal, or mineral in person.
3. The meaning of this clause is not clear.

an account of the regulations they impose, and in the city of Nombre de Dios the regulations shall be controlled by the mayor, or, if he cannot ⟨control them⟩, or is absent, or is otherwise prevented, ⟨they shall be⟩ in ⟨the control⟩ of the chief magistrate of the city.

If by reason of your office you can and must take legal proceedings against any person or persons, you must be accompanied for the passing of a sentence by one of the judges of the said Court, who will be nominated by the president and judges; or, in the city of Nombre de Dios, by the mayor, or, if he cannot ⟨nominate one⟩, or is absent, or is otherwise prevented, the chief justice, so that you may not pass sentence without being so accompanied.

Before and until you begin to use your office, you shall present these instructions before the president and judges of the said Court in whose district you expect to be present, in conformity with all that is said above. If you wish to move from your seat and desire to go and reside in another pueblo where a chancery is located, you may do so, provided you take the same care to present these instructions to the president and judges there and stay within its confines. In Nombre de Dios you must present yourself before the mayor, or failing him, a magistrate, according to the conditions set out above.

In view of the trust that is placed in your person, you shall exercise all due care and diligence.[4] Madrid, the eleventh of January, 1570.

I the King.

By order of His Majesty, Antonio de Eraso.

[Seven rubrics]

Letter 1

May 15, 1571

S[acred] C[atholic] R[oyal] M[ajesty]. The viceroy has done what your majesty commanded, with much care and dili-

gence, so that now the geographer[5] is preparing to start, and the painters are beginning to do their job. I am taking charge of this with all the due diligence that such a difficult enterprise requires, entrusted to so many, and accomplished by no one.[6] I hope that God will be pleased to favor and assist me, that I may succeed in serving Your Majesty. I do not write in any more detail about all this, so as not to burden Your Majesty, but I am doing so with some members of the court,[7] who will inform Your Majesty, as they are in your service. For the present I am not sending any details of all the notable things because time is short. I shall advise Your Majesty and send them as I have been commanded. May Our Lord protect the Sacred Catholic and Royal Person of Your Majesty many years with increase of more kingdoms and realms as we your subjects desire. Mexico, 15 May 1571. Your most humble subject and servant of your Majesty, whose royal hands I kiss. Doctor Francisco Hernández.

Letter 2

May 15, 1571

S[acred] C[atholic] R[oyal] M[ajesty]. In my other letter I advised Your Majesty how the geographer and the painters were progressing, that Your Majesty's orders may be carried out. What I am writing about now is that the geographer, with my encouragement and equipped with some other necessary things for the expedient[8] description of this land, and that the painters have served me quite well and have begun to paint the natural things. I hope, and may God bring the end that I desire, to serve Your Majesty successfully. I will ensure that any notable things that I find are offered to you, or I will take care that they are sent to you, as I have been commanded. As far as the office of protomédico is concerned, I am going to bring to it the restraint and moderation that such a new land demands. To give Your Majesty some account of what is happening about it, I understand that

---

4. A formal phrase that Hernández frequently echoes in his letters to the king.

5. Francisco Domínguez, who was eventually replaced by Enrique Martínez.

6. Hernández's sense is not entirely clear. He may mean that such an enterprise has never been achieved (or even undertaken) before, that his enterprise has not yet been accomplished, or that it is not something that will be accomplished by only one person.

7. I.e., the court of the king.

8. Hernández speaks several times of Philip's desire that the project be carried out, or written, with all brevity (*con toda brevedad*). Hernández's meaning seems to require a suggestion of timeliness: the descriptions should be finished in reasonable time and be "brief" only in the sense that they are not filled with extraneous information.

some of the judges of the royal audiencias say that they have to hear an appeal of the cases that are brought before me, maintaining that Your Majesty decreed the contrary by express law,[9] and waiting to see Your Majesty's mandate to me. They say I must be accompanied by one of the judges from that audiencia; and the city, which has to defend many licenses and titles that have been issued, says that what I brought to this land, I have no authority to use, but only Your Majesty's protomédicos do. This will thwart the exercise of my office and in great measure confound the interests of the state, contrary to Your Majesty's express laws. For this reason I beg Your Majesty to remove all these obstacles, to be pleased to dispatch your royal edict, in which this royal audiencia is ordered to do what Your Majesty has already commanded, and go no further than that. May Our Lord preserve the Sacred Catholic and Royal Person of Your Majesty many years with increase of more kingdoms and realms as we your subjects desire. Mexico, May 15, 1571. Your most humble subject and servant of your Majesty, whose royal hands I kiss. Doctor Francisco Hernández.

Letter 3

[November/December 1571]

Sacred Catholic Royal Majesty. The natural history of the Indies is proceeding with all proper care and diligence, and thus in the eight months since the work began, more than eight hundred new plants, never seen before in these parts,[10] have been depicted, with large figures on large paper, all true to life and representing all the parts and proportions with greater and fresher exactness than ever before.[11] I have written of their very great virtues, and of their incredible and immense usefulness, in Latin and Spanish, something that could easily occupy someone for his whole life. As I under-

stand it, this will be such a grand enterprise that there will be no need to bring to the Indies medicines from Spain, nor to Spain from Alexandria,[12] and that not only will the whole world rejoice, but it will be astounded, and Your Majesty will gain even more renown and eternal fame, more than princes of old ever received from their victories and empires. Let us suppose that you are Alexander, and name me Aristotle because of what you have commanded me to do in these parts. Your Majesty could multiply Alexander by twelve, and that would still not be enough. There are so many things in the new world, with so many wonderful virtues, all of which I see, I touch, I test, I draw, and I describe clearly and precisely in Spanish[13] in a not unpleasing style, and which I am beginning to prepare to transfer to Spain. God knows that I speak true, that I am up all night every night thinking of ways to serve Your Majesty more successfully and speedily and less expensively, and thus I have conceived a thousand designs by which before my death this benefit to the world may be placed in the hands of Your Majesty.

But all great and new things always provoke opposition and jealousy, and this work has not escaped either, and thus there is further work, which has robbed me of no little time in the service of Your Majesty, which is my continuing concern; for which reason, if it pleases Your Majesty that this project continue with the same felicity with which it began, it is vital that I be favored with your royal inspiration and encouragement by way of command to the Viceroy to permit me to remain here, and when it is most appropriate, to grant me all the favor and assistance that have been given to me until now, and more if service to Your Majesty, as well as the project entrusted to me, should require it, and that I bring together in my house people who have the relevant expertise, to show them plants so that they may help me to

---

9. I.e., that Hernández should not hear appealed cases independently of the court.

10. I.e., never seen by Spaniards, but see the next note.

11. Hernández's emphasis on the novelty of the illustrations suggests either that his depictions are better than any ever devoted to botanical illustration or that his are better than surviving Mexican images of the same plants. As the Spanish have never seen these plants before, they cannot have depicted them, so it seems most likely that Hernández is merely emphasizing or exaggerating the high quality of his images.

12. Spain did import drugs from Alexandria, but the rhetorical parallel developed in the next sentence is more important than Mediterranean trade.

13. Hernández wrote principally in Latin, but, as he says in this letter, he has written about the plants in Spanish, too. What survives of his work on natural history in Spanish and in his hand is only one part of a volume (two "books"), now BN MS 22,439.

establish the medicinal virtues and tell me their experience with them.

The geographer set out a month and a half ago to describe New Spain according to my instructions; he will be sending to Your Majesty what he was commanded to do.

The Viceroy has seen the number of plants that have been done, together with the text,[14] which is a good volume: I do not think they should be subjected to the risks of a sea voyage until they have been translated, and thus they will not go today with the fleet: I intend at least to send Your Majesty some interesting samples of plants.

As far as my convenience is concerned, the expenses here are enormous; the favor that Your Majesty confers upon me, though very great, is insufficient to support me, nor could I desire more to serve Your Majesty: I beseech you to order that I be given some financial assistance, for I am obliged to employ more experts in your service. May Our Lord preserve the Sacred Catholic and Royal Person of Your Majesty many years with increase of more kingdoms and realms as we your subjects desire. Your most humble subject and servant of your Majesty, whose royal hands I kiss. Doctor Francisco Hernández.

Letter 4

April 30, 1572

Sacred Catholic Royal Majesty: I am going ahead with the descriptions, experiments with, and depictions of the natural things of New Spain with all the assiduousness and industry of which I am capable. Thus, as I trust in God, Your Majesty will see from my work just how much there is and how useful it all is, as I understand now that I have finished writing about it, so much so that the Indies could provide medicines for the whole world without the need to ship them from any other place at all. I have completed two books, each one roughly comparable to Laguna's Dioscorides,[15] and the third one is nearly finished: it is in Latin, so that this great gift of Your Majesty's may be communicated

to all nations because this is the common language. It is also being written in Spanish, for others, so that everyone may have and enjoy it. Much more might have been done if I were to have been given the necessary encouragement and that at the right moment, even though it will be ⟨only⟩ about a year since the work began. Furthermore, the Viceroy, who adheres strictly to Your Majesty's orders, does not recognize the importance of this project. I beseech Your Majesty with love and humility, for my only desire or intent is that Your Majesty be served speedily, as enjoined upon me, that the Viceroy might be given all the encouragement and inspiration necessary, to prevent my failing to serve Your Majesty. If this is granted to me, I will have the work on New Spain completed in two years. If not, it could take twenty, which inevitably means delay, and if I fail to complete it, it would be difficult to finish, not to mention exhausting the funds in ten years.[16] I did think of sending some things with this fleet, but I thought better of it because of the scant assistance and shortage of time, and because what would be leaving from here is domestic and established there,[17] so that it may be cultivated and conserved in that region, and because the kind, the quantity, and the manner of sending them may not be worthy of Your Majesty; but this cargo will go without fail in the future. The geographer is coming along with his description of the land; it will be definitive and accurate; what he has completed so far is not enough to be conveniently sent; perhaps it could go with the plants that have been done already. I am now pressing the Viceroy, that the protection he gives me here may be accorded to me everywhere in New Spain, because I need to travel widely to bring this project to perfection; I do not know when that will be. Your Majesty may be pleased to order this, and to grant me some financial assistance, for, as long as I am in Mexico and not busying myself with anything but service to Your Majesty, the favor that Your Majesty grants me is very great, but it is scarcely sufficient to sustain me on my travels throughout the land, where I will be for a good six months, because things are so expensive and the value of money is so

---

14. Apparently meaning that the viceroy had seen the illustrations as well as the text, though the phrasing ("the number of plants") is slightly odd.

15. *Pedacio Dioscórides Anazarbeo, acerca de la materia medicinal y los venenos mortíferos* (Antwerp, 1555).

16. A good example of Hernández's repetitious style and errant syntax. He appears to mean that if he does not finish the project himself, it will be difficult for someone else to do so.

17. *Domestic* means native to Spain; *there* means Spain.

low, and I will be in serious need of a great many supplies. The books of plants that are finished are not going to be risked on a sea voyage until they have been translated, and shown to the Viceroy. In addition, it will be essential that Your Majesty give me the authority to oblige the doctors to meet me once or twice a week to give them plants for testing, and to see and examine the plants' virtues and nature, for in the absence of such authority this enterprise will not last long.

I undertook to finish this project in five years; it is necessary that Your Majesty grant an extension up to nine or ten, though if I could accomplish everything in a single year, there is nothing in the world that I would rather do.

When it pleases God that I may depart for Peru and the other provinces, it will be necessary that Your Majesty grant me the same protection that I receive here, to enable me to do my duty prior to embarking, because there painters and astrologers are scarce, as I have been informed, and where there are any, they will be more expensive beyond comparison. It will be necessary that Your Majesty command that I be given the ones I have here, or some of them, with the provision that in all those territories I be given the same favor that I have been and continue to be given here.

The office of protomédico I am scarcely performing, although there has been a serious need for it, for it has been declared on appeal to be contrary to law in this royal audiencia; I have been accompanied by Dr. Villalobos.[18] What is worse, they have had six months and still have not decided if one who has been ordered to produce his credentials actually has to produce them or not, or if I am to send them or not, which was fortunate because I could not send evidence of your decision; I do not know if they have them for the sake of your jurisdiction or something else, or because it seems to them thus; I beg Your Majesty for authority in this land that I may do my duty, and, that the jurisdiction of Your Majesty's protomédicos be protected, let them be ordered not to admit any appeal contrary to explicit and justified law, especially when it is also fair and learned.

I have also petitioned Your Majesty for the title of Doctor of the Royal Chamber, more for the authority than for any real activity that Your Majesty might have commanded me to carry out, and so that they may not say that I, serving Your Majesty in this capacity, have not earned this title because I am unworthy of it. If it is God's will that I return, I do not think my health or my age would enable me to occupy the position: Your Majesty would be better served in this than I would, since, as everyone knows and my works testify, I serve you with care and warmth, for as long as Your Majesty is pleased to grant me favor, however many days remain to me in this life. Mexico, last day of April, 1572. Sacred Catholic Royal Majesty, may Our Lord keep the Sacred, Catholic Royal person of Your Majesty, with increase of more realms and domains, as your subjects desire. Your most humble servant and subject of Your Majesty, whose royal hands I kiss. Dr. Francisco Hernández.

Letter 5

September 22, 1572

Sacred Catholic Royal Majesty. I received the letter from Your Majesty dated Madrid, 24th of May of this year: I kiss the royal feet of Your Majesty for commanding me to come here with all the necessaries for the history that by your royal mandate I came to these regions to compose; and for Your Majesty's memory of my works, that I am granted this favor. I will do what Your Majesty commands by sending whatever I do with great secrecy,[19] leaving a copy in translation here, and thus I will send what I can when it pleases Our Lord that the fleet sets sail. I have so far drawn and painted three books[20] full of rare plants, most of them of great importance and medicinal virtue, as Your Majesty will see, and almost two more of terrestrial animals and exotic birds, unknown in our world, and I have written a draft of whatever could be discovered and investigated about their nature and properties, a subject on which I could spend my entire life. I could do even more if I were given the assistance I desire. This care

18. Pedro de Villalobos, an experienced and prominent judge with whom Hernández enjoyed "cordial but fruitless" relations, as Somolinos says (162).

19. One of several allusions to the need for secrecy, a multilayered concept for Hernández.

20. Hernández usually distinguished between volumes (the physical objects) and books (the conceptual units into which he divided his work).

and pain I think have been part of a long and serious illness, from which at present the Lord as by a miracle has spared me, because my works remain to be finished, and Your Majesty to be served, and from which I am at present convalescing.[21] Thus because of the extremely weak state in which I find myself, I cannot give Your Majesty in this letter a more detailed account of the whole, entrusting it if Our Lord be pleased with the fleet, which, I am informed, will depart soon. May God preserve Our Lord the Sacred Catholic and Royal Person of Your Majesty many years with increase of more kingdoms and realms as we your subjects desire. Mexico, the 22nd of September 1572. Sacred Catholic Royal Majesty. Your humble subject and servant of your Majesty, whose royal feet and hands I kiss. Doctor Francisco Hernández.

Letter 6

December 12, 1572

Catholic Royal Majesty: On one of the ships that set sail from here in October of this year, I sent a letter to Your Majesty in which I did the same as I have done in all the others I have offered, complying with Your Majesty's wishes by giving an account of what I have done in the matter of the history of the natural things of the Indies and the rest of what Your Majesty commanded me to do when I came to these parts. This work, as Your Majesty will have been informed by the viceroy Martín Enríquez, turns out to be much greater than some people imagined could possibly be sent. I am sending something of what I have been doing. So far I have completed some four medium-sized volumes, containing for the most part things that are very important for human health and well-being. There remains so much, and of such importance, that if Your Majesty is to be served well and the work brought to that perfection and glory that is required, I will need more time than the five years allotted me. The Lord knows that it is my desire to return to Spain and there serve Your Majesty, to see out my old age in peace, and that I request this extension against my natural inclination and desire to serve Your Majesty, not to mention my passion for the work, which is

my consuming interest, but taking due note of my duty rather than my personal welfare, I should say that it would be best if Your Majesty would grant an extension of another three or four years, seeing that much of the time is eaten up by travel, illnesses, and having to go through the necessary procedures with Your Majesty's viceroys and officials, and in view of the sheer immensity of the project, which could never be brought to its true height in any shorter time. Your Majesty will order whatever is your pleasure, which I will acknowledge as to what I understand is agreed, and I will comply as is my duty with your royal pleasure.

Also, it will be essential that Your Majesty order more letters to be sent to me like those I brought for the Viceroys of New Spain and Peru, mandating the presidents and governors of the audiencias of New Spain, Peru, and Guatemala and other representatives from the rest of those parts where I shall be traveling, that they support this enterprise with the requisite care and duty, the same as was supposed to have been done in New Spain, for although the viceroys may be so ordered, they do not exercise anything like the care mandated specifically by Your Majesty.

Likewise when I depart for Peru, because I understand I will not have painters and a geographer assembled there, and I will have to pick up people for those purposes as I find them en route, ⟨I beg⟩ that Your Majesty order that they give me here painters and a geographer for there, and that they are young and strong, so that they will be fit to make the journey willingly, and serve Your Majesty.

It is also crucial for the perfection of this work that Your Majesty order that the Canary Islands, Santo Domingo, and China be described in writing, which I am drawing up,[22] and that pictures in miniature of everything natural be sent, which can be done easily, with an account of their virtues and qualities, supplied by native and Spanish doctors. I can have it painted over here the way I want it, in my style and manner as no one else could initiate or complete this. Your Majesty will have a model, which the world will admire. I dare to say this because all of this extraordinary evidence of the works of God and of the secret treasure of these lands and of their benefit will be in Your Majesty's hands.

---

21. Whatever this illness was (a kidney or urinary disorder, probably), it remained with Hernández for the rest of his life.

22. Any of Hernández's writings on the first two are lost; his essay on China survives in Hac. MS 931, fols. 17–49.

The geographer continues very well with his exact measurements of the longitude and latitude of the provinces and principal pueblos of New Spain; he is sending Your Majesty whatever he does of any note. May Our Lord keep Your Catholic and royal person many years with increase of kingdoms and realms as Your Majesty's servants and subjects desire. Mexico, December 12, 1572. Your humble subject and servant of your Majesty, whose royal feet and hands I kiss. Doctor Francisco Hernández.

Letter 7

March 31, 1573

S[acred] C[atholic] R[oyal] M[ajesty]. In my letter to Your Majesty that went with the fleet on the second of January this year, I mentioned that it would be desirable for the completion of the history to write about China, Santo Domingo and the Canaries, that all the natural things of those parts be painted in miniature, or at least the more important things, with all their constituent parts and colors, and that their virtues and temperaments be described from the accounts and experiences of the natives, and that it be sent to me so that I may make the style consistent and have it drawn my way, and add it to the rest. Also that letters be written to the presidents of all the Indies, the same as those that were written to the Viceroys of Mexico and Peru, that they may come in to this project as Your Majesty has ordered, for without documents from Your Majesty, they will not cooperate. And that my term may be prolonged by three or four years, because New Spain alone will take six years to complete: there is so much to do here. And that it be ordered that I be given here in Mexico some Indian painters, who will go voluntarily, for I will have none awaiting me in Peru, and ⟨those I do find there⟩ will be incomparably more expensive, and that I assemble everything necessary before I head there.

What I may now advise Your Majesty is that four volumes of paintings of plants have been completed recently, in which there are 1,100, and another in which there are 200 animals, all exotic and native to this region, and scripts in draft and almost half of the descriptions in fair copy, of the nature, climate of the places to which they are native, the sounds they make, and their characteristics, according to the Indians, whose experience stretches over hundreds of years here. I have relied both on the evidence of other curious persons and of the doctors of this land and my own experiences, beyond what can be deduced using the rules of medicine. In all this, great care has been taken that no plant is painted unless I have seen it ten or more times in different seasons, smelled and tasted all its parts and asked more than twenty Indian doctors, each one individually, and considered how they agree and differ, and unless I have subjected it to the rigorous methods of identification and examination that I have developed here for this project.[23] I thought to send them to Your Majesty with this fleet to fulfill the mandate with which I was charged for the conciseness[24] of this work, but it has proved impossible because the fair copy of the script is not completed, principally because it is being written in Spanish and Latin, and because every day the ⟨descriptions of the⟩ plants are brought nearer to perfection with the addition of parts that are missing in many of them: such as the flower, seed, fruit, and such like, which cannot be painted until nature has produced them and they have appeared; thus one must wait for the right season and the right weather; also, the precision and style of the manuscript continue to be corrected and perfected: I take it for granted that these five books, with some more, will leave from here in one year[25] and I will strive with all my power to make sure that they do. Much more could have been achieved if people here had taken some account of Your Majesty's desire for expediency rather than the strictures of the edict, and if more support had been in evidence, and fewer delays than has been the case, as I know all too well to my cost, for then I would not have had to spend so much time, or to worry so much about preparing ⟨the work⟩.

If it pleases Your Majesty that the important part, on New Spain, be finished soon—and here I think is the major part of what there is in the new world, on account of this region's diverse climates, vastness and fertility—agree to let

---

23. This appears to be the first reference to Hernández's separate treatise (now lost) entitled "Method of Identifying the Plants of Both Worlds."

24. Again, this word carries the sense of "in due time."

25. That is, with the next annual fleet.

me have, freely[26] and not temporarily (which to me is a great nuisance) the interpreter they have given me, and that the painters[27] they have given me, then, be paid and that some reward be given them, because they help me on a regular basis. In this way ⟨those I have⟩ may be among the best, and not, like the ones I have at the moment, among the most useless in Mexico, since for something that has to appear before Your Majesty and has to endure, it is most proper and necessary.[28] And ⟨grant⟩ that three herbalists be given to me, or more if more are needed, regardless of the limit laid down in the edict, for over there ⟨in Spain⟩ no one understands the size and difficulty of this undertaking, going through a world as large as this with a fine-tooth comb. The number of ⟨herbalists⟩ I ask for is still not enough, but it is even worse if I have only one, as now. I would not request this except that this project is my sole work and occupation,[29] and I would rather not be idle for lack of plants.[30] If it be done at all, it is right that it be done well. And ⟨grant⟩ that the Viceroy orders, with some urgency, all the governors of New Spain to send the best people who can be found in their provinces, that they pay the Indians for their travel and labor, and that when I judge that the time is right to travel across the land of New Spain, that I be given resources for the expedition, proportional to my needs, because the costs will be great and will exceed the amount that Your Majesty has hitherto made available for it, and that if before my departure I have further expenses, I may be recompensed from the day of my departure and, if it should be necessary, that I be given a scribe—for there is a lot of text, and a translation can remain behind here. For all of this I do not ask for even a penny, unless you deem otherwise, for I have worked myself like an Indian day and night on nothing but this work. I would like to be given due credence for what I say is needed, thus in the above-said as in the proper remuneration of the Indians, for nothing in the world could persuade me not to speak the truth and speak with conviction, in order that this work shall not be unworthy of the fore-

most prince of the world, by whose mandate and benevolent will it is done. If this is granted to me, I prefer, at the risk of losing Your Majesty's grace, to finish it at the latest within two years from the time these resources might reach me, and possibly earlier. This will save the royal treasury much expense, which for these two years will be slightly more, while many things from here will be transferred to Spain, as I pass through the land and have at my disposal other means necessary to the perfection of the enterprise and intent of Your Majesty. If this is not granted me, it will cost incalculably more time and money, and it could even happen that I fail in this enterprise, despite my love and determination in the service of Your Majesty to bring an expedient end to the work that I have begun, and although I am still going, I know for certain that if I were not following this path, I could not serve Your Majesty in this land according to my desire and Your Majesty's wishes. May you be pleased to mandate what you will; having done my duty, my desire will be fulfilled. If Your Majesty is pleased that it is thus and takes effect, agree to order the same to the presidents of the other royal audiencias so that I may be accommodated everywhere I may travel, and that I may be given what I need wherever I go, wherever there is expected to be a shortage of things I need, and that the time in the provinces and parts of these Indies be distributed according to what I may judge to be necessary for the service of Your Majesty, without anyone's imposing limitations on me or putting impediments in my way.

The geographer measured a part of New Spain in one year of traveling, and if he had persevered, Your Majesty would have been well served and I would have benefited a great deal from his history, which Your Majesty said I should obtain, but at the end of a year, he refused to return, saying that he did not want to go on my commission. I suspect Your Majesty's viceroy was not pleased, and I warmly agreed with the decision, or perchance took up the chase, either to give the geographer satisfaction and honor at my expense, or to let him have his way, or to have you pay for his commission.

---

26. I.e., "at my disposal."

27. Two painters, whose work Hernández clearly did appreciate, are named in his will (below); it is not known how many other painters worked for him, or when.

28. Hernández thought of his work as an enduring legacy to the king, to Spain, and to the world.

29. Implying that Hernández, concentrating on his history, was not performing any of the functions of the office of *protomédico*.

30. The phrasing suggests that the herbalists habitually came to Hernández with plants to show him.

The evidence that this is what has happened is that I have not been able to send you what I have finished, though he should be (I believe) more grateful to you today than any man; that any man so poor should have dared to do such a thing, to undervalue a salary of a thousand ducats each year. What is more surprising, as the Viceroy told me this past December, is that although Your Majesty ordered the royal audiencia to mark out the land, they must have forgotten that he was seconded to me, and that I know what this was about. In February I gave him notice of another geographer who would do very well: he did not like that, so it was my turn to say that Your Majesty had commanded the royal audiencia that it had to be done, and that the audiencia believed that they must give the task to Sancho de Zavallos, who had done it before. I said that if any edict repealed mine, it would be cause for congratulation, but that, if not, what Your Majesty had mandated be kept for the support of the history and that no harm should come either to me or to it. He said I should stick to my commission; I told him that it had to be agreed by Your Majesty, that it was already mandated to be done, so that the same thing not be done twice, and the cost needlessly increased. The other morning the geographer agreed to this as I gave it to him, a thing entirely new, principally because of what had passed the previous afternoon; but so many inconveniences have arisen that he has yet to sign the agreement, nor does he have a way to sign, because I, having certified that he will be sufficient and that I myself have seen him work practically and gain experience in the field, I handed him over outside here to an Augustinian friar for examination, who approved his credential and his oral account. Then I had him examined by Your Majesty's accountant, whose finding accorded with my understanding—which was to his advantage—and with all this he said that he had to send me a certain account, which is the one by Zevallos, who he thinks should go, even though he is not ⟨authorized by⟩ the document from Your Majesty that I have, so I may go back a fourth time to reexamine him. Thus it could be that the Viceroy may write to Your Majesty (if he has not already done so) to say that there is no one else who can do it, but this one does not want to

go because of my commission that Your Majesty ordered. In this way he will be cut out of my history, even though he is necessary for this task, and he will be doing serious harm to it and to me; he should be doing me the honor to complement my works and services, which he has done feebly in his unhelpful dealings with me. I beg Your Majesty not to permit him to go on doing this, for without him the history will suffer, and I will have to suffer for his failings through no fault of mine, which would not matter, before you choose to send him one of these two options—either Your Majesty sends someone from Spain, someone in whom you have confidence, who would cost less, because you know that Zevallos earned a salary of 1,000 ducats, with other expenses each year, that he might do what I ordered here and in Peru, according to the royal edict that I have from Your Majesty, and that which has to do with the history I am writing: and if there is anything else to be provided for, that it be taken care of, according to the reasons that are so true and necessary for these things to be carried out. May Your Majesty be pleased to judge my work on its own merits and not otherwise, because I understand I have so annoyed the Viceroy, being so punctual in asking him continually what he might think is necessary to complete this document with the expediency that Your Majesty has ordered and charged me. Also, things like this always attract imitators and detractors, even though they are to be treasured in centuries to come.[31]

As for the protomedicato, which I exercise by Your Majesty's command, the royal audiencia recognizes my title, but there is a law prohibiting my holding it, which hinders my proper execution of this duty, even though it is so necessary because of the many excesses against this profession committed here, and so my office is in vain and meaningless. Furthermore, the city has taken upon itself to visit the confectioners who belong to Your Majesty's protomédicos: I beg you to issue an order that no harm will come to them, for it is illegal and against the common practice in Your Majesty's kingdom and provinces, where everything is done and carried out according to Your Majesty's orders and in concert with obedience to Your Majesty's statutes and orders. May

---

31. Apparently a non sequitur, but a reference to the *Natural History*. The fear that his work would be subjected to imitation and

detraction seems to have haunted Hernández. See his *Epistle to Arias Montano*, lines 128–29, in "Spain, 1790," below.

Our Lord keep Your Catholic and royal person many years with increase of kingdoms and realms as Your Majesty's servants and subjects desire. Mexico, last day of March, 1573. Your humble subject and servant of your Majesty, whose royal feet and hands I kiss. Doctor Francisco Hernández.

Letter 8

November 10, 1573

Sacred Catholic Royal Majesty: I have been traveling through New Spain for many days to bring the natural things to perfection, which, by Your Majesty's mandate, I have written about and depicted, adding many other things that I am every day discovering, things of great importance and weight, and I am putting all in order so that I can ship to Your Majesty six books or volumes, or perhaps seven, of depictions and history. Thus Your Majesty can order the most useful things, and whatever else seems necessary, to be shipped from here to Spain for the benefit and health of the state. The geographer too is covering and marking out the land as the Viceroy advised Your Majesty seven months ago; and because the books will certainly go when I say, and in them will be seen the care and attentiveness with which I serve Your Majesty, beyond what the Viceroy Martín Enríquez, here in New Spain, knows and could tell Your Majesty, and what is more, I obey Your Majesty, as I have written at length in other letters, so in this there remains nothing more than to acknowledge the immense favor Your Majesty has bestowed upon me by commanding me to do this, a duty that I shall perform with all my power; neither more nor less than I am ordered to do, regardless of other rewards and special favors, which I have received from the hand of Your Majesty. May Our Lord keep Your Catholic and royal person many years with increase of kingdoms and realms as Your Majesty's servants and subjects desire. Yyauhtepec, 10 November, 1573. Your humble subject and

servant of your Majesty, whose royal feet and hands I kiss. Doctor Francisco Hernández.

Letter 9

March 20, 1575

Sacred Catholic Royal Majesty. I have finished ten volumes of paintings, and five of text about the plants, animals, and antiquities of this land;[32] I understand from the Viceroy Martín Enríquez, who has seen them, that he is writing to Your Majesty: I intended to send them in this shipment; but considering that I have nearly come to the end of the time that Your Majesty commanded me to be in these parts and considering how much there was to be done in New Spain, it will be completed and polished in one year from today if God pleases; and because there is a great need for my presence in Spain, in order that this great benefaction and favor that Your Majesty has done for the republic, that the books remaining to be printed be not lost, it seemed to me more sensible, more convenient, and better for the safety of the books, and of more service to Your Majesty, if I put them on the ship that we are currently awaiting, rather than send them today, especially as the interval is so short. As for Peru and other new territories, God knows that I wish I were younger and healthier, as I have the resolution and the will, to beg Your Majesty for more time and spend the rest of my life serving on this project, grateful to Your Majesty and bringing benefit to the world. But I have neither youth nor health, because I have exerted such great efforts of body and mind, that I am robbed of my health, and now I am nearly sixty years old,[33] and cannot hope to live much longer. Having done what I have done here, I can leave the rest undone elsewhere; either it is quite like, or very close in form and virtue to what I have already described, or else it is not very important;[34] but because it is Your Majesty's will that what remains must be tracked down, I have laid such foundations

32. It is difficult to know for certain just how many volumes and books Hernández had completed at any given time, because his conception of his "history" was not limited to plants and animals but, as here, could include the *Antiquities* and may have included other works.

33. If we take Hernández at his word, his date of birth must have been mid-1515.

34. I.e., Peru is unlikely to have any natural resources that cannot be found in New Spain. It is conceivable that Hernández derived this opinion from Acosta. His rhetoric demands that the importance of Peru is played down, because he has made up his mind not to go there.

for the project and given them such an order, that the door remains open for those who may follow me to finish that work with ease. For the remainder of this year I still have to look over the text and add whatever my checking and rechecking may turn up, translate it into Spanish, and into Náhuatl for the benefit of the native population, collect seeds and hope that the plants delivered to Your Majesty prove robust enough to propagate, and I hope that they will prove to be as beneficial as possible in a different climate. Because my time will be up in mid-September, which is close to the time for my departure, and a whole year is needed for all these things to be done and corrected, without denying the assistance that has been granted me by command of Your Majesty, without which all of this would have turned out deficient and imperfect, it is important and very necessary that Your Majesty be pleased to grant me an extension, which gives me time, and which covers my salary until I am back in Spain. And still the geographer has not yet finished his survey, which is continuing, and even though I may have gone, my project remains incomplete until an Indian who is translating my books into Mexican finishes them. If I leave, they will never be finished, so ⟨I must stay to ensure that⟩ what is done must not be lost, especially in view of the benefit that will result for the native population. If it pleases Your Majesty that the salary that I receive now should not be stopped, until such time as I can ensure that Your Majesty sees my work and thus may assess it, I should be enormously grateful, since in the meantime I may not suffer from need nor relinquish the position in which Your Majesty has placed me, particularly as I have renounced my own interest and convenience in order to serve Your Majesty more perfectly, as God is my witness, for this is the major purpose and value of my work. I have always attended to all those neglected interests that present themselves in this land, and they are many, spending for these purposes the salary for which I am grateful to Your Majesty, and I have not received a penny in reimbursement for my journey to New Spain or for my extra expenses—which have been huge—in the service of Your Majesty, and have employed my son who is with me day and night, without whose help I would never be able to complete such a vast work in such a brief time, all of which I will give to Your Majesty in a year from today, God willing, or slightly later. For this, I beg Your Majesty's consideration. May Our Lord keep Your Catholic and royal person many years with increase of kingdoms and realms as Your Majesty's servants and subjects desire. Mexico, the 20th of March 1575. Sacred Catholic Royal Majesty. Your humble subject and servant of Your Majesty, whose royal hands I kiss. Doctor Francisco Hernández.[35]

Letter 10

October 22, 1575

Sacred Catholic Royal Majesty. By the mail carried on the last ship, I responded to Your Majesty, and I wrote there that fifteen volumes would leave without fail with the fleet that is now in port; thus I say in this letter only that I am writing down my experiences, together with other things that are essential as I put the finishing touches to my work, and adding small details as well as more complex things, which I have to do here, before I leave, and I am organizing everything according to the mapping[36] of the land.

For this reason I humbly beseech Your Majesty to permit me to leave on the next fleet[37] to arrive from Spain, for by then I will have accomplished everything I can possibly do here. My health is not good enough to allow me to travel to other parts of the Indies, and my return to Spain is important if my writings are to be put to good use.

Likewise I beseech you, because ever since I came here I have been paid less than my due, and I have also spent my own money on Your Majesty's work, that you may be pleased to command that papers be drawn up to enable me to be reimbursed, and that they be sent with my sailing permit allowing me to leave Mexico; by the foregoing I mean attached to the document, because I have not received a penny, and there has been no change in my salary, either

---

35. On the cover of the manuscript is a note in the king's hand: "I have read this and written to the Viceroy telling him that this doctor has frequently promised to send these books, but he never does send them; he is to pack them up and send them on the first ship for safe keeping."

36. Hernández's word is *graduación,* meaning measurement and marking.

37. I.e., not the one that is in port now.

here or in Spain, and there will ⟨still⟩ not be ⟨any change⟩, it seems, until I have left here, and I am there, and you have seen my work. After all is done, it will be up to Your Majesty to judge all this according to what you think, and to send me some help toward these costs, that I may leave and hasten my leaving, and then I will bring my finished translation of, and commentary on, Pliny, and other things that will please you and will be a benefit to the nation. May Our Lord keep the Sacred, Catholic Royal person of Your Majesty, with increase of more realms and domains, as Your Majesty's subjects desire. Mexico, 22 October, 1575. Your most humble servant and subject of Your Majesty, whose royal hands I kiss. Dr. Francisco Hernández.

Letter 11

February 10, 1576

Sacred Catholic Royal Majesty. I have written even more than the fifteen completed volumes on plants, animals, and minerals of this land, which are extremely useful and valuable to the health of everybody, for we know how very expensive medicine is. The reason that they were not sent on the last fleet was that I was thinking I would leave on this one, and circumstances being what they are.[38] And afterward over here it seemed opportune that I postpone my departure until the next one might come, so that I might experience all that which I have written about, and have observed in the hospitals, which I have visited freely, with no personal interest at stake, other than what anybody walking around the city would experience, thus I could continue to inquire and perfect everything, and clear off all that remained for me to do. They will leave with the present fleet now in port, God willing, because the fifteen volumes that I have finished will have become sixteen by then, and they will be accompanied by the history of this land, which is not complete yet, but which will please Your Majesty[39] when I

return with this work, which will be, God willing, with the next fleet, if Your Majesty gives me permission to ⟨wait until then⟩. This will only make it better, because the nature of this work means that it will cover more and be better written if I remain here. Because of my age and my ill health, I cannot go to Peru. I do not even know if I will be able to get back to Spain, where there is a great need for my presence, particularly for the printing, for otherwise all this will be lost, as will everything else that ⟨I have done here⟩ in the service of Your Majesty.

The extension that was sent to me arrived with the condition that I send the books on the last fleet, and the Viceroy seeing that it was my service to Your Majesty that detained me, that it was thus not my fault that the books were not sent, they will go without fail with the fleet now in port, furnished with the appropriate document; Your Majesty's officials have done no more. I implore Your Majesty, now that the books are finally going, and I am always working and always have worked in Your Majesty's service, day and night, and I will never fail you as long as I have life, please to grant me an extension until September 75 [*sic*], when I will be with you in Spain, and then you will judge my works and their utility.

When it is Our Lord's will that I may leave here, I will bring with me sketches and translations of everything, the natural history and the topography of this land with four other works very necessary for the completion of the natural history, which are finished in draft, which are: method of identifying the plants of both worlds; table of illnesses and remedies of this land; the plants native to this world and the virtues attributed to them by the natives; and on the antidotes.[40] Also the thirty-six books of Pliny that I have finished translating, and the commentary,[41] all of which will please you, with the help of no human hand—only God's— save that of my son, who has earned Your Majesty's reward. In all that I have done, I have attempted to incur as little

38. It is not known what "circumstances" are meant here; the epidemic of *cocoliztli* did not begin until June.

39. The "history of this land" presumably means the *Antiquities,* which, so far from pleasing Philip, was one of those works earmarked for censorship. See Georges Baudot, *Utopia and History in Mexico: The First Chroniclers of Mexican Civilization (1520–1569),* trans. Bernard R. Ortiz de Montellano and Thelma Ortiz de Montellano (Denver: University Press of Colorado, 1995), 507.

40. Of these works, only the table of illnesses and remedies (the *Index medicamentorum*) can be identified with any confidence as one that has survived.

41. Hernández's work on Pliny was already under way in the 1560s. He finished translating the thirty-seventh and last book of Pliny's *Natural History* a month after writing this letter (see the following letter).

cost as possible, and I put up a lot of my own money; indeed I have spent more than 20,000 pesos in my curing in the city, putting myself completely at your royal service, all as service well given if I should succeed in doing my duty and completing my work. I think likewise that when I return I will bring with me the history of plants translated into Náhuatl for the benefit of the native inhabitants, and into Spanish for the convenience of those who prefer that to reading it in Latin, and also some living plants and many simple and compound medicines from this land, so that Your Majesty may begin to reap the benefits of these labors.

I beg Your Majesty to send the extension as I have requested, and the permit allowing me to depart, and the declaration of the document for my present and past departure, and to command that I be given some financial assistance that will enable me to leave. May Our Lord keep the Sacred, Catholic Royal person of Your Majesty, with increase of more realms and domains, as Your Majesty's subjects desire. Mexico, 10 Feburary, 1576. Your most humble servant and subject of Your Majesty, whose royal hands I kiss. Dr. Francisco Hernández.

Letter 12

March 24, 1576

Sacred Catholic Royal Majesty. I have delivered to the royal officials, so that they can send them to Your Majesty, with the fleet that is now ready to leave New Spain, sixteen large volumes on the natural history of this land, of which the last two are not completely full, because what remains to go in them is not quite finished, which explains why it is missing from what is being sent to Your Majesty.

The work, which has cost me my health and life, promised much benefit and is now beginning to show some, and the devotion and care with which it has been written, and the nature of my service, Our Lord God knows and Your Majesty will be able to judge. I have been the first and last author[42] at Your Majesty's mandate and expense, and I have accomplished this novel and most difficult enterprise.

These are not clean copies, nor are they polished, or in order, so they will need one final going-over before they can be printed; in particular many of the images are mixed up because they are in the order in which the paintings were made. These go in the history and antiquities of this land, and the actual size is rendered in the paintings.

The table with its etymologies is going, in which Your Majesty will find the number of the painting on the left-hand side, and that of the description on the right, except when the number of the painting is found in the description, and vice versa.

I cannot match each description with its corresponding image until the work is printed, to prevent damage to the paintings from the emendations to which manuscripts are always subjected; nor will every plant or animal from this world go here yet: because some of those I selected were not painted properly, and others are not well represented by ⟨their⟩ European ⟨equivalents⟩.

Some things are depicted twice or more, either as a precaution, or because they were painted in different regions and at different stages;[43] but it will be easy to choose the most appropriate one at the time of printing.

The descriptions treat, concisely, the forms of the root, branches, leaves, flowers and seeds, or fruit, its nature and degree, taste, smell, and virtue according to the evidence of Indian doctors, gauged by experiment and the rules of medicine, the region and areas they come from, and even sometimes the climate in which they are found, the quantity applied, and their manner of cultivation.

The writing is done, as are three additional works; the paintings only in miniature, and with that desire in the extreme, I pray that the Lord deliver the work safely into Your Majesty's hands.

They will be of service to this world and that alike, because they will promote universal health as well as reduce the high cost ⟨of medicine⟩, and because as demand gradually grows they can be delivered to Spain and acclimatized in a place appropriate to their quality,[44] and thus the Lord may be praised through his works.

---

42. I.e., he did the work single-handedly.
43. I.e., different stages of the life cycle.

44. I.e., their humoral quality, their "nature" and "virtues."

I am still today finishing writing about additional discoveries, and I am putting the final touches to the books that are still in rough draft, and producing fair copies of four other books that will be of service to you. I am also translating them into Spanish and Mexican, and obtaining firsthand experience in two hospitals, where I began curing only when there was no one else left in this land with any competence to do so. I am also gathering seeds, plants, and medicines both simple and compound from this land, which I shall send to Your Majesty. I shall likewise be preparing the books of topography of this land, antiquities, and the conquest, which I have done, and the thirty-seven books of Pliny, which I have finished translating and annotating, together with other matters of physic and medicine, which will be of service and pleasure to Your Majesty, and which will be delivered, complete, as soon as the next fleet from Spain arrives here, if Your Majesty will grant me permission for this.

I beg Your Majesty to send me such permission, for this is in the royal interest, for then the majority of this ⟨description of the⟩ land will have been completed. However, my health will not support the journey to Peru and I do not even know if it will hold up long enough for my return to Spain. I am afflicted with chronic ills, and yet my attendance and my life will be necessary there to perfect and print my books, and have them put to their proper use, as well as other things in the service of Your Majesty.

Because the prorogation writ, which was sent to me by the last fleet, came with the condition that the books were to go with the fleet before that, and the Viceroy agreeing that it was service to Your Majesty that delayed me, and that it was thus not my fault that the books were not sent, they would have gone before now, as they are going now. I beg for this document according to your wisdom. Your Majesty's officials are in agreement with this proposition. Since the books are going, and I have always labored, and I continue to toil in your royal service night and day, and I shall never fail to serve you as long as I live, I beseech Your Majesty to be pleased to have an absolute and unconditional prorogation sent, effective from September 75 [*sic*], so that up to the point of my arrival in Spain, I may be honored and rewarded by Your Majesty (whose sole favor I enjoy apart from that of God) according to your judgment of my works, in which I have had no more personal assistance than that of my one son, who compiled the table and dedicated it to Your Majesty and a few other things that he did that were essential to this work, and without whose help I would not have been able to achieve what I have done, for which it would be most just if Your Majesty be pleased to grant him some reward.[45]

In all of this I have kept the costs down as much as possible, making use of the salary that Your Majesty granted me, in large part, and not having more than 20,000 pesos to spend. Other efforts have used up much more in this land in exchange for your employing me totally in the service of Your Majesty for the consummation of this work, which I will consider time well spent if I can be certain that I have met some of the expectations placed upon my labors, which have been carried out at Your Majesty's expense and mandate.

I also beg Your Majesty to declare the edict that was sent to me for assistance with the costs when I leave Mexico, since it is as just that it be understood also for what is already done, since no other compensation beyond my salary has been paid to me, and also some assistance with expenses be given me to facilitate my departure, and that the Viceroy of this land be commanded not to be concerned about the amount spent so far, but to calculate the expense after I have left.[46]

May Our Lord keep the Sacred, Catholic Royal person of Your Majesty, with increase of more realms and domains, as we Your Majesty's subjects desire. Mexico, 24 March, 1576. Sacred Catholic Royal Majesty. Servant and subject of Your Majesty, whose royal hands I kiss. Dr. Francisco Hernández.

---

45. This paragraph is a slightly revised version of a part of the previous letter.

46. Viceroy Enríquez in a letter dated March 30, 1577, announced the departure of Hernández, "carrying with him 22 volumes, in addition to the 16 that he has already sent, and he is also bringing for Your Majesty two chests filled with sixty-eight sacks of seeds and roots, eight casks and four boxes containing trees and plants, which Your Majesty ordered as the tangible result of this expedition: he wanted to make sure he gathered everything here first, because he has taken such pains with it. He deserves the thanks and recompense of Your Majesty for his labors, because he has been of great service and taken great care, as his works will testify; the effort has cost him his health."

Hernández's Petition to the King

[Early 1577?]

Sacred Catholic Royal Majesty:—Doctor Francisco Hernández declares: that he has resided by order of Your Majesty for nearly eight years in New Spain, during which time he has caused the natural things of this land to be depicted and described better and more accurately than had previously been possible, and caused the land to be surveyed exactly, and he has written the history of the western regions with their states and customs, images of their gods, sacrifices, and other antiquities, and because the natural history of this world is conjoined to that one, he has completed a translation and commentary of the thirty-seven books of the *Natural History* of Pliny, in nine volumes,[47] and furthermore he has described the plants of the islands of Santo Domingo, Cuba, and the Canaries, subject to the little available time he could spend in these places, and the plants of this land[48] that grow in New Spain, distinguishing between those that are native and those that have been transplanted, and how to recognize the plants from here and from there. Item, another treatise of sixty natural purgatives both native to this region and imported to it,[49] which he used in experimental trials to cure the sick in two hospitals, not in his own interest nor in that of virtually anyone else at all, but all in the service of Your Majesty and your ministry; in addition he has succeeded in adding to the illustrations, which have been sent to Your Majesty, flowers, fruits, and virtues, which have been taken and investigated here, with many more new drawings and descriptions to add to the books that Your Majesty has already; and beyond what concerns the Indies, he has completed other books, which he is sending from here, which will please Your Majesty and be of benefit to the nation.

As for the plants that Your Majesty ordered to be sent to Seville, of the fifteen that came planted in barrels, there are six that are alive and among them the balsam, which is very important, and the tunas, which is germinating. Almost sixty different types of seed remain sown and entrusted to the *alcalde,* together with one that is live, which are the lilies of this land, which have survived the rigors of time, and others there are that go to seed in spring, and which will all be sent, at your Majesty's command, to be sown in that region.[50] Medicinal drugs are being sent as well, which are used in experiments, and whose effectiveness can be seen in this land.

All that remains, that Your Majesty may be served and the nation favored with this benefit that it has begun to receive, is that Your Majesty be pleased to order the printing of these books, and that all be published (for a translation is also coming in the Mexican language for the benefit of the natives of that land, which cost me no little effort, and it is still being translated into Spanish) and that without delay, because of his age and poor health, and the long time that the printing will require; it is important that it be begun now, because if that cannot be, nobody will know how to put it in the right order and make proper use of it,[51] and thus the nation will be disadvantaged. It will not be possible to make good this loss however many years go by, because a great number of doctors and Indian artists who contributed to this and made sense of it have died in this latest plague.

---

47. Today, BN MSS 2,862–2,871 and 6,656.
48. Spain.
49. No such treatise is known to have survived.
50. Meaning Seville?

51. A loaded remark: the *Natural History* was organized in an order that would make little sense to most Europeans. It certainly made no sense to Recchi. Hernández thought that his organization of the descriptions was essential to its usefulness.

THE WILL OF FRANCISCO HERNÁNDEZ

There are two copies of Hernández's will—or rather, two wills, as Somolinos surmises (285). One is preserved in Madrid, Archivo de Protocolos, 1017, fols. 329–333r. A transcript of the will of May 8, 1578, appears in P. Barreiro, "El testamento del doctor Francisco Hernández," *Boletín de la Real Academia de la Historia* 94 (1929): 475–96.

The Will of Francisco Hernández, doctor

In the name of the most holy Trinity, Father, Son, and Holy Spirit who are three persons and the one true God, and of the most glorious Virgin Mary, mother of God and our protector, amen. Let it be known to whomsoever shall see this last will and testament that I, Doctor Francisco Hernández, His Majesty's Protomédico of all the West Indies, native as I am of the town of Monte Alban, being at present in the city of Madrid at the court of His Majesty, being ill and confined to bed with the illness that Our Lord God has been pleased to visit upon me, and being of sound mind and judgment and unimpaired memory, fearing death, which is a natural thing, and desiring to place my soul speedily in salvation, believing firmly and truly in the Holy Catholic faith and all that pertains to the Holy Mother Church of Rome, which is governed and enlightened by the Holy Spirit, in which I profess

to live and die, and as I make this profession invoking the grace of the Holy Spirit, I hereby make and ordain this my will in the following form and manner:

First I commit my soul to God, who created and redeemed it with his precious blood, and my body to the earth where it will remain interred until the Day of Judgment, and I desire that if the will of God be pleased that I lead this present life at this court, that I may be buried in the church of St. Martin in this city of Madrid in the tomb that my executors consider proper, and that for accompaniments my body shall be accompanied by the cross and clerics of the church of St. Martin and of the church of Santiago where at present I am a parishioner or of whichever parish I may be in at the time of my death, and the council of the most holy sacrament of the said church of St. Martin. And I desire to be received by one of that brotherhood, and that the said brothers be given alms as my executors deem apposite at the door.

61

I desire that six masses be said for my soul: the passion of Our Lord twice, the Holy Trinity twice, and the Immaculate Conception of our Lady twice.

I desire that my goods be dispersed for each one of these obligations a half real with which I divide my goods.

I desire that, in the event that His Majesty does not recompense the Mexican painters in the amount that I requested, that to each of the three, namely Pedro Vásquez, and Anton and Baltasar Elías, to each or to his heirs be given thirty ducats[1] from my estate.

I desire that, if His Majesty does not make recompense to the Indian doctors of Mexico they take according to my intent twenty bulls of composition[2] and hereafter those that can take it be paid alms of two reals each, that they will not be more than 300 ducats, counting each bull as worth 5,000 maravedís, and other such to compensate the Indians who were engaged to bring me herbs and who were either dissatisfied with their remuneration or not remunerated at all, and by this let it be understood that all others who worked in this enterprise should be compensated, it being the case that there are so many of them and so varied that they cannot ⟨all⟩ be identified, that these would take bulls up to the amount of 400 ducats, and let it be understood that I do not speak of what should be paid to them, except that they should be given two reals each, counting for each 5,000 maravedís, with the exception of the three or four painters who are identified, and known to have given their assistance there, but it is my desire that they be given 30 ducats to compensate for lack of payment to them; in case His Majesty does not desire to recompense them, only and thus it is my will that four or five of the regular assistants be selected and each one paid eight Castilian ducats, it being understood after payment is made to the former three or four painters and then four or five more be selected according to what is herein stated.

I desire that care be taken to find out if the Castilians in Seville were troubled for the amount of 27,000 maravedís, by looking in their book, and if it turns out that this is true, that they be reimbursed from my estate. Pedro de Aguilar will affirm if this is the case, or in his absence the Tapias family, or Benito Luis, public scrivener of the city of Seville, my factor.

I desire that if by chance Diego López de Montalbán does not wish to pay the pesos that he owes me, about eight in all for each of the litter bearers who carried me, it is my will that whatever Diego Caballero says should be paid from my estate be paid, he being resident in the city of Mexico. Those pesos should be paid by the said Diego López de Monta[lbá]n.

I desire that whatever His Majesty owes me of my emoluments be covered.

I desire that alms be sent to the brotherhood of the most holy sacrament of the town of Ajofrín that they obtain indulgences from the bull of that brotherhood, thirty ducats.

I declare that I have in the town of Ajofrin and in the city of Toledo certain fees, to recover which I authorize Diego Martín, resident of that town, and I give him power over the documents and securities, and I commission him to provide for my two daughters, legitimate and illegitimate, whom I left in the monastery of Saint John the Penitent in the city of Toledo. I desire that he pay their expenses, and his own charges for this work, and salary, in accordance with what was in the documents and the collection of the fees which I claimed as my goods.

I wish and it is my desire that to His Majesty King Philip our Lord be left the sixteen volumes of plants and animals of the Indies that His Majesty has in his possession today, and the description of New Spain with other paintings of plants and animals that were added in all, the sketches and tables and paintings on wood[3] and the volume that contains five supplementary books, and the three volumes that were translated into the Mexican language,[4] and I beg His Majesty to take notice of how much time I devoted to the above-mentioned, day and night for the seven years that I

---

1. Currency in use in the sixteenth century was based on the maravedí. The monetary units mentioned in Hernández's will and letters include the real, which was worth 34 maravedís, the peso (165 maravedís), the escudo (330 maravedís), and the ducat (375 maravedís).

2. Bulls of composition: historically, these were what the Comisario General of the Crusade gave to those who possessed another's goods when the owner could not be determined.

3. This is apparently the sole allusion to paintings on wood.

4. An affirmation that a translation into Náhuatl was actually made. No such translation is known to survive.

spent in New Spain in the royal service, and I have an unmarried daughter who would be deserving of bounty and thanks.

I wish and it is my desire that all and any of my books that may be printed be dedicated and addressed to his majesty since they came into being for the most part by his grace and favor.

I declare that Juan Hernández my son brought livestock from the Indies—his own property—although this was counted and included in the body and total of my estate as [1,000?] pesos at eight reals each. I desire that twelve pesos be given for each of them, taken from that body and total, and further I desire that they be given in recompense from the sale of my books, because the rest of what may be left to his siblings be distributed among my heirs. And it is my desire that if they my said heirs make objection to the contents of this clause concerning what is given to my son the said Juan Hernández, I desire that this be remedied thus: that there be recompense of the twelve pesos that it would seem to the objectors not to be so distributed. I attest that this is in accord with the laws of this realm.

I desire that, for the ease of my conscience, the heirs of Juan Martín, pruner of trees, resident of the town of Ajofrín, whom Juan de Torres my executor will identify, be given 150 ducats.

And to complete and conclude this my will, desire, and bequests contained herein, I appoint and establish as my executors Juan de Torres and Diego Mon, residents of the town of Ajofrín, as far as concerns that which must be completed in the said town, and Juan de Herrera and Juan de Valencia, cleric created by his majesty, for what concerns the completion of my testament in this court, to all whom and each one I give one *solidus* and grant all my power so that after my death they complete and conclude this my will, desire, and bequests contained herein, and that they enter and take my estate and sell my remaining goods for charity or outside, and for that completion I give them whatever powers are necessary.

I declare that according to the order of the church of Santa Madre I was married legitimately to Juana Díaz de Pan y Agua, my legal wife who is now deceased, and during that marriage we had and gave birth to our legitimate children the abovementioned Juan Hernández and María de Sotomayor our children, and as such I name and declare them.

I declare that I have an illegitimate daughter, who has lived many days since my said wife died and who remains unmarried. I also being unmarried and both of us free therefore to enter into matrimony such that we could contract a marriage, I desire that in this my completed will, desire, and bequests, the said Francisca Hernández my daughter be given a fifth of all that remains of my estate, which I can dispose according to the law, which I desire with such obligation and condition that if she is married or joined in marriage all the above-mentioned be given to her as dowry, and that if she dies without issue the above-mentioned reverts to my heirs, my children and their heirs, and if the said Francisca Hernández enters a house of religion, in such case the said fifth shall be given to her as her dowry in accordance with the custom upon entry into monasteries in the city of Toledo with, further, the veil, dowry, and collation that it is customary to give all such nuns and furthermore what exceeds the said fifth shall be taken and inherited by my legitimate children and it is my will that the convent where the said Francisca Hernández my daughter may become a resident nun, desiring to belong to the religious and the order whose vows she will profess and where she shall be cloistered, and what remains of the said fifth shall be paid in a redeemable pension and of the proceeds my daughter the said Francisca in each year 5,000 ⟨pesos⟩ for her needs and the rest my heirs take, and by this be understood that my said daughter takes this, and not the abbess, the nuns, or the convent, and when the above-said dies, I desire to leave at that time and my heirs inherit as inheritance the said 5,000; as my goods for such solely the said Francisca my daughter has to be usufructual of the said 5,000: in each one year every day of her life as it is stated here.

I declare that at present I owe no debt to any one person, but for the ease of my conscience if anyone shall declare that I am in his debt and can show legitimate proof that I am in his debt, my executors shall discharge the debt with all due diligence.

And, all that is said is completed and concluded in this my testament, I declare that for the remainder of my goods, chattels, and rights and actions, I leave and institute by my legitimate heirs in all to the said Juan Hernández and María de Sotomayor, my legitimate children, that they may have and inherit by means that take place according to law, in equal parts.

And I revoke and annul and deny any other will or testament whatsoever, codicil or codicils, and orders that have been made before this date in writing or by spoken word or any other manner, and declare that they are invalid and not to be accepted or believed. This testament that I hereby make and give, is that which I desire to be valid as my testament or codicil or any document that this is my sovereign will, and stands firmly as the last desire that I express. In confirmation of which, before the public scrivener and witnesses in the city of Madrid this eighth day of May, 1578, in the presence of witnesses Pedro de Palacros, maker of armor, and Diego Bautista and Pedro de Rueda, ordained priest, and Francisco Rodríguez, servant of this doctor, and Francisco Vasquez, servant to the Count of Alba residents of this city, and being in the court of His Majesty and the said gentleman offering this will, I the scrivener declare in good faith that I know him and inscribe his name in the register, Doctor Francisco Hernández. This all took place before me, Alonso Pérez, scrivener, all the sentences that say thus, and any emendation above or below the lines is valid only where I sign my name.

I Alonso Pérez de Durango, public scrivener to His Majesty and citizen of the city of Madrid and of this earth was present for the above-said and in the presence of these witnesses, and I wrote it and I sign my name that is it is true.

Alonso Pérez de Durango, public scrivener

THE ANTIQUITIES OF NEW SPAIN

Hernández compiled two versions of his books of antiquities. The principal changes introduced in the second version concern the ordering of the texts. For discussion of the relationship between the two, see Jesús Bustamante, "De la naturaleza y los naturales americanos en el siglo XVI: Algunas cuestiones críticas sobre la obra de Francisco Hernández," *Revista de Indias* 52, nos. 195–96 (1992), esp. 314–25. The second version is preserved in manuscript at the Real Academia de la Historia in Madrid, MS 9-2101. Three published editions of the *Antiquities* exist: a facsimile of the Latin manuscript (Mexico City: Talleres Gráficos del Museo Nacional de Arqueología, Historia y Etnografía, 1926), and a Spanish translation prepared by Joaquín García Pimentel, published as *Antigüedades de la Nueva España* (Mexico City: Pedro Robredo, 1945), reprinted in *Obras completas,* vol. 6, with Pimentel's terse introduction and, in places, detailed notes.

It has been known for a long time that Hernández borrowed heavily from three similar sources: Toribio de Benavente Motilinía, *Memoriales;* Bernardino de Sahagún, *Historia general de las cosas de Nueva España;* and Francisco López de Gómara, *Historia general de las Indias.* Juan Eusebio Nieremberg, apparently not realizing that this was what Hernández had done, included the description of the Great Temple of Tenochtitlán in *Historia naturae* (Antwerp, 1635) and attributed it to Hernández, who had translated it, word for word, from Sahagún. Hernández's purpose was to compile, as the king had ordered, an ethnographic account of the people of New Spain, so he consulted the available sources and produced an anthology in which his own hand is evident. Hernández translated his Spanish sources into Latin and added his own interpolations, which are most obvious when he refers to his own work on natural history. The manuscript's heavy revisions of Sahagún (especially) show that Hernández did more than merely copy his sources. Above all, the selection itself is his.

Just two chapters (the second and third of our selections) have been translated into English before: they appear in parallel texts in Miguel Guzmán Peredo, *Medical Practices in Ancient America/Prácticas médicas en la América antigua,* translated by Joseph Doschner (Mexico City: Ed. Euroamericanas, 1985), 151–59.

General Description of All the Indies

(1.1)

This fourth part of the world, virtually unknown[1] to antiquity and thrown open at the end of our era under the auspices of King Charles, is divided into the upper and lower West Indies.[2] Almost in the middle it narrows into an isthmus,[3] which divides it in two, and from there extends long and wide to the south and north. The Isthmus, not unlike an arm, faces east on its oblique side and the upper part of the south, and extends between the northern sea and the southern. Where it begins it is very wide, but farther along, near its coastlines, it descends smoothly southward. Then, turning toward the eastern equinox, almost as wide, it proceeds for a long space. After a longer tract, in which it gets more of the rising sun, it becomes narrower and where it is narrowest the Lower Indies stick to it, like an Amazonian pelta.[4] Two small but famous cities overlook different seas: Nombre de Dios to the north, which means Name of God,[5] and Panama to the south, seventy-two miles away. This is the narrowest point of the Isthmus, but at its widest it is 1,000 miles, at Colima, which is in 20° latitude, to the Palmas river, whose mouth is half a degree farther from the equinox than the summer line. The Upper Indies between the east and the west face toward Asia and Europe and extend as far between these as the Frigid Peninsula in the region of Labrador is distant from the snowy mountains in the Province of Quivira,[6] popularly understood to be 6,900 miles. And the snowy mountains are 40° above the equinox, the Frigid Peninsula 61¼°, more or less. Where they are inclined more to the west, where the western side begins, the peninsula of California projects to the south, a little smaller than Italy. The coast of California, unlike Italy, is not divided by various arms of rivers, except that it ends in one single promontory, below the summer equinox, opposite the promontory of Corrientes in the province of Jalisco. These two peninsulas, rather like the Adriatic, enclose the Red Sea, which is longer, as it runs by 320 miles of coast, but it is a little narrower. At the innermost part of this sea the river Miraflores penetrates more than the Po: which is called the Estuary, which discharges the rivers Axa, Tetonteac, and Tigua. The side that faces south overlooks the northern sea and the southern. Where it washes in the north and its coastline turns northward, opposite the coasts of the lower Indies, it does not go forward more to the east than the lower, and they are defined, both almost by the same meridian circle. Between one coast and the other the northern Ocean comes in, and while it goes farther forward to the west, because the coasts come together gradually, the coast curves more, most of all at the islands of Haiti and Cuba; principally when it reaches the proximity of the Gulf of Mexico; here the coasts of the Isthmus and the upper Indies project out to the promontories of Yucatán and Florida and the island of Cuba, which closes the mouth of the Gulf, as far as they curve, which opens an entrance for 240 miles to the Gulf (the distance from Yucatán to Cuba). And although there is another way[7] between that island and the Florida peninsula, however much more it is curved open, it is drawn together by a seething current,[8] which flows between Yucatán and Cuba perpetually to the Gulf of Mexico or the Sea of Cortes; a secret of nature that is still unknown. The Florida Peninsula is 25° and that of Yucatan nearly 21°. These two give the Gulf of Mexico its circular shape. The inner parts of it belong to New Spain because of Fernando Cortés, from whom the Sea received its name, not from the people defeated by Spanish troops. The eastern side resembles Iceland and the British Isles, its limits being the two promontories, Raso and the Cold.[9] This is 4,800 miles distant from Iceland, 6,600

---

1. See Pimentel, note, *OC* 6:49. He considered that Hernández was not referring to any discovery of America before Columbus but that he was maintaining a distinction by which the Antilles ("West Indies") were excluded from the denomination "New Spain."

2. I.e., continental America and the Caribbean islands.

3. By "isthmus" Hernández means, essentially, modern Mexico and Central America.

4. A shield. The allusion is to Virgil, *Aeneid,* 1.490.

5. δεούνομα in MS.

6. The snowy mountains (in Spanish, Sierra Nevada) are in California, but the province of Quivira seems to have been in present-day New Mexico.

7. The Florida canal.

8. Understood by Pimentel, *OC* 6:52, to refer to the Gulf Stream, but this passage is a textual crux.

9. It is not clear which promontory Hernández means by Raso. López de Gómara, his principal source for this chapter, speaks of the *cabo frio* (cold peninsula) without identifying it.

miles from Ireland, and as much from the Peninsula of Thorcyrolandia.[10] The snowy mountains and California are the terminal points of the western side. The space in between is 2,400 miles. The Lower Indies are more properly called golden than the Asiatic Crimea.[11] What place is so placid that there is no abundance of gold? Almost all the shapeless mass of them is situated in a straight line from the Equator to the south. On this side a small part remains; if not attached to the Isthmus, they are surrounded by sea: by the Arctic to the north, by the southern sea to the east, to the west by the southern, which is commonly known as the south. 440 miles south is the Strait of Magellan: this is the length of the Strait and where the Indies meet it. These on the wide side, from the Isthmus to the promontory whose name is Anegado, to eight degrees from this side of the equinox, are thrown in the way of the north and, as they advance to the south, they gradually extend to right and left between the two oceans, until at the equator they prolong their coastlines. After turns to the north, they reach out more toward the eastern sun than the western, across from the Cape Verde Islands off Guinea and the region of the Nigerians and Senegalese, no farther than 2,000 miles away. But from here they extend farther, except where they face toward Africa, the coasts gradually recede (because from the promontory of Saint Augustine to the other Cold Promontory the coastline is almost straight) and after that they come closer and stretch more gently, until they reach the strait of Magellan, where they are about nine miles (which is the width of the Strait) from the fifth world.[12] The coasts of these measure in circumference about 16,300 miles. In length, from the Promontory of Vela, which is 12 degrees this side of the equator, to the Strait of Magellan, 52½° farther, it measures 4,800. The maximum width is 4,000 miles and that is between the promontories of Saint Helena and Saint Augustine, both in southern latitude at 2° and 8½° respectively. And if from these the Lower Indies did not project south, they would have the exact shape of an Amazonian pelta. The Isthmus, to the west, touches the higher side at 8° this side of the Equator, with a transverse mountain range, and should be noted for many things; since here for 100 miles the Seas of Viana[13] and San Miguel are separated. The former, in the southern Ocean, famous for what happened there and for its name, is 6° distant from the equator. The latter, in the north, the more famous, because in it was the first victory on the continent and there arrived the first colony of Spanish and took first possession of the Lower Indies in the name of our Invincible Catholic King; and the famous victory of Martin Fernández and his brave men at the river of Darien, which was no less momentous than that of Otumba in the Upper, and continued by the exploits of Vasco Nuñez of Balboa in the Gulf of San Miguel, and lastly because here Carlos Panquiaco gave the first fruits of the Indians of this Continent, to God.[14]

How Mexican Women Give Birth, and the Double Bath for Children

(1.2)

When the newlywed woman reached the seventh month of her pregnancy, her close relatives, after eating and drinking, would discuss the choice of a midwife, with whose art and advice the delivery would be safe and easy. Then they would go to one whom they knew to be the most skilled in the city and the most diligent in the practice of her art, so that she would care for the health of the woman in labor, and assist her at the moment of childbirth, and they begged her assistance with fervent supplication. She replied with reasons that she would do so, with all the diligence and care of which she was capable, all for their satisfaction, the health of the child, and the health of mother. And after frequent visits to the pregnant woman, she would not only take her to the baths known as temazcal[15] in their native country, which they used a great deal for pregnant women, mothers of young children, and convalescents, but she would also lay

10. Greenland, possibly.
11. See Pimentel, *OC* 6:53.
12. Unidentified; possibly Tierra del Fuego.
13. Unidentified: Pimentel, *OC* 6:54, concludes that Viana could be the Gulf of Urabá or the Gulf of Darien.

14. See López de Gómara. Panquiaco was a Mexican ("Indian"), apparently the first to be baptized. He was under Balboa's command.
15. Steam bath. The Náhuatl word is derived from *tema* (to sweat in a bath) and *calli* (house).

down a set of rules for living that were to be observed care-fully and religiously at the time of delivery. The midwife thought these would help to ensure a safe and easy delivery and would be helpful immediately afterward. A woman bear-ing her first child would sometimes be so debilitated by the delivery that she died: she would then be numbered among the goddesses in heaven, and her name inscribed in their roll, and later worshiped with a cult dedicated to goddesses, and she would be buried with solemn funeral rites. But if the birth went well, the midwife would talk to the baby, as if he were already capable of reason and could understand what was said to him. She would invoke the gods to ensure that his birth gave him a prime place among the gods, and access to a good augury at his birth. She would ask what fate or destiny had been assigned to him from the beginning of the world. As she cut the umbilical cord, almost shedding tears, the midwife predicted menacing disasters, and she foretold what unfortunate circumstances and toil had been reserved for his lot. She washed the child, with customary little prayers, greeting the goddess of the sea, and afterward she would joke and say comforting things to the new mother and console her for her pain. Furthermore, the family thanked the midwife for her diligence and congratulated the young mother on the birth of her child and then pro-ceeded to dandle the baby. Four days after the birth was the time for the child's second bath and for him to be given a name. The family prepared drinks and a variety of things to eat, according to custom and in celebration of this bathing. In addition, a small shield, a bow, and four small arrows appropriate to the child's age,[16] and a small mantle like the Mexicans' cape [were given to the child]. If it was a girl, a *huipilli* and *cueitl*,[17] girls' clothes, as well as a case, a distaff, and a spindle—and all things concerned with sewing—would be given to her. When everything was ready, and the relatives of the parents came to celebrate this bathing, they would send for the midwife. After the rising of the sun, she would place a bowl full of water near the middle of the patio and, holding the naked infant with both hands, placing the above-mentioned weapons somewhere near, she would say,

"My son, the gods Ometecutli and Omecioatl, whose realm is in the ninth and tenth heavens, have begotten you in this light and brought you into this world full of calamity and pain. Take then this water, which will protect your life, in the name of the goddess Chalchiutlicue." At that moment, tak-ing water in her right hand, she sprinkled some on the head of the baby, adding, "Behold this element, without whose assistance no mortal being can survive." Then, she sprin-kled some more of the same water on the infant's breast, say-ing, "Receive this celestial water that washes impurity from your heart," then, sprinkling water on his head again, she said, "Son, receive this divine water, which must be drunk that all may live, that it may wash you and wash away all your misfortunes, part of your life since the beginning of the world: this water in truth has a unique power to oppose misfortune." At the same time she washed the baby's little body all over, exclaiming, "In which part of you is unhappi-ness hidden, or in which part are you hiding? Leave this child; today he is born again in the healthful waters in which he has been bathed, according to the will of Chalchiutlicue, the goddess of the sea," and then she raised the child toward the sky, adding, "Great Teuel and Omecioatl, creators of souls, I offer this child unto you, whom you have formed, and sent into this brief life of toil, that you will receive him and give him your strength." Then lifting him a second time, the midwife said, "I invoke you too, goddess Citlallatonac, and conjure you to give your strength to this child," and lift-ing him a third time, she said, "O celestial gods, I call upon you and implore your divinity. Blow through this child, I beg of you, to generate in him the divine power that emanates from you, that he may enjoy celestial life." Yet again, lifting him for the fourth time, she said to the sun and the earth, "Greatest father of all, and you, earth, mother of all things, see what here I offer softly unto you, this child. Receive him, both of you, and as he has been born to mili-tary life, after he has shown illustrious signs of valor, grant that he may die in battle." The midwife then took in her right hand the shield, bow, and arrows, and raised them all aloft. She spoke thus to the sun, which is another Mars to

16. The arrows are small because the child is small.
17. These two words are left in Náhuatl in the Latin MS. Sahagún

mentions both but describes neither. *Huipilli* is a short-sleeved woman's shift; *cueitl* is a skirt.

these people: "Highest sun, receive these arms of war, dedicated to you, with which he may obtain felicity in heaven, granted to soldiers who fall in battle, to enjoy incredible delights." While all these things were going on, by the light of four flaming torches, the child was given a name, which was repeated three times, and three times she said, "Take these arms, take these arms, my child! With these you shall please and serve the highest light." Then they turned to the food, near the place where the child had been washed, grabbed the food, and as they left, swallowing at the same time, they shouted, "It is important for you, newborn baby, to go to war, to die in battle, so that in the end you will go to heaven, to serve the sun, and to live a life of peace and happiness, among the bravest of men who lived, lost once they fell in combat." With these words they demonstrated that every boy was destined to go to war in obeisance to the sun. Once these things were done, the midwife returned with the child to the house of his parents, with torches preceding them, burning until the fire was consumed, when they would go out completely.

The Bath for Girls

(1.3)

Newborn baby girls were customarily bathed in a similar manner, though the midwife would also utter different supplications. Then, wetting her hand, she would place it on the lips and say: "My daughter, open your mouth that you may receive the goddess Chalchiutlycue, her who is adorned with emeralds, under whose aegis it may be granted that you enjoy this light." Sprinkling the chest with the same hand, she quickly murmured to her, "Receive the water that cools, cleanses, and strengthens." She raised her hand to the head and added, "Welcome Chalchiutlycue, icy goddess of the waters, and perpetually mobile as one whom sleep can never overcome. May she succeed in entering your bowels, and staying with you, that you may remain vigilant and that you may never sleep badly." Sprinkling water from her hand, she added, "Theft, leave this baby girl." Then, putting the water below the groin, in a low voice: "Where will you hide, ill fortune? Depart from this child, expelled by the powers of this fresh water." When these things were done, she took

the baby inside the house and laid her in the crib, uttering the following prayers: "Oalticitl, parent of all, ruler of the ninth heaven, who created this child and brought her into this calamitous world, I beg you—for no other deity is concerned with guarding and sustaining newborn infants—to take her to your breast. To you also, god of the night, Yohoalteuhtli, who preside over sleep, I beg you to watch over her and allow her to sleep in peace and tranquility." Then she spoke in a high voice over the crib, saying, "Mother of babies and guardian of children, welcome this newborn baby to your breast and protect her." It was customary for all the relatives, when newborns were placed in the crib for the first time, to greet her and call on the universal mother of all mortal beings, and ask that the baby be kindly welcomed, and they would celebrate the day with great joy and mirth.

Death, Souls, and Burial

(1.15)

They held it as a certainty that souls are immortal, and they were convinced that incorporeal souls inhabited one of three regions, to wit: heaven, hell, and earthly paradise. They said that those who fell in war have conquered the sky, where the sun presided, as have those who were taken prisoner in battle and were sacrificed on the altars of the gods, whatever form of death might have befallen them—which differed according to the feasts and the gods to whom they were sacrificed. They believed that heaven was a flat and wooded place ruled by the sun, and thus, on leaving, one was greeted with loud voices and uproar, the clattering and clashing of shields and arms. Only those killed by [enemy] arrows could look upon the sun, for it was not licit to raise the eyes any other way in contemplation of it. They said that this place consisted of beautiful woods filled with different kinds of trees, domesticated animals, and the songs of a multitude of the most beautiful birds. They have not the slightest doubt that any living thing that is offered by them will arrive without the loss of a single particle of the oblations, which would be received and accommodated for their use by the inhabitants of the sky, to whom they were consecrated.

These were transformed after the passage of one year into birds covered with various feathers, and roamed through the sky and the land, like the *hoitsitzilim,* sucking the dew that has collected in the corollas of flowers. It is also said that among those who were received into the earthly paradise were those who had been shipwrecked, and those who died after being struck by lightning, those who died of leprosy, mange, and rash and the Indian disease which the natives call *nanahuatl*[18] (which infected the entire globe) and those who died of dropsy. This earthly paradise bore all sorts of fruits and earthly delights. There were never any problems in this place of eternal spring, where the climate was most beautiful. In this place the earth yielded up squashes, corn, chili, and all kinds of blite, orach, vegetables, and fruits. It was also said that those who lived in these regions were the gods who brought the rains and were commonly called *tlaloques* in the native tongue, and were to be placated with blood drawn from young boys. Those who died of such causes, that is, infected by plague, wretched and publicly known, were never burned but were interred instead, with a wand placed between their hands and some chenopod seeds on their jaws, tinting the face blue and adding strips of paper all around, which they put on the neck and the rest of the body as an ornament peculiar to the gods. All the rest, whoever they were and however their souls may have departed from their bodies, were thought to have been cast into hell. As for sacrifices, fasting, prayers, effusions of blood and other things with which they placated their gods, they believed that these could only obtain a transitory thing, but the seat occupied by the souls devoid of bodies depended only on the manner of death.

In this way they said to those who parted from the living, with eloquent and quiet speeches (in truth these people are quiet by nature and, untutored as they are, skilled in speech). They said that they had already traveled through the course of their life and, having put out this light, they believed that they were going to where the gods seemed to be; to wit, to a hideous place of perpetual darkness, which no endeavor could evade. They had lived already for the benefit of the gods and had traveled the course that the gods had assigned them. And although life was thus narrowly circumscribed, it was not permitted to defy destiny or subvert the constant order of things. Already the gods of the underworld called them to the abode of the dead, and one had to obey them leaving one's home, the sweetest wife, the loveliest children, and the kindest friends. And once a dead man was reunited with his kinfolk, they said that this was the work of that god and the nature of things, which no mortal being could avoid, for mortals were born already condemned to die, which thus had to be universally and calmly accepted. They said many more other things of the same sort, which could be conjectured from the rest. This done, they drew together the legs of the dead man, and wrapped him all over with paper called *amatl.* They sprinkled the neck and head with cold water, adding that as he had drunk it during his life, it would serve him in death to travel on his longest journey. Consequently, they put it in a small cup among the linens and cloths that accompanied the body, which varied according to the kinds of death and the quality of the dead.

They put other papers in on top, adding that the time would come when they would be of no little use. They burned and reduced to ashes all the clothes and ornaments that he had used in life, since he would not need them now that he was dead, except to protect him from winter and the intense cold of those regions he had to cross.

They placed beside him also, as companions on his journey, a gold-colored dog, with a few threads of cotton tied around his neck, since they believed that without the aid of this none could cross the river of hell. Once that river was crossed, one had to give those papers as a supplicant to Pluto, god of the underworld, with other loose threads and torches included in the funeral vestments. A dead woman's clothes were kept folded and wrapped until the eightieth day after her death, when they would be burned. This would all be repeated on each anniversary for four years, and only then were the obsequies completed. But these absurdities did not stop even here, for they affirmed that after entering the darkness of hell, they still had to encounter new hells, and, mounted on the dog, to traverse new rivers as they came to them. They added many other, equally infantile things, which strike me as too silly to write down, so I pass over them in silence.

---

18. Venereal disease.

THE ANTIQUITIES OF NEW SPAIN 71

Once the corpse was suitably adorned, they seated it in a chair and surrounded it with flags if it was the funeral of a lord. They killed slaves and placed their hearts around the corpse, which was burned and reduced to ashes, then buried. A common man's corpse would be placed the same way, but on his forehead they would put foodstuffs and one-third of his goods (if he had any), and then they would bury him. They burned bodies in accordance with the rites associated with fire. The task of burning was entrusted to two old men who, while two more sang chants, pierced the body with lances as it lay in the fire. Then they sprinkled water on the ashes and the bones, and finally buried them in a round grave, but just before doing so they placed an emerald in the mouth if it was a nobleman, or a much less valuable *iztlin* stone if it was someone of lower class. They believed that these stones replaced the heart of the dead. The eminent would be accompanied by elaborate paper effigies adorned with feathers of many colors; twenty slaves would be immolated while other slaves pierced them in the neck with arrows, the day on which the lord was burned, so that wheresoever he was going, he would be accompanied by servants as he was in life.

Mexico City When the Spanish Took It

(1.21)

The city of Mexico comprised 60,000 buildings or more when Cortés first took it. The temples, royal palaces and courts were built very skillfully with stone and timber; the rest were long, narrow, and lacking doors and windows. The city was built on a great lake that filled or half filled some public and private streets with water, but hardly touched others. Each house had two entrances, one giving on to the street on dry land, the other giving on to the canal; in the former, pedestrians could walk, and in the latter they would be transported in barges,[19] and in this the city resembled Venice or Antwerp. The lake of Mexico was divided into two parts, one salty, the other blessed with fresh water, and the city's foundations are better on the freshwater side, but although it may be called "fresh," the water is completely useless for drinking, even though springs and rivers with the sweetest and most pleasant water flow into the city, whether it is the floods that come from the mountains encircling the city (in effect it is situated in a great valley) that provide copious but stagnant water,[20] or because of all the filth that gets into the lakes in neighboring cities. For this reason, the purest and most healthful water comes to the city from the spring of Chapultepec, in tunnels and aqueducts. The city was also divided in two parts, and at one time was ruled by two kings. One part was called Tlatelulcum, meaning "pile of earth." This was dedicated to Saint James in name and deed. The other was Temehtitlan, or "place of the cactus that grew from a rock," which afterward would be called Mexico, or navel of the maguey, and to this day it enjoys this name among the Spanish. Entry to the city is by three roads on dry land; the rest is occupied by the lake. One road leads from west to east for two miles, another from north to south for five, and the third, finally, from south to north for two miles. The lake seems covered with barges floating from here to there to the city, bringing the necessaries of life to the neighboring and surrounding populations, which, counting only Mexicans, still come to more than 50,000. The two lakes are 100 miles long and 50 miles wide, but the circumference is 150.[21] Within it there are about fifty settlements, and in no small number of them, we know, 5,000 buildings have been counted, and in others actually more than 10,000. The part that is salty is abundant in niter and salt because it is the nature of the lake bed, not for the other inane reasons that some people dream up.

Mexico City about Fifty Years After It Was Taken

(1.22)

This city, rebuilt on the lake that we have said was the original foundation, is distant from the meridian of Toledo in longitude 97°45'; it has an elevation north of 19°30'

---

19. As Pimentel notes, *OC* 6:88, the word in the MS is *monoxylis*, a boat made from a single piece of wood, usually a hollowed-out tree trunk (a *linter*), as described by Pliny, *Natural History,* 6.26 105.

20. A crux. See Pimentel, *OC* 6:88, for the presumed sense of *prohibito* as prevention of movement.
21. Obviously wrong, but it is not clear what Hernández was calculating.

advancing four of our miles.[22] In great part it was ennobled by strong, large walls, worth being seen by the Spanish, besides other humble dwellings for the Indians, which are thought to number 20,000. The public streets measure 1,500 feet long and 50 wide. Very wide marketplaces, huge royal palaces, numerous temples, and monasteries, famous for their sanctity, doctrine, and their large numbers of men and women. The city abounds with hospitals, schools, and colleges. It is made greater also by the viceroy, the royal audiencia, the magistrates, the archbishop, the most skillful craftsmen, who can make anything, and cultivators of the fine arts and sciences—in short, all the greatness one could meet in the most prosperous cities of Spain. What can I say of the very extensive jurisdiction, of the most delightful gardens, of the crystalline sweet water springs, of the fertile wheat fields, of the abundance of livestock, and numerous types of fish, of metals, gold, silver, bronze, and also of the incredible salt gem that is a copy of all the other minerals, of the balminess of the pleasant climate in perpetual spring, of the quantity and variety of fruits and vegetables in every season of the year, of the beauty of the native women, of the elegance, celerity, and strength of the horses, and of very many other things that I judge will have to be passed over in silence, as much because to leave them out is safer than to say only a little about a very famous city, as that I do not want it thought that I describe the city as a friend, rather I depict it as an impartial judge or censor, on its own merits and in its natural colors.

The Climate of Mexico City

(1.23)

In my opinion Mexico City has a climate that is intermediate between cold and hot, but rather humid because it sits on a lake. During the winter the inhabitants have no need to light fires, nor are they bothered by the heat during the summer; and it is sufficient just to move into the sun if they feel cold, and if they feel too hot, even in the height of summer,

to move to the shade. In May the rains begin, and they last until September; the temperature in these months is about the same as ours in spring; thus virtually all the plants flower and bear fruit. The four following months tend to be cooler, then from February the warmth gradually increases as it does in summer. The air is to a large extent salubrious, but thanks to the humidity arising from the lake, which I have already mentioned briefly, rottenness sometimes predominates. The spots or exanthems that usually accompany fevers are peculiar to this city. The sheer strength of the patient can sometimes overcome them, provided there is a skillful and assiduous doctor in attendance. In addition, a pain in the side, which is truly serious in this region, kidney and bladder infections, dysentery and diarrhea are all fatal here. Foodstuffs are more moist and copious than pleasant to taste, even when they taste much like those that one is accustomed to. Fruits from here, indigenous like ours, are eaten practically the whole year round because they are so plentiful. For the sheer natural abundance of nature (nutrients, for I do not speak of gold, precious stones and silver) and the number of markets, there can hardly be any city on earth that rivals Mexico. What else? One could say that because of this exceptionally rich and fertile soil, there is never a dearth of anything; all sorts of things thrive and grow luxuriantly and fruitfully. Horses and homes, households and highways (all those words beginning with the same letter that have become proverbial in the Spanish language) are particularly beautiful.[23]

If you live in Mexico you can naturally become homesick, miss your native land and your own people, and if I may say so, miss the superior intelligence of the Spanish. The Indians are for the most part feeble, timid, and mendacious; they live from day to day, they are lazy, given to wine and drunkenness, and only lukewarm in their piety. May God help them! But they have a phlegmatic nature and are notable for their patience, which enables them to master even the most demanding of arts, which we do not even attempt, and to make exquisite copies of any work, without having to be

22. In the title of this section, "about Fifty Years After It Was Taken": meaning about 1574, when Hernández was writing this work, as Pimentel notes, *OC* 6.88, 133. Hernández mentions that year in book 2, chapter 13. Regarding "four of our miles": the meaning of the Latin is unclear.

23. Hernández wrote: "equi, domus, viae publicae ac infantes" [horses, houses, public streets and children], rendered by Pimentel as "los caballos, las casas, los caminos públicos, los caballeros." The MS shows that "feminae" had been in the author's thoughts, too. Like Pimentel, we know nothing of any relevant proverb.

taught. But plants do not have deep roots, nor is anyone's mind constant and strong, and the people who are born now and who in their turn begin to occupy these lands, are either of Spanish descent, or come from an ancestry of diverse races; if only they would obey Heaven, not degenerate until they adopt the customs of the Indians. But I digress.

Those emerging from any illness at all have difficulty recovering. In summer the rains begin, and in the calm time of the winds, mainly the northerlies, the country gains vigor. The richness of Indian wheat and of ours, of legumes and other cereals, is inexhaustible. It is amazing that in a distance of as little as three miles one encounters so many variations in temperature; here you freeze and there you boil, not because of the weather, but because of the topography of the valleys, where adequate, almost temperate air circulates. All of this means that these areas produce two harvests a year, nearly three, because at the time that one is extremely cold, another is predominantly hot, and in some other place spring temperatures softly caress people and other living beings, and it stays that way for quite some time, if the area is wet and balmy air keeps the heat off.

What shall I say of the wonderful natural properties of so many plants, animals, and minerals; of such different languages—Mexican, Tezcoquense, Otomi, Tlaxcalteco, Quexteco, Tarascan, Chichimeca, and so many others that can scarcely be listed and that vary within such short distances; of such variety of customs and rituals of the people, of the clothing they wear, the ways in which they decorate and ornament themselves, which human understanding is barely capable of grasping even when we have provided as much help as we can, so that, somehow, we can present some idea for those who are absent, when the true image can be understood only by those who are here and have the experience of seeing it and representing it for themselves.

Wonders of New Spain

(1.24)

It is astonishing that in the province of Yucatán a demon should be accustomed to conversing familiarly with any Spaniard, and to being present at his meetings, and that his voice really can be heard. In the same area you can see ruins of buildings that were constructed with wonderful skill; similar ones are found around Mitla, not far from the city of Oaxaca, and others not far from Cuernavaca, of which it is reported that they never stayed the same size, and that contact with anything, however small, caused them to move and shake, but now (so they say) they are immobile, because thanks to the ravages of time and the negligence of the Indians the stone that contained the secret of the power of this magic and miraculous structure is now lost. Innumerable human bones have also been found, not just in one place, but mainly close to Texcoco, of incredible size, together with jawbones five inches wide. There is a lake near Ocuila, not far from the country of Cuernavaca, inhabited only by fish known as axólotl,[24] and this lake always looks extremely clear because of the care of the many little birds at the water's edge: if anything foreign falls into it, the birds pick it up as quickly as possible and remove it. There is a stream near Cuernavaca that, even to the keenest sight, appears not to flow down but to rise to high ground. Also, in the open fields near Tuxtla, some cercopitheci, both small and large, have divided ⟨the territory⟩ among themselves in such a way that they do not cross the boundaries that they have made, nor do they enter any other fields. The sun frequently beats down in some places and yet others nearby it never touches. In Teccispan, not far from the country of Yautepec, a spring spontaneously gushes up above the height of four men, and thus repels everything; it pounds anything thrown into it, spits it out, swallows it, or devours it. And what shall I say about the many volcanoes found mainly in Nicaragua, Jalapa, and Los Angeles, where perpetual fires burn as they belch out terrible clouds of smoke, mixed with soot and ash? And what is more astonishing is that they are covered with snow all year round, and that intense cold up there battles incessantly with ardent heat, and that when they erupt sometimes, they throw up a fantastic quantity of black, liquid pumice and ashes. They have destroyed and smothered neighboring towns. The land shakes all around and sucks men in through the cracks, and even the widest rivers, which

---

24. Not in fact a fish but an amphibian, described below, in T 9.4.

have been there for three or four days before being thrown into confusion, but the towns and their inhabitants have been destroyed in their entirety.

There is a mountain near Tlapa, whose slopes, on contact with the feet of just one man, quiver way off into the distance. When leaves and a few other things fall into certain rivers, they petrify immediately. There are some springs that give water in summer but dry up in winter. The spring at Huastepec, with the sweetest and most healthful water, and which from its source widens into a considerable river, after only a short distance becomes contaminated and is polluted with sulfurous water that is unfit to drink. Further springs, sweet and brackish, hot and cold, turn up at regular intervals. What shall I say of the many differences in salt found condensed in these regions, and of the waters that ferment and boil at the very source, of springs that dry up during the rains and afterward pour out masses of water, of others that gush underwater, and whose lymph, mixed with clean water, tastes very sweet? Others that gush here and there can cook meat and melt iron; they have the power to lift enormous stones; one group of men, most of them hunchbacked, crossed the Conchas river. There are many other things like these, which if I had more leisure time on my hands (for now in truth I am writing hurriedly), would be described more fully: as for the many marvels that pertain to plants, animals, and metals, they are described with the greatest care and precision of which I am capable, in my *Natural History*.

The Nature, Customs, and Clothing of the Mexicans

(1.25)

They are of medium stature, reddish skin, large eyes, broad forehead, very open nostrils, smooth necks, but this is due to the efforts of the fathers; they have black, oily hair that is soft and long and grows on parts of the body that are usually covered by skin, but otherwise they are not very hairy or may be completely hairless. The few of them who are born blond are considered monstrous, as are those who are frequently born among the Spanish. They paint their bod-

ies with different colors, mainly when they are going to fight or take part in the dance, in which case they also cover their arms, head, and thighs with feathers, fish scales, wild animal skins, skins of tigers [sic] or similar quadrupeds, or birds. They pierce their ears and noses, chins and lips, encrusting the body with gems, gold, or silver, or with the talons and beaks of eagles, the teeth of animals, or the bones of large fish. The men, and the rich, wear all these things, or precious stones, or gold, but still imitating the various forms above mentioned, which they consider will terrify their enemies while making themselves seem more fierce. They wear sandals to protect the soles of their feet. They cover the genitals and anus with a loincloth, and otherwise go naked, except for a piece of linen like our cape, draped over the right shoulder, the other one remaining bare, not unlike the women we call gypsies who roam through Spain. It is customary for the richest, on festival days, to cover themselves with numerous layers of colored cloth, while going virtually naked the rest of the year. As we have said, the men marry at age twenty, but in Pánuco they remain celibate until their forties. It is permitted to divorce women, but not without a legitimate reason. The men are so terribly jealous that they are always beating their wives. They go unarmed, unless they are preparing for war, and so those who have suffered some injury are permitted to provoke their rivals. The Chichimeca do not admit foreign merchants, but the rest, for the most part, do business with them. They are dreadful liars and cheats, and for this reason their transactions are conducted in cash for imports, and for like goods, payment is in kind. They do not easily endure hunger or labor, despite the fact that in other parts they live on nothing but corn tortillas and chilis. They are gentle and extremely tolerant, which is why they are so outstanding in many arts, as I have said, even if they lack teaching. They flatter submissively, and obey when they are obliged by force or fear to do so. They obey above all their kings and lords, which appears to produce pusillanimity. They are highly religious, but they kill and eat men. They are given to luxury particular to men, and they are not ashamed of their prodigious lust, nor do they punish so great a crime. They have faith in auguries and sorcery, and believe that the future can be known, so they venerate fortune-tellers, those people who believe they can question what must remain in doubt, when there is nobody other than the supreme God who can give a certain and true judgment of the future. The married women emulate freely the fashion and appearance of their husbands. They do not wear shoes; in fact they content themselves with underskirts and skirts alone.[25] They let their hair grow long; some dye their hair darker with a certain type of mud, to make themselves more beautiful and to kill some persistent creatures that hatch on the scalp, which they sometimes, disgustingly, eat. Married women gather their hair at the back of the head and tie it with a knot at the front; but virgins and spinsters wear their hair loose at the back and the front. It is said that they use as a medication, to pull their hair out by the roots, mostly the very longest, and to stop it from growing back, the oiled dung of ants, as I have heard, but they leave their eyelashes and eyebrows alone. They consider it beautiful to have a small forehead covered with hair, and almost no neck, which, so that they can carry a load, they flatten at birth, because then the skull is very tender, and this shape can be retained by newborns lying in their cradles.—They get married when they are only ten years old, and have a great inclination toward luxury. They have children when they are still at a tender age, and they try to have very large, pendulous breasts, to ensure that their babies can feed easily most of the time. They bathe, and wash their faces, believing that thus they achieve beauty and grace. This they do with the milk of the *teconzapotl* seed, which the Haitians call "mamey," and which they also use to repel mosquitoes, with which many of the peoples of New Spain are cruelly plagued. They treat themselves with herbs, and not entirely without cursing and begging for the assistance of demons, so that it sometimes happens that they secretly abort. For the rest they have strong heads, perhaps because they are always out in the open and they wash often in cold water, indeed during a hot bath, which to other people would be dangerous. They are not given to working unless obliged and compelled to do so; occasionally they take part in dances, but only if the

king orders it or religion demands it. They do not have any liking for wine, and as is the case with many other nations, they are more temperate than the men. With one hand they hold the cotton, with the other the bobbin, which, resting on the rim of a small vase with a little curved piece cut out, can then be spun with great industry and speed; they rub three fingers on the right hand frequently with powdered *cicatl,* which smoothes out the threads of cotton, with which they sew and weave mantles, as well as many other kinds of clothes.

Markets

(1.27)

Every neighborhood has an open space where, every five days (or more frequently), markets are held, called tianguis, not just in Mexico City but also in other cities and pueblos in New Spain. Of the Mexican ones, the market of Tlatelolco is the largest, with a capacity of nearly 60,000 people, and then that of Tenochtitlán. In these two almost never does a day go by without a throng of men and women gathering to buy and sell various things. Merchants of both sexes set up in their own assigned places, which no one else may occupy; in addition to these enormous markets (such is the multitude of the native population that gathers in them), the public streets nearby are brimming over with goods: there you find firewood, charcoal, and red clay pots that are every bit as elegant as anything produced by our people. There are hides of deer and other animals, dried and treated, with or without hair, and dyed with a variety of colors. From these they make sandals, bucklers, shields, breeches, cuirasses, and sheaths for wooden weapons. Also, there are skins of all kinds of birds, softened and filled with herbs; various kinds of salt, and cotton cloth of different colors, from which they make bedspreads, cloaks, loincloths, rugs, napkins, tablecloths, chemises, shifts, skirts, and many other things of this kind. They also sell linens woven from the leaves of palm, gladiolus, and maguey, and from feathers and rabbit skins. They weave with white

---

25. Hernández left *nahoas* and *cueitl,* which we render as underskirts and skirts, in Náhuatl in MS.

and colored cotton thread. Also, they have species of edible birds, whose feathers are used for clothing, and whose wings are used by bird hunters, and all for dancing and dances known as nitoteliztli. Those worth seeing most are made of wood, feathers, and gold, which Indian craftsmen use to make all the most elegant, distinguished images. They are extremely skillful in these arts, and most patient in this type of work. Also displayed and sold in the markets are marvelous pieces made from silver, or engraved in metals, or cast in bronze; hexagonal plates that have three parts in gold alternating with three of silver, attached to one another but not stuck on in any way, but cast, strengthened, and soldered in one fusion; amphorae in bronze with unattached handles; fish with alternating gold and silver scales; parrots with moving tongues, heads, and wings; monkeys with prehensile hands and feet that make a bobbin turn as if they were spinning, and others holding an apple or some other fruit that they seem to be eating. Our craftsmen could not emulate any of this, but they should offer great admiration for such notable workmanship. Nor for that matter are they inferior to Spanish craftsmen in setting, carving, or drilling precious stones. They sell, then, feathers, gold, silver, refined minerals recommended for curing different kinds of illness, tin, lead, brass, pearls, and a thousand kinds of shell that at one time were preferred as a considerable dowry and to adorn and lend dignity to attire, but that now are little appreciated and considered valueless. And very many other things, extremely diverse, and at times also really insignificant and unimportant, according to what fashion dictates, since in truth such is the genius of people and so disposed are they by Nature that what some esteem highly is by others scorned and dismissed. And what shall I say of the herbs, leaves, flowers, roots, and seeds that are used in medicine and food and that are still found in the fields by people who, impelled by the seriousness of illness and hunger, do not pay doctors for them? And what of those ointments that are put up for sale much like our perfumes, or of things called syrups, distilled liquors, and of so many compound medicines (despite the fact that they mostly use simple medicines); of such medicinal plants as they know and offer for sale, also suitable for killing and repelling bedbugs, lice, fleas, mosquitoes, and flies? And from what

things do they not extract food in order to sell it? It is a rare animal that their palates spare: even to the point where they will use the most poisonous snakes for food, after they have cut off their heads and tails; dogs, moles, dormice, worms, lice [sic], mice, lake moss, and although I would rather not have to say this, lake mud, as well as other things of the animal and plant orders that are horrible and disgusting. They sell there, besides, deer cut up or whole, sheep cooked in water, the meat of oxen, rabbits, hare, moles, dogs and cuzatli of the species of weasels; which they catch, raise, and fatten at their homes and finally, eager for gain, they bring to market to sell. There are so many taverns in which the townspeople consume and devour an amazing quantity of meat, when in addition there is such an abundance of fish, both raw and cooked, of corn cakes, and corn tortillas; so many eggs from different kinds of birds; great quantities of corn, cooked, uncooked, and on the cob; the same goes for roots, beans, kidney beans, and vegetables. For sale there are innumerable types of fruit, both indigenous and from Spain, dried and fresh, and what is valued above all the rest is cacao, which will be discussed at greater length among the plants. What shall I say of the various different dyes, unknown to us, which they make from flowers, fruits, roots, leaves, bark, stones, wood, and other materials that it would be too tiresome to list in detail? Also much honey, be it the kind that requires the industry of bees or that which is prepared by human hand, from the sap of sugarcane, corn, maguey, and other trees and fruits. They also sell oil from chia, which protects statues of the gods from damage caused by rain and bad weather, and is used as a flavoring, though it is more common to use butter, lard, grease, and fat in preparing food. They also sell torches and spatulas of [a stone called] iztle. Who does not know the different kinds of wine they blend, which will be discussed in their place? It cannot be said how many and how various things are put up for sale, how many craftsmen are present, how many people throng the market places, with how much care and attention the Mexican governors and Tlatelulco officials, their assistants and ministers deal with everything they think needs to be regulated. Omitting nothing, we have resolved to place all this before the reader as an image of those things that are found in the markets.

Things Familiar in Europe That the Mexicans Lacked Until the Spanish Conquered Them

(1.28)

They had no system of weights and measures. They did not have metal money, instead bartering or using cacao seeds. They also knew nothing of the use of iron, in whose place they used wood, stone, or sometimes bronze. They also lacked candles and used torches instead of lamps. Their boats, except their canoes, were all made from hollowed-out wood like long skiffs. They did not have our wine, although they did have many other kinds that taste very good but go straight to the head. They also had no horses or donkeys. As for writing, all they had were those images of things that the Greeks call hieroglyphs, but with these they could express abstract ideas. They had almost no idea of any kind of decency, comfortable clothes, shoes, underwear, caps, tunics, or anything else that covers the body except for their mantles, which not even everyone was permitted to wear. They had no airborne steel weapons, defensive weapons, shields, knives, machines of war, doors, windows, meat of oxen, sheep or our goats, wild boar, pork, and virtually none of our fruits and vegetables. They had little in the way of just laws, or statutes for the good governance and regulation of the republic, nor most of the necessary arts. Most lamentable of all, they knew nothing of the worship of the true God and the doctrine and practices of the true religion, nor anything else that must be considered essential for the happy and innocent life of the soul and the body. That these things were lacking is not because the region was hostile to all good things (in my judgment), as I have found from experience, but because of the idleness of these people who, so many centuries after the creation of the world, have remained in such simplicity.

Knowledge of the Heavens and Heavenly Bodies, as well as Meteorological Phenomena and Celestial Omens

(2.1)

It is rumored that they have discovered the multiplicity of the heavens, but they know next to nothing about the sun, the moon, Orion, Venus, the Great Bear and the Little Bear, and other stars in which they believe divinity resided—that is, with the exception of a few common observations and some old wives' tales, and so, ignorant of the causes of things, they wretchedly revere eclipses and meteors and anything else like that, while at the same time they are terrified by them. But they took meteors and phenomena generated in the heavens, such as lightning, comets, shooting stars, fiery whirlwinds, meteors, pillars of fire, snow, clouds, frost, winds, and similar things to be omens. Thus they believed that white clouds on a mountaintop presaged hail, and dense clouds indicated rain. Frost falling like drizzle presaged a good crop for the year. The rainbow meant calm and the very end of the rains, and the twinkling of the stars, the fortunes of kings and queens.

The Doctors Called Titici

(2.2)

Among the Indians, men and women alike practice medicine and are called *Titici*. These do not study the nature of illnesses and the differences between them. Instead, without knowing the cause or accident of an illness, they are accustomed to prescribe medicines, but without recourse to method in the treatment of the illnesses that they must cure. They are merely empirical healers and use, for any illness whatsoever, only those herbs, minerals or animal parts that they have received, passed from hand to hand, as a birthright from their elders, and this they also teach to those who follow.

Practically all that they do is to prescribe a diet for their patients. They never cut anyone's veins, not even when, through an incision in the skin, they take out blood and burn the body. Wounds are treated with simple medicines or by covering them with their flours; with these things they are usually helped, but only rarely are compound or mixed medicines used. There are no surgeons or pharmacists among the titici, but rather only physicians, who by themselves dispense all manners of treatment. And it is amazing how ineptly and artlessly they do so, and how dangerous this is for the people. For not only do they oblige recently delivered women to take steam baths, they also instruct them to bathe themselves and their newborn children in icy water after these baths, which they call temax-cálli. But what am I saying? They sprinkle icy water even upon those who have fevers with eruptions and other types of outbreaks. Such actions are no less imprudent than when they rub their patients' bodies with very hot things, replying haughtily to anyone who would question them that heat is defeated by heat. They use extremely strong and even poisonous pharmaceutical remedies, without controlling or countering them with any kind of preparation. They do not examine sick people right away, nor usually before they have been given medicines that dissolve a humor or are purgative. Neither do they know how to adapt a remedy to a humor that has to be removed. For that matter, they never talk of a crisis, nor of required rest. They do permit, naturally, young women who have just given birth to use cold and astringent medicines, to strengthen the kidneys, they say, when it would be better to open the uterine tracts to provoke the terms. With the same things they cure fleshy growths of the eyes, as well as the French disease, and stiffness caused by lack of humor in the joints, not entirely unsuccessful in this last case, perhaps owing to dryness. And it even happens that they apply very hot medicines to inflammations of the eyes and also, to a great extent and quite contrary to nature, to swellings; and they indiscriminately use cold, glutinous, or astringent medicines without taking any account of how long an illness has lasted or which part is affected. And thus, even when they have a marvelous array of healthful herbs to choose from, they do not know how to use them properly, nor exploit their real value.

The Mexican System of Writing, Numeration, and the Calendar

(2.20)

Like the Egyptians, they use glyphs instead of letters for the things they want to represent, and they paint them on paper prepared from the pulp of various trees, as we have shown elsewhere. They carve them also on stone, bronze, leather, and walls, and they weave them into their garments. The volumes of their writings were folded one on top of another and doubled over like clothes, but very few are extant today. They do not pronounce some of our letters, which we use all the time in speech and writing. These are B, D, F, G, H, R, S and L, but this applies only to speech. I refer only to the Mexican language, for there are others in New Spain subject to different rules, which I may describe if I ever have enough time. In truth there is hardly any province that does not have its own particular language, even if it is just a short distance from the others. Of all of them, however, the dominant and most common language of communication among the people of New Spain is Mexican, in which—here I leave it to grammarians of this language to teach it—we encounter different ways of counting months, years, and so on; an elegant and rich vocabulary unsurpassed even by Greek; common verbal inflections do not employ just one mode for both genders, like Hebrew, and names of holy days, months, and years. It seems amazing that among such uncultivated and barbarous people, one scarcely comes across one word that does not have a considered significance and etymology, for almost all their words have been adapted to things with such precision and care, that the name alone is enough to indicate the nature of any important thing.

INDEX MEDICAMENTORUM

Hernández compiled an index of native remedies in use in New Spain. The index is organized in the classical Theophrastan manner, by parts of the body, beginning with the head and moving down. There are four texts of the index: that of Juan Barrios, in Spanish, printed in *Verdadera medicina, cirugía y astrología* (Mexico City, 1607); that of Archivio Segreto Vaticano, MS Riti 1716, also in Spanish but significantly divergent from Barrios; one found in Madrid, Universidad Complutense, Facultad de Medicina, MS 6.151 Her; and the index to the Rome edition, which reduces the text to a table of page references, specific to the printed edition, which is therefore omitted here.

Wherever possible, we provide cross references to the plants, animals, and minerals mentioned in this index. Some plants exist in so many varieties that identification is impossible, and some of the Náhuatl names are garbled beyond recognition.

Juan Barrios, *Verdadera medicina, cirugía y astrología* (Mexico City, 1607)

For headaches from a hot cause

Dissolve the leaves of the quilamolli[1] in water. Also put the leaves and the fruit of the tomato in water and rub these, or those of the cozolmécatl[2] on the forehead. One can also use the spines of the hoitztlacuatzin.[3]

For migraines or chronic headaches

Put the dissolved leaves of the tzocuilpatli[4] plant in water along with the leaves and fruit of the tlameme. Rub these with the juice of the former, or of the yyauhtli[5] or the leaves of the cozolmécatl[6] or the spines of the tlaquatzin,[7] which are placed on the forehead. In order to purge the head, take the vapor of the texaxapotla[8] through the nose or take the

---

1. *T* 8.26.
2. *T* 6.57.
3. Spiny possum.
4. *QL* 2.2.2.

5. Mountain yyauhtli is described in *QL* 2.1.41.
6. *T* 6.57.
7. Spiny possum.
8. *T* 2.3.

amount of two reales of the ixpatli root,[9] or take the juice of the quauhíyac[10] through the nostrils. The juice of the tlalcuitlaxcolli[11] or thetlalcuitlaxocilli may also be taken.

For sleep

The resin of the xochiocotzoquáhuitl[12] should be placed on the nostrils, or the leaves of the tlápatl[13] or its fruit should be placed on the head or the leaves of the cozolmécatl[14] should placed on the pillow. One can also use the leaves of the picietl.[15] The juice of this plant can be taken through the nostrils or in the form of a drink made from the root of the pinahuizxuchitl, as well as that of the pinahuiztli.[16]

For heart problems or epilepsy

Take one ounce of tecopalquáhuitl,[17] or one ounce of xiuhnanhuapatli, which are two species. The first is to be drunk, the other, which is of a whitish color, should be taken with one real of water or with the root of tlalzamecaxóchitl,[18] or by eating half an ounce of acaxaxan[19] or the juice, or a decoction of the above-mentioned. One can also inhale the vapor of burned hoactzin[20]—the smoke from the burning of its feathers—or use a bezoar stone[21] weighing six grains, or a decoction of *borjas* or of melissa[22] or one real of the dung of the tzopílotl.[23]

For a runny nose

Tecomahaca[24] is placed on the corners of the mouth in the form of a plaster. One can also use pitzáhoac tlacopatli. One makes a rosary of this root and places it around the neck, and also uses the juice and oil of the bulbs, or the root, of the cuentictlanelhuatl,[25] which are eaten or placed on the head, or the root of the quauhmecapatli,[26] which is cooked and the broth drunk. One can also use a decoction of the holcuatzan[27] or drink a broth made from this substance as well as the broth of the quauhtlepatli,[28] which is drunk for fifteen days or by breathing the vapors of picietl leaves.[29]

For easing the mind

The tecomahaca[30] is placed on the head in the form of a plaster, or one can eat the root of the tomahuac tlacopatli,[31] or take the juice of its bulbs, cooked very well, or take the juice of picietl[32] through the nostrils.

For headaches with a cold cause

Take the vapor or smell the burning leaves of the texaxapotla[33] plant, or the leaves of the tzocuilpátli plant[34] or the gum of the copal tree, or take in the aromatic herbs of the roots or branches, or eat some of the yyauhtli plant,[35] or take the weight of a real of nahoitéputz root,[36] or the gum of the xochiocotzoquahuitl,[37] which is placed on the corner of the mouth, or drink two reales of the root of yxpatli[38] or eat the mashed fruit of huitzxuchitl[39] and place it in the nostrils or place the pounded leaves of the ecapatli[40] on the head.

---

9. Not described separately, but mentioned in the chapter on nahoitéputz (*T* 6.12).

10. *QL* 1.2.34.

11. *T* 8.67.

12. Liquidambar styraciflua (M 3.57).

13. *QL* 3.2.28.

14. *T* 6.57.

15. Tobacco (see "Five Special Texts," below).

16. Pinahuihuitztli is said to have the same property (LMS 7.32).

17. Incense tree.

18. *T* 7.6.

19. M 1.106

20. A bird with a call that sounds like its name (Animals 2.50).

21. Described in the chapter on the mazame, *T* 9.14.

22. *Melissa officinalis* L., also called apiastrum, because bees are attracted to it.

23. A bird also known as aura (Animals 2.112).

24. *QL* 1.2.16.

25. Coen (or coentic); Lovell (see "Seven English Authors," in "England, 1659-1825," below.

26. *QL* 3.2.43.

27. Perhaps olcacatzan, an alternative name for cozolmécatl.

28. One of the oleanders, several of which Hernández described. Most likely *QL* 1.3.29.

29. Tobacco (see "Five Special Texts," below).

30. *QL* 1.2.16.

31. Sloane (see "Seven English Authors," in "England, 1659-1825," below).

32. Tobacco (see "Five Special Texts," below).

33. *T* 2.3.

34. *QL* 2.2.2.

35. See *QL* 2.1.41 (mountain yyauhtli).

36. *T* 6.12.

37. Liquidambar.

38. One ixpatli (medicine for the eyes, however) is described in *T* 6.26.

39. Lovell (see "Seven English Authors").

40. Hernández described seven varieties of ecapatli, none of them said to cure headaches.

Archivio Segreto Vaticano, MS Riti 1716

For bad condition of the body and cachexia

Root of acxoyátic[41] drunk in suitable liquid six oboli after fasting, or petals of cempoalxochitl[42] drunk in water, and in wine, or root of nahoitéputz[43] weight of one dram, drunk, or decoction of the root of phehuame,[44] drunk. Or powder of tlalquequétzal[45] drunk. Or decoction of tragorígano[46] drunk, or decoction of root of quauhmécatl[47] drunk.

Intestines, colic, and pain in the liver

Decoction of ahoapatli[48] in clyster, or root of chichimecap-atli[49] drunk, or root of coayelli[50] ground and drunk, three drams to ten ounces of water. Or, mecaxóchitl[51] drunk with cacáoatl, or, decoction of tlaltochitl[52] drunk. Or decoction of root of tepatli[53] drunk. Or root of tzahuéngueni[54] drunk two drams. Or, root of acocotli[55] drunk one ounce. Or, decoction of leaves of acueyo[56] drunk, or, made into a clyster; or, coaquíltic[57] drunk, or, root of coapatli drunk in water half an ounce; or, gum of holquáhuitl[58] applied to the anus, or rub balsam on the place where it hurts and lick there three or four drops in the hand. Or, decoction of the root and wood of sassafras[59] drunk, and applied in a clyster; or, root of tzonpantli[60] drunk, or seed of zacachíchic[61] infused, in a clyster. Or, root of axixtlácotl[62] taken, two drams, or ancoas[63] blended and rubbed with coconut oil and applied to the part; or axoaitl drunk. Or, leaves of chichicpatli[64] pounded and drunk in water one handful. Or, root of yellow tomato[65] mixed with *siliquastro,*[66] or, two drams of that drunk, or its hot decoction. Or, root of cuitlázotl[67] drunk one ounce; or, infusion of the trunk of coatli[68] cut in rings and soaked in water, this infusion to be drunk. Or, root of the spiny tomato[69] applied in a clyster, or, root of coanenepilli[70] drunk three ounces. Or, leaves of cozolmécatl drunk in wine. Or, decoction of huacuica made in a clyster made from oil in which the leaves of picietl[71] have been infused; or, seed and roots of tlacochichi[72] taken in water one ounce. Or, rub the part with grease of axin;[73] or, a possum's tail ground and drunk in appropriate liquor one dram. Or a dark emerald[74] carried in the arm, or applied to the part that hurts. Or, the stones[75] tlalayotic and quetzalitztli attached to the wrist, or placed on the part that hurts.

Lientery, or belly flux

Bark of quauhíyac drunk.[76] Or, outside bark of coconut drunk, or yyauhtli[77] drunk. Or, tzontollin[78] its root drunk, or, root of tlalcacáhotl[79] drunk one ounce; or leaves of cacapolton[80] drunk; or root of tlaelpatli half an ounce drunk.

---

41. N 15.40.
42. LMS 3.69.
43. T 6.12.
44. T 5.36.
45. Lovell (see "Seven English Authors").
46. QL 2.2.24.
47. N 15.43.
48. T 5.1.
49. LMS 3.21.
50. Sloane (see "Seven English Authors," in "England, 1659–1825," below).
51. Stubbe (see "Seven English Authors," in "England, 1659–1825," below).
52. Tlilxóchitl (vanilla)?
53. Hernández described what may be this plant. He inadvertently repeated his description near the end of his manuscript.
54. QL 3.2.67.
55. M 1.25.
56. LMS 3.5.
57. T 6.9.
58. N 15.29.
59. QL 1.2.27.
60. Also known as mazaixtli, under which name Hernández described it.
61. QL 2.2.29.
62. N 15.38.
63. OC 3.200
64. T 2.18.
65. "Five Special Texts," below.
66. Presumably *Capsicum annuum* L.
67. QL 2.1.17.
68. Probably 21.30
69. "Five Special Texts," below.
70. T 8.58
71. Tobacco, "Five Special Texts," below.
72. M 4.93.
73. T 9.5.
74. T 10.7.
75. These are plants, not stones.
76. In title of this section, "Lientery, or belly flux": that is, lienteric diarrhea, characterized by the passage of undigested food. "Quauhíyac": QL 1.2.39.
77. QL 2.1.41.
78. LMS 3.16
79. The small peanut, M 6.93.
80. QL 1.2.36.

For difficulty in childbirth

Apply to the mother's aperture suppositories soaked in balsam, or made from this liquor; or, decoction of root of phehuame drunk. Or, powder of tlalquequétzal or its decoction drunk. Or, pods of vanilla given to drink with mecáxochitl; or bezoar stone drunk, seven grains. Or, possum's tail ground and drunk, one dram with water of pond cilantro.

To restore wounded flesh

Powder of leaves of cozolmécatl[81] scattered within [the wound].

Against spells

Root of coanenepilli[82] drunk; or, root of zocobut[83] drunk. Or, stone iztehuílotl[84] carried about one's person.

To stop hair falling out

Root of acxoyátic[85] six oboli drunk.

To find out if the sick patient will recover

Root of zozoyátic[86] ground and placed in the nostrils, if the sick person sneezes it is a sign of health, if not, the contrary.

---

81. *T* 6.57.
82. *T* 8.58.
83. *T* 7.57.
84. A crystalline stone.
85. N 15.40.
86. M 6.24

ON THE ILLNESS IN NEW SPAIN IN THE YEAR 1576, CALLED COCOLIZTLI BY THE INDIANS

Another brief text, Hernandez's description of the dreadful disease that swept through parts of New Spain in 1576 may have been only a prologue or a summary of a longer work, now lost. That, at least, is the hypothesis put forward by Somolinos in his introduction to the Spanish translation, *OC* 6:475–80. The Latin text is in Hac. MS 931, fols. 50–51. This text was neglected until Muñoz "discovered" it in the 1780s, but even then it was not published, because Gómez Ortega intended to put it in the fifth volume of the Madrid edition of Hernández's *Opera*.

On the Illness in New Spain in the Year 1576, Called Cocoliztli by the Indians

The fevers were contagious, burning, and continuous, entirely pestilential, and in a great many cases, lethal. The tongue dried out and turned black. Intense thirst, sea-green urine, or vegetable green and black, but from time to time the color would change from deep green to pale. Frequent and rapid pulse, but faint and weak, sometimes almost none. The eyes, and the whole body, yellow. Delirium and convulsion were reported. Behind one or both ears a hard, painful swelling appeared, accompanied by pain in the heart, chest, and stomach, shivering, distress, and dysentery; the blood, obtained by venesection, was green or very pale, dry, and completely lacking any serosity. In some people, gangrene invaded the lips, the pudenda, and other putrefied parts of the body, and blood ran from the ears; in many cases blood ran from the nose as well. Almost nobody who suffered a relapse could be saved. Many who suffered nosebleeds (provided the bleeding could be stopped) were saved, but the rest died. Those suffering from attacks of dysentery (if it happened that they were treated by medication) for the most part were normally saved, and even the abscesses behind the ears were not fatal, if they went down a bit, except when they grew spontaneously, or were drained by cauterizing with needles, and even in immature abscesses the liquid part of the blood flowed out, or the pus was eliminated, which meant also that the cause of the illness was eliminated. Furthermore, the urine of some was both profuse and pale, autopsies showed that the dead had very swollen liver, blackened heart emitting a pale yellow liquid and later, black blood, black and semiputrefied spleen and lungs; atrabiliousness could be seen in their blood vessels, the dry stomach and the rest of the body, wherever it was dissected, was extremely pale. The principal victims of this epidemic were the young, and occasionally the old, who despite being infected with it, frequently managed to overcome it and were saved. This plague began in the month of June 1576, and was still not over in January, when we wrote this description. From New Spain it invaded all the cold regions in a circle of about 400 miles, and was somewhat easier on the warmer regions (that is, it attacked rather less) infecting different areas in turn, beginning with those occupied by Indian tribes, then places where Indians and Africans lived, then those with a mixed population of Indian and Spanish, and later still, those areas occupied by Africans, and now finally it is attacking the Spanish. The weather was dry and calm, though rocked by earthquakes; the air, impure, full of clouds, which did not produce any rainfall, but provided a real breeding ground for rotting and corruption. The Indians were great lovers of wine, and indiscriminately ingested chili and corn—which generated profuse bile, blood—as well as other substances, not just bad, coarse juices, but also the most sordid food. A few were saved whose stomachs appeared very distended. In the beginning, in a few cases, blood was lost without extremely serious illness, but then, for a very few, it rapidly extinguished vital energy. Gentler medication was prescribed, such as that obtained from the drumstick tree,[1] or if the ingredients were unavailable, one ounce of totoycxitl, a half ounce or up to two of cacamotic, a measure of two drams of the powdered root of coanenepilli, which in addition to gently purging bilious and atrabilious humors, provokes urine and counteracts the toxin, and later actually theriaca magna, with which drink numerous people were miracu-

lously saved. But if the illness persisted, dissolving unguents were the next recourse, rubbed over the whole ventral area; the patient would drink barley broth, the pith of cultivated celeriac, the root of coanenepilli, and fennel seeds, and from time to time cococtlacotl chipaoac and atochietl would be used as well, which we have described in more detail in our history of the plants of New Spain, in order to open all the orifices through which the poison, which was also evacuated by the urine, could be expelled. Those unnatural swellings—even the immature ones—behind the ears could be stopped with an application of a red-hot iron, and the pus that flowed from the ears was cleaned up with cotton and rose honey. We provided a great help against the affliction of dysentery, not just relying on the current popular medicines, but also the juice of sour pomegranates with rose flower water, rose honey dashed with plantain, alum, and the so-called Egyptian ointment; all these ingredients were mixed together over the fire, and introduced into the patient's bowels by means of a tube once a day, ten or more times. Soothing poultices were applied to the heart, the air was perfumed, and bitter cabbage added to food to expel decayed matter. Some set great store by cooked atochietl, or the root of a plant known as quauhayoachtli, both of which plants we describe in our history. Others used chopped chilis with the so-called atole; there was no shortage of people who to the great detriment of the sufferers washed their bodies with cold water and rubbed their foreheads with the juice of cooked coatli, also giving them the juice of iztacpatli to drink; finally, almost nobody, with such a shortage of remedies and a lack of doctors, not to mention even a lack of food, stopped trying anything that came to hand. But for our part the medications that we have said were most useful, we tried to test by proper experiment and administered them with the result of enormous improvement in health and the happiest outcome. We made this clear to others, so that they in turn could apply these remedies against this most terrible of plagues.

---

1. The text adds that the purgative was known as diaprunis simple or (in Spanish) *diacatólicon*. This was normally made with tamarind, rhubarb roots, and senna.

THE CHRISTIAN DOCTRINE

Hernández's 1,791-line Latin poem on Christian doctrine (Hac. MS 931, fols. 58r–86r) has been almost entirely neglected, along with most of the other writings preserved in the same manuscript volume. The poem is essentially a missionary document, but we have little idea about its actual use, if any, in Mexico. It is a tool for converting Mexican adults to the Catholic faith, but it combines conventional Christian concepts with images that could be expected to resonate with an audience familiar with Aztec symbols. Nevertheless, Hernández does not opt for much symbolic or metaphorical language. In manuscript the poem is preceded by a proem written by Pedro Moya de Contreras, archbishop of Mexico, and a personal friend of Hernández. Moya de Contreras added a few marginal notes, mostly summary headings, to the first few pages of the poem. Hernández addressed an epigram to him, too (BN MS 22,438, fol. 172). The proem, notes, and epigram are omitted here.

After a thirty-four-line prologue, *The Christian Doctrine* is organized in three unequal parts: (1) the articles of faith; (2) the seven sacraments; and (3) the Ten Commandments, which are followed by a rendering of the Lord's Prayer to conclude the poem. In our translation of the poem (after the prologue) we have attempted to render Hernández's verse in iambic pentameter, for although this was not the form he used, it is a form more suited to English verse. We have left the poem lightly annotated on points of theology. Elías Trabulse's intelligent introductory commentary on the text, in *OC* 6:409–26, is the only published treatment in existence, as far as we know.

The Christian Doctrine

Book 1: The Articles of Faith

Whoever prepares to follow that road
Which winds between perilous rocks,
On straitened paths to the airy abode
Where splendid choirs angelic dwell;
5   Whoever seeks to unite with the saints,
And merit a seat upon high,
With them to praise God in eternal delight
And reflect on the illustrious figures,
The radiant Family enthroned apart;
10 Desiring so, hear they this song,
Born of this humble rhapsodical heart,
Which unlocks the secrets of love.
In this verse is nought that glitters or shines:
Plain words must address the devout;
15 How to live, and how armed, in these lines
I sing, and our duty inspire,
What to seek, what they have whose hearts are filled
With love of Christ, who bear with cheer
The burdens, torments, trials of this life,
20 Knowing ascent draws ever near.

O Thou, Supreme Wisdom, Omnipotent
Creator of all that lives in this orb,
Vast sphere which you embosom! The blessed
He who sits at your right hand, may He
25 Bless this endeavor, that those by the Lamb's
Precious blood redeemed, wrested by his grace
From hell's dread jaws may rise to dwell at last,
Bless'd in th' ineffable sublime of Heaven,
For ever to adore the radiant light,
30 The prime work of God, Jesus Christ Our Lord.

I here set down what Christians must believe
With resolute will and with ready mind:
In the beginning there was but one God,
Father at once of existence entire,
35 Who was pleased to make all things from the void,
And all to encircle in one vast sphere:
By his grace and omnipotent virtue
All beings are nourished, restored, conserved,
For his mercy grants to each living thing
40 Its birth and death and time upon the earth.
To God we must reach out with all the soul,
With all our senses and capacities,

So at our end we may become as one
With good supreme and ineffable beauty.
45 It is not sufficient within us to bear
The true light. Our duty demands that we
Show it to the world without petty fear
Of mundane taunt. And should the raging tyrant
Ever threaten death, torture, and the rack,
50 Do not quaver! The saints call out to you,
Await you in the golden great beyond.
The true splendor of this heavenly faith
Illuminates the path we mortals tread
To arrive at our true home; and holy
55 Mother Church defines it and engraves it
In the soul, for all that God reveals is
Revealed to her, from his exalted height.
Though God is one in simplest purity,
Yet you must believe that in him he has
60 Three distinct persons, even in his one
Indivisible divine essence; that
These are the persons of Father and Son
And Holy Spirit, equally imbued
With wisdom consummate and infinite power.
65 Although these three are the one Lord our God,
Each one is intimately different:
For the Father was of no other born;
The Son proceeds from the Father, begotten
By him; whence the Holy Spirit emanates,
70 Clasping them round in passionate embrace.
That in the beginning, before the start
Of time, this divine process was so, teach
The sainted fathers, and holy scripture's
Text affirms, as they explain the triune
75 God's one essence. And thus, although the Son
And Holy Spirit are, like the Father,
Omnipotent, yet the power and the force
Proceed from him, who is the fathomless
Eternal fount of goodness to the Spirit,
80 And infinite sapience to the Son.
The father is all powerful and wise,
Lord of all the heavens and the earth;
Nothing his divine empire can elude:
Every thing he rules, disposes, governs.
85 How can we give him condign gratitude?
Who will be able to tell of those deeds,
Those miracles that, in the name of Christ
Performed are, by the faithful of the Church?
And who is not accorded the Supreme
90 Creator's assistance, who humbly begged?

Badly will the proud and the ingrate fare,
Who do not know his love and total power,
Those drawn one day from nothing, those whom
    Christ
With every drop of precious blood redeemed.
95   Religion commands us to believe that
God the Father created, from the blank
Void of nothing, the heavens and the earth,
Without material preexisting form,
Moved not by obligation but by good;
100 That he formed likewise water, and the seas,
The fire that flicks its flames into the air,
And from these varied elements conjoined,
The massed throngs of innumerable beings,
And formed he then the race of humankind,
105 And last of all, sublime angelic hosts.
    It is an article of faith that Christ
Jesus is the divine Son, Lord of Heaven
And Earth, the life, the health, and nourishment
Of men, those lost that first and fatal day
110 Of sin. Intoxicated by the sweet
Fruit, Adam tasted, and committed thus
The greatest sin of disobedience,
Provoking wrath divine, and for his heirs
Meriting the pain of eternal death.
115 Moved then by his love of his creations,
God chose (oh, prodigious, ample goodness!)
That his immortal Son become a man,
Virgin born, to live among us on earth
And at the last to salvage us from death,
120 Suffering cruel, bitter death for us.
    Disdain now, if you can, the heavenly
Favor of Jesus, or deny the sublime
Grandeur of him our all powerful Lord,
Who so loved men that he became a man,
125 Him whose nativity and painful death
Pay for all our lives, our health, our strength,
Without whose assistance our entire globe
In horrible perdition would succumb,
Him we call Jesus for he is our Savior,[1]
130 And for exalted sacrifice we call
Him Christ, proclaimed Messiah, the Anointed.
    With all our being this God-Man mystery
We must believe, for in it is comprised
All of the faith and doctrine of the Church.

135 Jesus it is reveals that faith, that doctrine,
And on the rock unmoving builds it firm.[2]
    Though the corporeal form of Jesus was
Nourished in the chaste womb of the virgin,
He was not of our human seed conceived,
140 But by the working of eternal grace,
A miracle caused by the Holy Spirit,
For, being mortal, Christ redeemed our sin.
    Truly good are the divine external
Works of the Trinity most sacrosanct;
145 That which from all three does not emanate
Comes not from one sacred person alone.
The sainted fathers say the origin
Of Christ is the Holy Spirit, which is
Love and mercy, and to this they ascribe
150 The favors, gifts, and all rewards bestowed
For our relieved succor and our counsel.
United in this ineffable mystery
Are principles unique to nature's power
And others that surpass the boundaries
155 Of our intelligence and mental strength.
Thus when we say that Christ's body was formed
Of virgin blood maternal, we accept
That the Divine Word assumed our nature
In order to confirm that God the highest,
160 As archangels in single chorus sang,
Engendered was, and that, body and soul
Conjoined, he raised the quintessence divine,
Not for desire of gratitude or gifts,
But he in his total, august grandeur
165 Had to enlighten us before our God,
That these prodigies excel nature's bounds.
    It is required also that we accept
The truth that Mary, virginally pure,
True mother was of God and man at once,
170 Then that the son to whom she gave such life
Is him engendered by the Eternal Father,
Before all time and of the divine essence.
Since none on earth discerns how such portents
Ever could be realized, you do not wish
175 To penetrate the mysteries divine,
But with submissive soul and ready mind
Hold as indubitable and as true
That which the Holy Church reveals to us,
Commands us to uphold and to believe.

1. "And thou shalt call his name JESUS: for he shall save his people from their sins" (Matt. 1:21). The name is derived from a Hebrew word meaning savior.

2. The allusion is, of course, to Saint Peter (Matt. 16:18–19).

180 It must not thus be said that Jesus Christ
Was adopted Son of God, or that this
Name honor and glory on him bestowed.[3]
Though such, once said, would others glorify,
It is not worthy of his majesty

185 Supreme; for Christ is the natural son
Of the living God, Him who created
The universe, man, and all the angels.
   Who can offer thanks for such great favors?
What adoration must we not offer

190 To the divine Son who wore flesh like ours,
To be united with us, and to share
Our miseries? Who from his heart, and from
Yet deeper within him will not desire
To raise an altar of reverence and

195 Love to him, lowly born for all our sakes:
On straw, in a manger, a poor infant
Numb with the cold, among beasts of the field,
Born to live among us, and to leave us,
By his life, of humility and work

200 And purity, the perfect example.
Certain it is then that there are those born
Of the lineage of gods, not of our own
Poor flesh and blood, when God himself was made
Man in the womb of the virgin Mary,

205 To rid us of our guilt and all its pains.
   I believe also that the innocent
Lamb Jesus, when Judea Pilate ruled,
Suffered cruel tortures, inhuman death,
Then took upon him all our sinful guilt,

210 The mortal sins against infinite God,
Gross sins meriting everlasting death,
And that he solely could erase them, who,
Man and God, suffered and died for them all.
   Faith in this mystery is necessary,

215 To meditate and feel with wondering soul,
How for our sake th' exalted Son most high
Would suffer death and insult on the cross.
Thus Paul, a man of strength to be admired,
Emphatically declares and does protest

220 Not to know any other thing but Christ,[4]

Christ hanging from the bitter wooden cross,
Ignited by his divine love of men,
Redeemed by his death, ever in his debt
For these his gifts, such grace and favor as

225 Were never known before. Thus such extreme
Reward must be imagined at the least.
The cruelest pains he suffered to save us
In body and soul, where from conception
Sacred dwelled immortal essence divine.

230 He died that thus Evil in serpent's guise,
Conqueror in that tree that bore the first
Fatal fruit, was vanquished on that other
Tree, the holy tree, the bitter cross,
And flew away at last, malign, debased,

235 To be united for eternity
With the grim shades of his grisly prison.
   Isaac is He, submissively prepared
For sacrifice by Abraham his father;
He is the innocent Abel whose brother

240 Murdered him with cruelty and cunning;[5]
He is the Paschal Lamb, eternal symbol,[6]
Who gives his life in sacrifice for ours,
Who knows the cold dark dolors of the tomb,
Though he is undefiled, and whole remains.

245   What great opprobrium, consider, reader,
What unspeakable affront, and what dread
Torments Christ was compelled to undergo
In cruelest torture on the infamous cross,
Inflicted, under Pilate in Judea,

250 Upon the basest, abject miscreants.
Observe gouts of his blood fall drop by drop,
The optimal complexion, and extreme
Sensibility of Jesus, and say,
If you can, conquered by the deceptive

255 Sweetness that sin offers you, that he be
Nailed again to that wooden infamy,
He who washes away all of your sins
With his beneficent blood, who opens
The closed heavens to men, and frees them from

260 The Enemy,[7] and forgives all our debt,
That debt immense, of all our crimes and sins

---

3. I.e., it is not the name but his essence that bestows honor and glory upon him.

4. "For I determined not to know any thing among you, save Jesus Christ, and him crucified" (1 Cor. 2:2).

5. The idea that the innocent Abel prefigures Christ is suggested twice, in Matt. 23:35 and Luke 11:51, and again more obliquely in Heb. 12:24.

6. The Paschal Lamb is the lamb slaughtered for Passover. One tradition held that Christ was crucified on the day the paschal lamb was killed (1 Cor. 5:7 and John 1:29).

7. The Hebrew word for "enemy" or "adversary" is transliterated into English as Satan.

Against th' Eternal Lord of Heaven and Earth.
  In Jesus see the example most pure
Of all the virtues. Is there anyone
265 In whom resplendent glow wisdom and love
As they do in Christ? Meekness, constancy,
And firmness? Oh! If it were given to me
To follow his holy path, recalling
At every instant all his steps on earth,
270 His days and nights, his death and sepulcher,
And how He, innocent, underwent all
That he suffered so that I could be freed
At last of all my sin, eternal bliss!
  Observe also how now the soul of Christ,
275 United with the Deity supreme
Eternally, and even while his frame
Lay in the dank tomb, still united was
With the Divine Essence, visited hell
With furious anger toward Evil wrought,
280 And snatched from there hell's valued prisoners,
Freed the souls of patriarchs and the just,
Releasing them from eternal torment.
  Christ, by his descent to limbo, reveals
That he extends his grace not only to
285 Those born after Him, but also to those
Born before, to men of all place and time.
Together they illume, his loving care
Assuring glory to the faithful and
Sempiternal peace. And his power o'er
290 The darkest forces, and his love's embrace,
Reaching even to the bowels of the earth,
Protects from the tremendous final death
This mortal and our sinful human race.[8]
  By his will and virtue, he rose again
295 On the third day, as the ancient prophets
Had foretold,[9] proving thus in manner sure
That he was man and God, for none could die
Unless he were a man, nor rise again
From darkest tomb to die again no more,
300 Unless at the same time he were not God.[10]
  All was fulfilled, the Holy Fathers say,
Who state and teach these lofty mysteries,

For divine justice radiates in glory,
Hope of our life eternal is affirmed,
305 And this mystery of faith is held to be
The fit crowning, wherein you apprehend
That there is new life, but you must remain
Free of sin's taint until your dying day;
Thus the knowledge of Christ resurrected
310 Lights up our souls and gives them peace and
   strength.
  He after rose to heaven before the awed
Gazes of the apostles and of his
Followers and of Mary, his earthly
Mother; and with the intrinsic virtue
315 Of his sacred nature the radiant air
He rived, toward th' exalted heights sublime
Beyond the choirs celestial and beyond
All of the angelic hierarchies
Until at the sublime throne he arrived
320 Upon which the glorious Father sits
And where, embraced by ineffable love,
He sat at the right hand of God the Father,
And thus the world, which serves as his footstool,[11]
With power and glory eternal he rules.
325   Thus are the sacred mysteries ordained
Of his life, filled with pain and sore insult,
To this end: that is, his ascent to heaven
In which his great grandeur is glorified,
But Christ Jesus ascended unto heaven
330 For, not mortal, his body could not hold
A fitting, permanent seat in regions
Most pure, which this our life cannot provide.
Here[12] the whirlwind of fatal destiny
Stirs up all, devastates, or transmutes it.[13]
335 Here none can be immortal or immune
From ills, or exempt from all earthly pains.[14]
He rose to occupy the throne on high
That his spilled blood merited, there to reign
In perpetuity triumphant over
340 The eternal mystic Jerusalem;
And likewise to be always united
With the Father, and to present to him

---

8. The sense is that our human race is both mortal and sinful.

9. The concept of resurrection occurs in Ps. 115:17, Isa. 26:19, and Dan. 12:2, but the Easter resurrection of Jesus appears to date no further back than Paul's account in 1 Cor. 15:3–8.

10. Despite the sequence of negatives, the meaning seems clear enough—that only a man could die but only God could rise again.

11. The image comes from Isa. 66:1, Matt. 5:35, or Acts 7:49.

12. On earth.

13. The usual biblical association with the whirlwind is its connection with the revelation of God—to Job, or to Ezekiel in a vision—and the ascent of Elijah to heaven in his chariot of fire (Job 38:1, 40.6; Ezek. 1:4; 2 Kings 2:1, 11).

14. A rare example in the poem of Hernández the doctor speaking.

Our humble prayers, our causes to defend.
He wished besides to show us that his reign
345 Is not of this world, as he had affirmed
In Judea before Pontius Pilate.
And furthermore, more valuable is
Celestial good than mere terrestrial gifts,
That thus, encircled by his love, our souls
350 To those same heights of heaven will follow him,
First with the mind and the desire, and then
Flying toward eternal light, and next,
Christ's death and resurrection, in the flesh
Death, but true life in the soul, teach us how
355 To rise likewise to heaven's lofty height,
And show the way to our true home, where bliss,
Felicity eternal, awaits us.
     What merit would there be in believing
In Christ, if we saw him on this our earth,
360 Already immortal, and could converse
With him, and hear his voice, and speak to him,
And if it were not possible to cast
The shade of doubt upon his existence?[15]
     By his ascent, at last, our hopes may grow
365 That we, his mystic family, may rise
To where he reigns; by his ascent he is
Our mediator before the Father,
To whom he counsels mercy, and obtains,
And from his hands flows free toward our souls
370 The flood of grace that gives them life and peace.
     From there he will come down for just one day
To judge men whom he redeems with his blood,
The living and already dispossessed
Of fleshly life, those who were or have yet
375 To live on earth. Two advents, then, must be
Believed; but while that first advent, in which,
Descending to the earth, the Word took flesh[16]
In virgin womb, was gentle, humble, quiet,
His second coming, the Day of the Lord,
380 That of tremendous justice, when the just
Shall separated be from the unjust,
Will be announced with trumpets' loudest blast,
And, terrified, the entire world will quake
Before impending divine judgment, when
385 Christ's majesty and glory radiate;
But no one knows the day, the hour, the age.[17]

First, at death, each one before the divine
Tribunal presents himself for judgment;
Then on the last day of the world, we go
390 To universal justice, final doom,
In which he weighs our merits in his palm
And punishes the vices and the crimes,
And be it thus, for not only our own
Trespasses are taken into account,
395 But sins also of others who arise,
And are perpetuated and renewed
Until the end of time, just as virtues
Ever after diffuse his radiance.
For this reason the Last Judgment will be
400 On the final day, when there is no place
For virtue or new sins or things forgot,
No secret will remain athwart the earth,
For good will then receive its full reward
And evil fall to odious disrepute.
405 Also then are the bodies resurrected
And for such judgment likewise they appear
And, since they are instruments of the soul,
For ever take their part in joy and pain.
     (And none should think that by a destined fate
410 The good are doomed to dolor or distress
While throngs of the unrighteous lead a life
Of pleasure or serenity, or ease.
Those also will be saved because although
A fit reward for all their works is due,
415 Evils once discovered will be erased.)
Justice terrible stirs in them such dread,
That the unrighteous will amend their ways,
While the righteous delight in expectation
Of final triumph, glorious recompense.
420   And although to the three Divine Persons
This judgment and this sentence correspond
And of the three is formed the tribunal
Sublime, which gives to each what he deserves,
Yet it is Christ, the Wisdom of the Father,
425 God and man in one, who came to the earth
To be arbiter supreme, that mortals
Called to such tremendous justice, could see
Him, speak to him and hear from his own lips
The sentence of eternal life or death.
430 It will be thus also that Christ himself,

---

15. Thus mystery is the test of faith.
16. The "word" in the Old Testament is normally spoken, not written. In an extension of this sense, the teachings of Jesus become the word, and so does Jesus himself ("and the Word was made flesh" [John 1:14]).
17. 1 Thes. 5:2 and Rev. 3:3.

Who one day suffered a sentence so cruel,
Shall hear and judge those men who condemned him
To die upon the cross between two thieves,
To whom he was the innocent Lamb who
435 Gave up his life in sacrifice, for he
Bestowed upon the world its health and life
Everlasting. When holy religion
Lights all the world and there are many who,
Benighted, blind, do not belong to it,
440 And the apocalyptic antichrist
Appears, that moment marks the end of time,
When the Lord has descended to judge us,
To give the righteous proper recompense,
To condemn the impious and wicked
445 And to hurl them to the eternal flames,
Where the throngs of malignant spirits will
Lament for ever more their blind revolt.
Then will shine forth the mildest law of Christ:
Joy to the good, to the evil dread pain.
450   The Holy Spirit is the third person
Of the Holy Trinity, which proceeds
From the Father and the Son, and is God
In one triune essence, with all wisdom
And infinite power: this must be believed.
455   I believe in the Holy Church, mystic
Spouse of Christ, which we do call Catholic
Because it is dispersed the world around,
Of which Christ is the invisible head
And near the end of time will be with her.
460 But the Church is twofold: one triumphant
And militant the other, one in heaven,
The other on earth; this victorious,
That fighting with the foes who lie in wait.
The figures of the Church are Noah's Ark,
465 Which from voracious flood escaped unscathed,
And Jerusalem, where sacrifices
Were offered to Jehovah, and the city
Was exalted by leaders and prophets.
    I believe in the communion of saints,
470 For we are the mystical fellowship
Of Christ and his mystical bride, the Church;
The sacraments give us ease, and the grace
Of Jesus sustains us all, and the favors
Which, thanks to Jesus' internunciate

475 Good offices, the Father wills to grant,
Come down to us like beneficent rain.
    I believe that the Church can pardon sins,
Which tie or untie knots that bind the soul,
But this by the grace of Christ, only if
480 Sinners contrite and humble renounce their
Sins, and promise never again to sin,
And thus they declare it with soul sincere.
    Also the resurrection of our flesh
Must be in us a certain hope, since our
485 Bodies, as the instruments of our souls,
Obtain with them their merited reward.
    Last, I believe that awaiting the just
Is everlasting bliss in Heaven, a life
Of ineffable joy that no human
490 Language can begin to describe, nor mind
Comprehend, a glorious life in God,
Who is peace and love, plenty and richness.

Book 2: On the Seven Sacraments of the Church

    With the favor of Christ, and of the Virgin
We have declared the mysteries of our faith,
495 Which he who is judged worthy of the name
Of Christian must believe. I now describe
The arms with which Christ's soldiers[18] can avoid
Wounds mortal to the soul, and can repel
The devil's fierce assaults upon the world
500 And human flesh. These arms together are
Devices that distinguish, signify
The faithful flock, and are symbols of all
That's known: the sacraments, I say, that by
The blood spilled from the breast of Jesus are
505 Granted to us as perennial founts
Of his eternal mercy and his grace.[19]
    In Latin, *sacrament* denotes the oath,[20]
Or mystery, yet the sainted fathers say
This word indicates all sensible signs
510 Which reveal and produce secret, sacred
Things. For the grace of Jesus, under the
Appearances of things or earthly signs
Concealed, succeeds, by virtue of this means,
The sacrament, in infusing itself
515 In the flesh and giving life to the soul.

---

18. See 2 Tim. 2:3–4.
19. The blood of Jesus as an image of grace is commonplace in the New Testament (for example, Heb. 10:10).
20. In classical Latin, *sacramentum* indicated an oath of allegiance or any other kind of obligation; in late Latin, a mystery, as in 1 Tim. 3:16.

In all the various whole of what exists,[21]
Some things are made or formed but to refer
To themselves alone; likewise others are
As signs or tokens—holy sacraments
520 Of Our Church are such tokens and such signs.[22]
Some of these signs originate in nature,
Like smoke, which reveals fire and flame below;
Others, fictitious, may be heard or seen,
And figure or signify natural things,
525 And others yet, by high divine decree,
Signify all at once that they engender
Arcane realities, and these are what
We call sacraments, those sensible signs
Of sacred purposes and causes (then
530 The grace that they bestow has such a name
Because we give our gratitude to God
And to him wholly do devote ourselves).
    From other rites the sacrament differs,
In which grace, though spoken of, is not made
535 Manifest, and which do not sole allude
To a present grace, but evoke the holy
Passion, by which we are granted virtue,
Or the radiance of the glory that
After death awaits us: refulgent beauty
540 Of the angelic choirs, in concert raising
Their praises up to God, and without shadow
Of any harm or prickle of desire
Enjoy complete and ever certain plenty.
    More of the institution of these rites,
545 The sacraments' just reasons and their causes,
Concealed from our knowledge cannot remain.
The first reason lies in our very nature,
For as it is imprisoned in the body,
Our mind sees no incorporeal forms
550 Nor any thing but what is apprehended
By our five senses. Fully cognizant
Of this our most terrestrial limitation,
Inexhaustible divine providence
Decreed that behind the dense veil of things
555 Visible would be invisible grace.
The second cause is that high Clemency
Reveals its gifts to souls in signs, that thus
Even hard and stubborn men would be moved
To seek and supplicate for such great graces.

560 God further desired that the sacraments
Should be distinctive signs of holy faith,
Common to all, thus all the Christian flock
Should be ablaze with love and piety,
And none could ever hide his faith but all
565 Should carry it, displayed to all the world.
    The sacraments consist of some matter
But their greatest strength resides in language,
An arrangement and apt order of words
That declare their sacred content, that thus
570 The sacred is revered, and that souls may
Behold in harmony of words and signs,
Divine secrets and their sovereign grandeur.

    With reason do we hold that there are seven
Sacraments, as seven are they that make
575 The perfect life:[23] first it is necessary
By holy baptismal water to be
Born in the light of the true faith; and then
By holy confirmation to renew,
Invigorate the faith and make it grow,
580 Then, having reached the appropriate age,
To nourish ourselves at communion
Most holy. When sin stains us, we are washed
Clean by the sacrament of repentance.
The extreme unction, which to the dying
585 Is dispensed, mitigates all of their pains
And proffers peace; the priestly order gives
To ministers authority to dispense
The sacraments of holy mother Church,
And matrimony sanctifies the union
590 Of spouses and the children born to them.
    And yet it must be noted that although
Even without holy matrimony
Eternal salvation can be attained,
And without priestly ordination or
595 Either communion or extreme unction,
A Christian soul can enter into heaven
(And if the soul is free of guilt, also
Without repentance, and when confirmation
Is lacking), but he cannot reach that goal
600 Of everlasting life without baptism.
And this despite the fact that mortal error
Requires a priest who will absolve it, and

---

21. Hernández's language in this whole paragraph contrasts the numinous with the concrete.

22. Perhaps the concept expressed here is itself a sign that Hernández is equally interested in theories of language and matter.

23. The symbolic significance of the number seven had biblical sanction, from the days of the creation (probably the source of the association with the perfect life) to the seven churches of Rev. 2–3.

That priestly orders are of more value
To the Church, and that holy communion
605 Is, of all the graces, the one supreme.
It must be known that from Christ's wounded flesh
Flow the sacraments and they come to us
Through the mediating ministration
Of priests, no matter who they be, even
610 If in them is absent the Church's true
Intent, or those related acts prescribed.[24]
For certain, whoever with impure hand
Or soul administers a holy rite
Ensures his everlasting perdition;
615 But conserves unscathed all the secret powers
Which the supreme power placed in him that we
Eventually, clean of soul and free
Of guilt, by virtue of these sacred cures,
May rise to heaven's celestial heights supreme
620 And humbly dwell there in the light divine.
    The sacraments' supreme rewards, thanks be,
Are blessing and a mark indelible,[25]
And even if the marking of the spirit
In the body, in realms ethereal
625 Seems to our minds impossibility,
As opposite to nature, who will dare
Deny that such a prodigy is wrought
By God, the mighty omnipotent God?
The famous miracles do witness this,
630 All validated by external things.
Thus, as John the Baptist poured the water
Over Jesus, the skies parted and sounded
From on high a voice;[26] thus, in tongues of fire
Came down the Holy Spirit to imbue
635 The twelve apostles with its sacred power.
    The faithful meditate what precious treasure
Divine clemency in the sacraments
Gives to us; with how much faith and ardor
We must seek them, and what terrible pains
640 Their absence would occasion unto us.
Truths are clearest to the Christian who
Recognizes and believes with sincere
Faith that the blood of the Lamb promises
Us those gifts in which God grants us his grace
645 And his assistance. Then although our souls

Are anchored in Christ, who is a living
And eternal rock, without sacraments
Or words of God who affirms them, soon would
They fall to their undoing and destruction.

650   This said, it is time briefly, pious reader,
For me to treat each sacrament in turn.
You see from there how not just any bathing
Receives the name of baptism—only that
Which by way of the sacrament and with
655 The language of ritual the ministry
Validates. This sacrament (also called
Re-marking, beginning of the mandate,
Lighting of the soul, sign of the faith)
Is a second birth by means of the lymph
660 And the Divine Word; submerged by the water,
The baptized are joined as one with the Word,
The solemn phrases are pronounced with which
The rite was instituted by Christ Jesus.
Thus though born in the wrath of God, it is
665 Given to every man to change, by way
Of this, a second birth, into the son
And heir of the Highest Being Supreme.
    It is then water, plain, common water,
That is the medium of holy baptism,
670 The ancient fathers' writings thus declared.
They prophesied by this means the flood that
Inundated the world, in Noah's time,[27]
And the exodus from captivity
Across the Red Sea, and the cleansing that
675 Was ordered in the rites by Nathan,[28] and
The holy place of miraculous waters
To which the prophets call us,[29] and the fount
That Zacharias and Ezekiel saw,
By whose waters our sins were forgiven.[30]
680 Water is the medium most fitting
Of the holy sacrament of baptism,
Because none lacks it, ordinarily,
And none has health or life without its aid.
As water cleans the body of all dirt,
685 So baptism cleanses the soul of sin
Returning it to pristine innocence.
    Water alone as medium is enough,

---

24. That is, even priests who are virtual charlatans will do in an emergency.
25. Possibly echoing Paul's "marks of Jesus" (Gal. 6:17).
26. Matt. 3:16–17 and Mark 1:10–11.
27. Gen. 6–8.
28. 2 Sam. 12:20.
29. Perhaps the pool of Bethesda (John 5:1–7).
30. Zech. 13; Ezek. 47:1–2.

Yet, whenever there is danger of death,
The chrism or holy unguent is required,
690 Whose valued effects are seen in clear signs
When the sacrament is most solemnly
Celebrated according to the rite.
And if by chance the wise minister doubts
Which water is proper and which is not,
695 He may take as certain and most secure
This norm: that nothing but ordinary
Water is the medium of baptism,
Which washes and purifies the body.
　　　Also, the form of this sacrament must
700 Be taught to all with diligence and care,
As much that they recognize the sacred
Mysteries as that, in their specific case,
They know the words that go with holy bathing.
He is immersed only when he who gives
705 Pronounces, on pouring the crystal water,
"I baptize you in the name of the Father,
And of the Son, and of the Holy Ghost."
Remaining of this rite to be defined
Is who administers the sacrament,
710 Who receives it, its divine origin,
And acknowledgment that at the same time
Our God is one and also he is three.
And if any say that in ancient times
Baptism was in the name of Christ alone
715 (However many deny such assertion),
Under this holy name enfolded are
The Father and the Holy Spirit both,
Who, with the Son, together are one God.
Whether the body of the one baptized
720 Be sprinkled or submerged, the solemn words,
The form of holiest baptism, are pronounced.
　　　This sacrament, 'tis certain, came to be
The day that Jesus was baptized by John,
When the voice of the Father rent the air,
725 Exalting the great glory of his son,
And the heavens parted and, descending
As a dove, down to Jesus came the love,[31]
Infinite love of God, the Holy Spirit,
And touching the body divine, the waters
730 Glistened as never, and from thence they gained
A wondrous virtue never known before.
Such was the origin, but the law that
Instituted it is the mandate of

The resurrected Jesus Christ, who told
735 His disciples, "Go through the whole world and
Teach the people, baptizing them thus in
The name of the Father and of the Son,
And of the Holy Ghost."[32] And from that day
Nobody could be saved without bathing
740 First in the waters of holy baptism.
In earliest times its celebration was
Entrusted to the bishop's power sole
Who administered the holy bathing
On certain holy and festival days.
745 It is conducted now by any priest,
And although in cases when death is near,
All Christians can impart it, man or woman,
Whosoever it may be, one who is
Pious and observant is most fitting.
750 A woman may not administer it
If a man is present, unless she knows
The service better. Thus may anyone
Conduct the rite except a heretic
Or any guilty of a wicked crime,
755 For he who bestowed simple elements
On this, the key that opens heaven's gates,
Wished, for our benefit, that it might have
Fit ministers in every time and place.
Likewise it is required that taking part
760 In this holy bathing are the guardians
Or godparents from whom children receive
Example and a pious education;
These guardians are but two, for proper teaching
Will not be changed by having many masters,
765 Nor do knots slacken, if not in the blood.
　　　Let it be known, without this sacrament
Of baptism none can be truly saved,
And that God does not desire that this source
Of life to children from them be removed,
770 And thus (according to the ancient texts)
This sacred rite in infants be observed
On the same day that they are circumcised,
That is one single week after their birth,
That if, before they die in Adam, they
775 Are born in Christ, now clean of soul and senses,
They can know later sacred mysteries
And be bred in the other sacraments.
And let it not be doubted that effects
So signal spring from baptism; not because

---

31. Mark 1:10–11; Matt. 3:16.　　　32. Matt. 28:19.

780 Infants of tender age can recognize
    Our faith for themselves, but because the good
    Offices of their parents will make good
    The deficiency of their children, thus,
    Although their souls do not yet have our faith,
785 Devoted love will give them strength and succor.
    For this same reason prudent Christians will
    Take care to lead their children to the temple
    Lest they, by dying early, forfeit heaven.
        And yet for adults,[33] on the other hand,
790 Receiving holy baptism must not be
    Hurried. The Christian doctrine first they learn,
    And duly are exhorted to the faith;
    When their conversion is complete, they come
    Closer to this divine mystery, and start
795 To enjoy the gifts, gifts with which the Church
    Nourishes her children, nourishes more
    Of those who derive from this sacrament,
    Erases sins and bestows bounteous grace,
    The origin and source of all that's good.
800 Besides, this prudent patience brings with it
    Priceless benefits, for it proves the will,
    The constant will of those who seek the truths
    Of baptism, which they do not request
    As custom to be followed or embraced,
805 But as the result of thoughtful judgment.
    Clearly, nevertheless, it will be rash
    In the face of death to defer it long.
        The baptized one must clearly understand
    All that the Church commands us to believe;
810 He must repent sincerely of his sins
    For having thus offended God with them;
    Present himself with humble, docile soul,[34]
    Fulfill the precepts of the divine Father;
    Contemplate how many heavenly gifts
815 From this one sacrament he has received;
    How he must look to thought and deed alike,
    Keep them as they were at the baptism,
    Clear of all guilt and free of all guilt's pains,
    Of original sin at the same time.
820   But some will ask why evils and sorrows
    Are not removed from those who are baptized,
    For if our first parents, when innocent
    Afflicted never were, before they fell

Into delinquency, neither should they
825 Be perpetuated in those who, by
    Means of this lymph, remain pure. But it is
    Not so, because baptism converts us to
    Mystic members of Christ. How then shall we
    Be immune to the pains and sorrows that
830 Jesus Christ, our head,[35] was forced to suffer?
    Our natural propensity to sin
    Is even food and motive of virtues;
    For heroes are in battle only forged,
    And he who enjoys the victory is
835 He who has fought the long, hard fight and won.
    Further, if this divine bathing expelled
    The sins of the flesh, we might then believe
    The body's good was good enough, and not
    That of the soul. And, finally, although
840 Encumbered with fatigue, we may inspire
    An intimate joy in our lives, for there
    Is nothing sweeter than to tread the path
    Of Jesus, and suffer the cross with him,
    And suffer with him death, and martyrdom.
845   Thus in this sacrament are given us
    Virtues and grace, and union with Christ.
    A sacred character is imprinted[36]
    In the soul that will never be erased
    For evermore. But once this imprint in
850 The soul is graven, no second baptism
    May be given, for it is contrary
    To all the doctrine and the practices
    Of the ancient Fathers, whom God inspired.
    Repeated it may be in doubtful cases
855 But then it must be said that such baptism
    Is given because the lack of it will cause
    Grave damage. It is thus that Jesus' grace
    Sanctifies us and opens heaven's gates.
        But when the Church imparts the sacrament,
860 It accompanies it with many signs
    And rites that everyone must recognize:
    First are the waters blessed, and at the time
    Appointed; the holy oil is dispersed
    In the waters; the one to be baptized,
865 His entrance to the temple barred until
    The whole has been consecrated and to
    Christ surrendered, the priest then asks him why

---

33. That is, adult converts to Christianity in Mexico.
34. "Docile" carries its radical sense of "teachable."
35. In the two senses of "leader" and "intelligence."

36. This image depends for its effectiveness among Mexicans on the relatively recent founding of New Spain's first printing press about 1539. It was the first in the Americas and predated the first press in Spain.

He has come, what gifts are sufficient,
And after the response, explains to him
870 The divine mysteries of the faith, and
Next placing salt in his mouth and making
The sign of the cross with his hands and arms,
He casts from him the curse of the first sin
To the bitter, old enemy, the Devil.
875 The body strengthened with the sacred sign,
The minister's saliva wets the nose
And eyes, and the one to be baptized, thus
Prepared, is led to the baptismal font.
The priest then asks, do you abhor the tempter,
880 The old serpent? the show and shining surface
Of this poor world? and in one God do you
Have faith, as holy mother Church instructs?
And last, do you desire to be made pure
In clearest baptismal crystal lucence?
885 The answer yes, the priest pours holy water,
Anoints at once the head with mystic oil,
And then invests him with a robe of white,
And last confers this gift, a sainted name.
As fittest athletes still must follow leaders,
890 And those who gain the laurels when they win
Do not oppose the fiercest foe unarmed,
Expect not the converted, by this rite
Become now faithful warriors of Christ,
To triumph o'er this world, the flesh, the devil,
895 If first their heads have not anointed been
With sacred confirmation's holy oil.

   With divine favor we shall now say who
Originated this holy unction,
Which animates the souls of the faithful,
900 And we shall say what was its matter, and
Who had the power to administer it.
Its author was Jesus Christ himself, since
No other but he could attain such power
To create such a valued sacrament,
905 Which maintains us and keeps us in his grace.
Its media are oil and sacred balsams,
The one a symbol of the strength that flows
From Christ, the others with a fragrance that,
Made stronger by this sacrament, and free
910 Of all corruption, spreads throughout the soul.
Its words of formula are these: "I make
The sign of the cross before you, and I
Confirm you with the chrism, which vivifies
And salvages." To consecrate this chrism

915 Unto the bishop falls, and on this subject
Saint Fabian declares that Christ our Lord
At the last supper instituted it,
And that, because it consecrates each one
Of us to the Maker, it must before
920 His divine power be sanctified, from where
This same to whom was given the faculty
Of confirming, must raise to God his prayers
Because he has in this most holy oil
An instrument divine of God's great grace.
925   There should be a godparent who instructs,
The oil should be dispersed in the waters,
And custom it should be among all good
Christians to confirm children when they
Reach the age of seven. All this although
930 We know that first this sacrament alone
Descended in the form of calls when in
Divine love the Holy Spirit embraced
The apostles, confirming them in grace.
Further, the confirmand should have before
935 Tasted and confessed his sins, and received
The symbolic slap, and the priestly sign
Of the cross, which imprints at once a mark,
A character indelible in the soul.
   To holy communion now we turn,
940 Which, at the last supper, ere he returned
To his Father in heaven, Christ founded
So that abandoned none would ever be
Whom he so loved, that he chose to assume
Their nature. Piety ineffable!
945 Oh ardent love, excellent charity!
In this are figured the holy passion,
The grace engendered by it, and rewards
Awaiting the righteous in ageless glory.
The matter is bread made from purest wheat
950 And wine with some water in admixture.
Its form consists in those words that are spoken
To consecrate the body and the blood
Of the holy Lamb who redeems the sins
Of the world, and by whose power the bread
955 Is transformed into flesh, the wine to blood,
Previous form annihilated, yet
By heavenly miracle retaining
Ever their accidents and appearances.
   I pass over the words of the sacred
960 Formula lest, by rhythms of this verse,
Subjects are altered or transposed, and so
Violate what the holy fathers ordered

To be kept intact. Because all are filled
With miracles, and sublime, and above
965 All human understanding, and although
The bread is converted into the body
Of Christ, and likewise wine into his blood
Converted by consecration, yet still
We confess that behind whatever part
970 Of such appearances was God and man,
Christ whole who as such in the heavens lives
And reigns. Then, after that, after dying
For us, he rose triumphant from the tomb,
Nor did his soul ever leave his body
975 Nor was the divine essence lacking there.
But double consecration is a sign,
Clear symbol of the sacred blood that spilled
And in this sacrament gives to the soul
Sustenance and drink, which recruit its strengths.
980   Nobody could deny the lofty gifts
That holy communion affords us,
If he will but consider how by this,
Flowing with goodness lives in Christ a sea
Of boundless grace. And if he contemplates
985 Its symbols, bread and wine that offer ease,
Though food and drink refer to life on earth,
Communion gives us life in and for Christ,
Among the saints it places and conserves us.
But all this is so only if, before,
990 Tested and purified is he who seeks
The sacred table to approach with thirst
For the celestial springs, and for the bread
Of eternal life, hunger to receive
And embody the Lord of heaven and earth.
995 Thus this first grace, which glows in those who wish
Their lips to touch the sacred body, but
Without risk of sin, is granted none
Save souls desiring with God to be one.
Communion does not just protect the faithful,
1000 It feeds their strengths, and venial sins rubs out,
Combats and removes mortal sins, and curbs
Appetite of the flesh and its dread furies:
In sum this august sacrament is sure
Token of everlasting life to come.
1005 If they are one day called blissful who watched
Jesus on earth enter beneath their roof
Or faintly brushed against his robe's mere fringe,

How much more so are those who now themselves
Glorious, receive and give him lodging!
1010   The body of our Lord in three ways can
In exalted communion be received:
Unworthily (God free us from disgrace
And the frightful evils that it calls forth!)
When one whose soul is stained with mortal sin,
1015 Comes near, to partake of the body pure,
Hiding sacrilege in his impure heart
Against the immense majesty of Christ.
Others receive the supreme gift with soul
Humble and pure, but only in the mind,
1020 Not in reality, yearning for true
Communion. The eucharistic gifts,
These do not enjoy, though efflux of grace
Envelops them also. But those who are
Worthily in the holy feast nourished
1025 By the body of Christ—what immense store
Of gifts do they receive! How divine love
Reverberates in them, transforming lives
And human actions into holy deeds!
But just as Jesus washed the feet of his
1030 Disciples ere body and blood he gave,
That they should be clean of the slightest spot,[37]
So whoever approaches the holy
Banquet makes sure beforehand that no sin
Stains him, so that the sacred body, which
1035 Has power to be the life and health of him
Who takes it, in mortal poison is not
Converted. No other rite gives support
Which both comforts and conserves the healthy,
And damages and dirties and weakens
1040 The wicked and the evil. Thus also
To the Israelites was the sacred Ark
Their strength and their protection, while to foes
Its presence caused affliction and grave woe.[38]
    Whoever comes to the divine banquet
1045 Will recognize two distinct kinds of table:
How on this table the bread is the body
Of God, adored and feared in heaven and earth.
He recognizes also if he feels
That in fraternal embrace his heart reaches
1050 Out to all humanity, if he does
Not nurse any hidden ill-will for one
Among those he should be loving. May he

---

37. John 13:5–17.
38. Probably a general allusion to 1 Sam. 4:1–6:21, which describes the seizure and subsequent return of the Ark of the Covenant by the Philistines.

Consider if it is the sinner who
Must wash before the holy penitence.
1055 He may be recognized as unworthy
Of such signal reward and may he love
With life and soul the God to whom himself
He surrenders. May he be prepared too
For the angelic feast with prayer, and fasting,
1060 And continence, and thus at last prepared,
Approach and take communion most supreme.
At least once every year the faithful must
Take communion to stay among the saints,
Each month and ev'n each day must he who yearns
1065 For gifts divine and in abundance full.
As the bread that sustains our weak bodies
Must be daily, so the most ardent souls
Must daily taste that other bread, the bread
Of everlasting life that allays all
1070 Hunger and weakness, but enables them
To live their lives in love and grace and strength.
But the doctrine of the holy fathers
Prohibits the laity from receiving
As wine the drops of this most precious blood,
1075 For causes that our reason shows us: since
The priest alone is empowered to take
Communion under both species, thus he
Alone the bread and wine may consecrate,
And dispense this most holy sacrament.
1080   Not only sacrament, the eucharist
Is also expiatory sacrifice
To the Eternal Father, for our sins,
As well as to our holy mother Church,
The propitiatory host is Christ
1085 Who sacrificed himself at the last supper,
And whom again the priest who celebrates
This sacrament offers and sacrifices.
The mysteries of our faith that we encounter,
The solemn rites in which they are figured,
1090 Of content so sublime, that the tiniest
Error or the most serious offense
Violates it—on these I will be silent.
    Consider now the sacrament of aid,
The rescuer of the shipwreck of the soul,
1095 The curer of the evil that besets
The soldier of Christ, antidote to bane,
Which threatens him with death. For to say it
Worthily, may the Lord give us his light,
Who tends and guards the health and life of men,
1100 Whom he created and his mercy saves.

Let us say then that only he repents
In truth who grieves from his soul's inner depths
For having offended the Supreme Father
And vows not to relapse in new disgrace.
1105 This virtue is called penitence, as is
The sacrament that prepares us for it;
The virtue is only encouragement
And preparation, as the sacrament
Erases sins with grace. The former is
1110 Repentance as an internal feeling,
External is the second called. In sum,
The contrite soul laments his sins to God
But filled with hope and guided by his faith,
Without which none meets God nor reaches heaven.
1115   The virtuous gift of penitence is divine,
Since there are those who even laugh and boast
That they insulted our Lord Jesus Christ,
And others still who dare not even hope
For pardon of their most atrocious sins.
1120 And for such serious sins the only cure
Is sincere regret and repentance. First,
The abolition of guilt is required
In thought, and deed, and word; and then one must,
For sins against the Lord committed, show
1125 Proper repentance, so that finally
He who has angered him so senselessly,
And many times, may turn to him anew
For amity and grace. We know the steps
From which such precious virtue is obtained:
1130 Before all, God, in his mercy, prepares
Us, looks for us, calls to us; afterward,
Illuminated by the splendrous faith,
Our upward gazes are turned unto him;
A great quaking the whole being invades
1135 On thinking of the inferno's fateful pains,
And the affliction of our being deprived
For ever of the face of God, to whom
Our souls are drawn. Later a certain hope
Consoles us, hope of pardon and of grace,
1140 Which leads us to a life of righteousness,
New life of righteous actions and morals;
And last, a true love of the divine Father
Who loves us so much, burns its flame in us,
And fearing like children to offend him,
1145 Thus we step on the felicitous path.
    Let us say what external penitence
Is, with the form and power of sacrament,
For sensible signs do exist in it

Of effects that its virtue has on souls.
1150 Providence wished that such a sacrament
Was instituted so that never would
Pardon for sins be lacking to us, which
God promised to the first fathers, for he
Detested their sins. Like the blood of Christ,
1155 Grace and forgiveness flow to all of us,
From Christ and from his blood, divine virtue,
Which purifies our stained souls, flows to us,
Erases sins committed after baptism,
And thus the foolish progeny of Adam
1160 Does not perish, for whom gladly the Lord
Suffered the passion and most bitter death.
Like baptism, external penitence
Is thus a true sacrament that cleanses
Our souls. This removes original sin
1165 And other sins besides. That washes off
Subsequent sins. This is shown by the priest's
Outward signs, and likewise the inward acts
Of one who rues his faults, and by what Christ
Said unto Peter: "What you loose on earth
1170 Likewise in heaven will be loosed and what
You bind here will there likewise be bound
According with your sentence and your word."[39]
     And so great are the Lord's mercy and love
Of us, that without limit or measure
1175 This sacrament can be repeated oft
To give life and health to the soul; which all
The faithful have to know because to none
Is ever lacking hope of forgiveness.
This sacrament is different in its mode,
1180 For others draw from nature or are made
By artifice, composed of different things,
But in this one the penitent's contrition
And humble, clear confession of his sins
With reparation for offenses past,
1185 And the return of stolen property
Are the medium. Even though these things
Parts of the sacrament could be well called,
Considered in another way, the sins,
The very substance of the sins, are like
1190 Fire from the burning wood that feeds the flame.
     This penitence reconciles us with Christ,
By erasing our sins and granting grace.
And if some say that absolution is

Denied to some or that some sins can not
1195 Be ever removed, it must then be known
That true contrition was lacking or that
With difficulty are some sins erased.
     This sacrament has justly and rightly
The three parts that are specified above,
1200 For we do sin against the Lord our God
In thought, and deed, and word, consequences
Of evil that we should shun, resistant
As we are to the good to which God called us.
The penitent regretting now his errors,
1205 With promise firm to obey holy law,
Required it is that he confess his sins
To the minister because he prescribes
To him the guiding principles to live
According to the divine will, and shows
1210 To him the secrets of sovereign mercy.
The penitent must feel sorrow profound
And abhorrence of faults with all the heart,
For he who dares offend almighty God
Must love him with the entirety of the soul.
1215 Thus contrite, feeling that at once is born
In him a keen desire to attain grace,
And forgiveness, an ardent wish to do
What must be done in order that he may
Come to the sacrament that purifies
1220 And saves, and lament all his grievous sins
Committed against God, with the whole being
And with the heart dissolved in salty tears.
     He who prepares to obtain such rewards
Must first of all examine all his faults,
1225 Regret them, give pardon for injuries
Received, and hold firm hope of divine grace,
Which never is denied to anyone
Who comes with contrite heart and humble soul.
Contrition unites us at once with God,
1230 Delivers to us amity and grace,
When just a little earlier we were
His enemies declared, of the inferno
Culprits, unfit to turn our gaze to heaven.
     Let us explain now the great benefits
1235 Which from this spoken confession do flow:
When contrition, at times too weak, does not
Succeed in erasing our gravest sins,
They can be pardoned by spoken confession,

39. Matt. 16:19: "and whatsoever thou shalt bind on earth shall be bound in heaven: and whatsoever thou shalt loose on earth shall be loosed in heaven."

Even horrendous crimes be washed away.
1240 Further, it protects us from future sins,
Fortifying and enlightening our souls.
If such valuable aid as God benignly
Gave us we now in one bitter day lack,
In how many diverse ways is our race
1245 Afflicted! How disturbing to the soul!
How many monstrous crimes would we commit!
No one would dare to place his confidence
In any other, nor could he feel sure
Of trusted guests, nor peaceful while asleep
1250 In company of his most faithful friend.
    Let us in brief define spoken confession.
Let us say that by this, moved with the hope
Of forgiveness, the sickness of the soul
Discovers its intimate, secret wounds.
1255 This rite began when Jesus Christ said that
In heaven would be forgiven all those sins
That on earth are remitted by the priest,
And there retained those that are here retained,
And telling his disciples to untie
1260 The ligatures of Lazarus,[40] and to those
Taking offerings to the temple that
They reveal their leprosy to the priests.[41]
In sum, the screeds of the ancient fathers
Confirm that God himself inspired the rite.
1265 Down on the knees, hands held up toward heaven,
The humble visage lowered to the ground,
With head uncovered, soul in reverence trembling,
The supplicant who has confessed his sins
Awaits his sentence from the priest and sees
1270 In him a heavenly power, and he entreats
God to forgive him and to grant him grace,
Grace that God enclosed in this sacrament
So that in it the keys to heaven are kept,
And that we should all know that without it
1275 None can be cleansed of mortal sin nor saved.
    Before all sin, and innocent of guilt,
None was obliged to holy penitence,
But afterward, it had to be practiced
Every year, or when danger of death
1280 Threatened, or if something had to be done
That does not correspond to guilt or sin,
Such as receiving holy communion
Or administering the sacraments,
Or when some fear well-founded us assails,

1285 Fear of forgetting sins we have committed,
And thus delays confession by a day.
    Confession must be prudent and entire,
If it is reticent or negligent,
Then the sacrament will be null and void,
1290 And the whole will have to be repeated.
Advisable it always is to cure
Our souls as soon as possible of all
Mortal ills with this holy panacea,
So that we do not live exposed to death
1295 And torments everlasting, which our words
Can never start to outline or describe.
    The minister most fit is he with power
To dispense this sacrament, by himself
Or a delegate of the priestly order,
1300 According to the jurisdiction, for
Those words, "The sins of whomsoever you
Shall pardon shall also by me be pardoned,"
Were spoken just to the apostles, from
Whom the ministers who in each place might
1305 Toil, impart there this forgiveness divine,
And only there dispense this sacrament.
For if all of the graces given us
By penitence originate in Christ,
Those who dispense them to us justly should
1310 Be those who offer us his holy body
As holy penitence will make us worthy
To take the sacred eucharistic host.
With zeal the ancient Church guarded those rights
Of ordinary priests; exact decrees
1315 Asseverate that they prohibit all,
Even bishops themselves, from transferring
Jurisdiction to someone else, except
When there are many faithful or some other
Serious reason requires it. Reader,
1320 Choose in the end for your confession,
A prudent priest and learned, and a man
Of probity without stain, who wisely
Directs your conduct toward an upright life.
    The priest may think that with sincere sorrow
1325 The confessor repents of all his sins,
And he reveres the Father, king of heaven
And for this precious gift he renders thanks,
Assistance begs against the poisoned darts
Of Satan's fierce attacks, and bitter wounds,
1330 Then there is not a day when he does not

---

40. John 11:44.

41. Probably not leprosy but impurity.

Meditate on Christ, his death and holy
Passion, and when he seeks not to reflect
On the saints' virtues and their blameless lives.
But if the penitent does not show true
1335 Repentance, then the priest will try to wake
In the soul sparks of sorrow for his sins,
And recognition of the divine gifts.
    To be reprehended without a doubt
Is the pride of those who apologize,
1340 Foolishly, shifting blame for sins to others.
Also condemned is the pernicious shame
Of one who dares not reveal sinful wounds
To the minister. Others are adrift
In such an ocean of wickedness that
1345 They cannot find what they must do and God
Has ordered them to do. They must be taught
How to examine their own faults, regret
And keep them in the forefront of the mind,
And taught to confess later to the priest;
1350 If they ensure that they confess as fully
As they can, it must be believed of them,
That once turned away they do not return,
A thing that at all costs must be avoided.
    To those who give signs of a wicked life
1355 And show themselves reluctant to confess,
May they be absolved with great caution, or
The priest may well defer the sacrament
Until a more opportune moment. And
If any, following the appearance of the crowd,
1360 Find it too hard to admit forgotten sins,
They must reminded be that there is none
Who recollects them all, that men sometimes
Know not even their own failings, and that
Not everything can be told to the priest
1365 In full completion and in words exact.
    The third and last part of this sacrament
Is restitution, which is also called
Definition, for the decree by which
It is ordained specifies that it must
1370 Completed be, fulfilled within a time
That is defined. To owners stolen things
Must be returned and recompense be made
For the damage done to them, and likewise
We have to pay for the things taken from
1375 The Lord our God, returning unto him
The love and honor we madly would not give.
Jesus Christ alone paid with his spilled blood;
But the first thing belongs to man and is

A debt that our poor powers cannot pass.
1380 Sin leaves a stain and guilt, which can be washed
By holy penitence alone, so that
Some pain that cleans upon us is imposed.
And if baptismal lymph removes such stains,
But holy penitence does not, this is
1385 The wise and just Lord's design, that if once
Clean, we dirty our souls and despoil what
Was once pristine, there may be then some pains
To show the sorrow it causes both us,
And Holy Church, likewise offended, in
1390 Visible manner honor fair be given.
Also he added such punishment that
Others would shrink from offending the Lord,
The punishment teaches them to fear guilt
And quake before the omnipotent whom
1395 They have offended. It is just, besides,
That Christ's divine semblance should radiate
In us, his mystic members, and with head
Encircled by a crown of thorns, we wish
To share his lacerations and his wounds.
1400 And also, if sin leaves guilt and a wound
And Jesus' vast piety cleanses them,
It is good that suffering cures our wounds
As a natural and apt panacea.
For though God is merciful, and the Lord
1405 Jesus Christ, who for our sake did assume
Human nature, cleanses our sins and guilt,
And frees us from the everlasting flames,
With fitting temporal penalties, men
Should still be punished as these transient pains
1410 Protect us from hell's infinite torments.
The reason for its efficacy is this:
That all flows from the death of Jesus Christ;
As also we succeed in deserving
By his precious blood, if we lead a life
1415 Of Christian virtue, full pardon for our
Sins, and last, the joy of felicity.
Whatever would spot the merit of Christ,
Would sooner shine with the brightest of lights,
For to that grace that his own merit earned
1420 Is added that which priests in us do pour
And so, by dying, conquest is achieved.
    One whose desire is to live in the grace
And amity of God must satisfy
Him for his guilt, even once-pardoned guilt,
1425 Mortifying himself in his gift and
Maintaining throughout life pains of his faults.

For offending God, his fellow, himself,
He must employ three medicines that cure
And combat them: very frugal food, gifts
1430 To the poor, and frequent prayer from the soul.
This is the piety with which the Lord
Views us, that unto others our merits
May reach, and in reciprocity, theirs
Reach out to us, in one community
1435 Of good for those who would have healthy souls.
      The priest does not neglect his exhortation
To urge the penitent prompt to restore
Things or honors robbed and will not absolve
Him unless and until he promises
1440 To do so, and the matter ascertains.
After that he imposes just penance,
Wise and appropriate to every sin,
And urges him to live a good, just life,
And the fountains of grace oft to approach,
1445 The living water offered us by Christ,
Where death is overcome and passions killed,
Sins are eradicated, life renewed,
And in divine love our souls are engulfed,
That we may know how Christ, so selflessly
1450 For our sake suffered cruel and bitter death.
      One first unction and the sacred water,
When we arrive in this world, reconcile
Us with the Lord, wiping from us the sin
Of Adam; one unction is then required
1455 When later we are about to depart.
This washes all our stains away and eases
Our return to the region whence the soul
One day came. This is a journey that we
Should never forget if we are prepared,
1460 Since anyone who meditates on death
Surrounded by the calm of night, and thinks
Again in the commotion of the day
Contemns it, and living a Christian life,
Looks forward to arrival tranquilly.
1465   That this is a sacrament none should doubt;
Although constituted of various parts,
It is one sole, and like the rest it flows
From the sides of Christ, from the bloody wound;
From the ancient Fathers' decree it is
1470 Clear that it cleanses the soul and must be
Considered a most holy sacrament.
      Its medium is the oil that the bishop
Has consecrated, symbolic of its
Wondrous effects: for it eases dolors,

1475 Returns lost health and vigor to the members,
The spirit comforts, strength restores, and thus
Provides a wholly new support to life.
Its form consists of the familiar prayers
Spoken by the priest on anointing each
1480 Member, a form established by the ancient
Fathers of the Church, which did carefully
Guard and practice it. And if this form is
Followed, all illness frequently will be
Absolved; but it expected cannot be
1485 That all grave illnesses will cease at once,
For God alone knows and determines them.
      Christ ordered this last unction and he bade
His followers to spread it through the world.
There is no need to give it to the hale
1490 Nor to those suffering from no serious ill,
Nor to those who have lost their sense or reason,
Nor to small children, innocents, who know
Nothing of guilt; neither to those who are
In mortal sin, unless they first confess
1495 To the priest and receive his absolution,
Which, by custom's imposition, must be
Preceded by holy communion.
And last, no one departs who does not see
With clearest eye that he has been anointed.
1500 It is not in the power of every man
To administer such a sacrament,
Only the priest, and then within his parish.
      Its merits are, in sum, that it gives us
The will to forge ahead, and it brings peace
1505 In body and in mind, when, with more rage
The Devil plagues us, and when at the last,
At death the serpent doubles his attacks,
With the result that, without Highest aid,
Our path of salvation would be imperiled.
1510   About the holy order now we speak,
For without this the other sacraments
Could never be fulfilled, or leastwise not
According to the proper rite. These men,
Illustrious men, with this ministry charged,
1515 Like those about to take the sacrament,
Revere the order, which sustains them all.
Its excellence is such that any man
Who holds this office represents our Lord.
Thus, God does not call everyone to such
1520 Great dignity, but only those who are
Predestined emissaries. No man moved
By flaming tongues of ambition's bright fire,

Nor any man who covets, dare aspire
To so sublime a charge, but only he
1525 Inflamed by love of Christ, and with desire
To serve his brothers better and the Lord,
For nothing worse is, nothing is more base
Than vilely to sell Jesus Christ for gold.
    The Church and all her ministers possess
1530 A double power: the holy order and
The jurisdiction, so the priesthood forms
One body mystical, which represents
The body of the Lord with distinct parts.
There is no doubt then that the holy order
1535 Is a true and high sacrament, by which
God on the priest confers the power to offer
Himself and his life to the Holy Lamb.
    The order is variety of men,
Diversely qualified, and with degrees;
1540 Tenor, and doctrine, and appropriate age
They must hold who aspire to holy orders.
Excluded from such service are all children,
All bastards, murderers, cripples and insane,
Because the priesthood serves the Church of Christ
1545 And all the faithful nourished by the Church
Inducted in the mysteries of the highest,
Led up to heaven's kingdom. Further, he
Belonging to this order has the power
To dispense all the other sacraments,
1550 The potency also, almost divine,
To consecrate the bread and wine, and thus
Convert them both into the living Christ.
    The laws of holy matrimony now
Let us explain, for this one sacrament
1555 Has to be counted as the solid base
Of perfect life for those who do not sleep
In solitary bed; lest any should,
Deluded by illusion's tempting call,
Be stained by lewdness vile, let us say then
1560 That matrimony is the tie that binds
A man unto a woman; which cannot
Be celebrated by those unfit, or
Disabled or illegitimate, but
Among those who are fit in all respects.
1565 It is a firm knot, indissoluble;
It is consecrated by Christ himself.
    Matrimony can be seen in two ways,

As nature's tie or purely human one,
And as a sacrament that exceeds all
1570 Terrestrial things and of such union makes
A holy bond. And as grace is the highest
Perfection of nature, thus matrimony
Is needed first to propagate our race
After this sacrament, which instituted
1575 Was by Jesus Christ—as clearly appears
In Genesis and in the holy councils—
As the knot that can never be untied,
Thus says the book: "Those whom the Lord has brought
Together, let no man put asunder."
1580 But when he said, "Go forth and multiply
And fill the earth," our Lord did not wish that
Everyone should be so obliged, without
Being so united, for the scripture
Praised the state of virginity above
1585 Matrimony, more perfect and more holy.
    It is full meet to say why man and woman
Should tie their lives together with this knot:
First to assist each other, then produce
Much valued offspring, heirs of heaven
1590 Who serve on earth and praise the Lord, their God.
An aid against temptations of the flesh,
This entails other gifts of great import;
And thus, seen as a holy sacrament,
Its excellence is greater, aims are higher.
1595 Marriage was there from our race's start,
The lineage of men extended long
Once God granted to it this dignity[42]
That thus the sphere of the earth would then be filled
With a race by his grace made noble,
1600 Faithfully obeying all his mandates.
That matrimony would a symbol be
Of his eternal love, God also wished,
And of that love with which Christ and his Church
Are loved, because no greater human love
1605 Than that between two spouses can exist.
    That matrimony is a sacrament
Declares the Church, and so Saint Paul confirms,
So said the ancient fathers in decree,
And so defines it the Council of Trent.[43]
1610 As such it is recommended to men
And mandated that they their spouses love

---

42. That is, once God granted to matrimony the "dignity" of a sacrament.

43. Concluded in December 1563.

With spotless love, as Jesus loved his Church
So much that for the Church he chose to die,
Suffering barbarous torture; and women,
1615   That they obey their husbands, as their heads,
As Christ heads the Church, his beloved spouse.[44]
For all which in this sacrament is grace
Given and is realized in it what is
Said by the holy Council: those whom God
1620   Has brought together shall always be one,
Faithful to one another, and so free
Of love illicit. How much better are
Our marriages today than those that were
Contracted in antiquity, is clear,
1625   For they refused the name of sacrament,
More wives than one the patriarchs took, and it
Was licit to reject some and take others,
All this for human ease and benefit.
By contrast today no man is allowed
1630   To have a wife or her repudiate
When another has been taken, although
Sometimes the laws will tolerate divorce,
For very serious and considered reasons.
      Of marriage children are the fruit, also
1635   At the same time its sign, safeguard, and strength.
For no man dares to unite with a rich
Or beautiful woman if he does not
Know her parents or if she has been forced.[45]
Neither contract a secret wedding nor
1640   Believe, by the deceitful demon's arts,
That any spouse must take at any time
A concubine t' indulge in lewd embrace;
Or think your wife is your slave, when she is
The companion with whom pure love unites.
1645   Thus in the end, when spouses leave this world,
They have holy matrimony's reward,
Together enjoying eternally
The love and glory of their sovereign Lord.

*Book 3: Of the Mandates of the Law,
and Sunday Prayer*

      The truths of faith that have to be believed
1650   To be united with God, good supreme,
We have attested, and we now declare
How much to us was given, the virtue of
Holy sacraments, since in this way each

And every faithful Christian may enjoy
1655   Knowledge of our faith and may come to see
With the mind's eye sublime mysteries divine.
Now will I sing the precepts of the law
Of God, if in my attempt he will grant
Enlightenment to me, that I may say
1660   What must be done to reach with zeal to own
The blessed life for all eternity,
And for ever enjoy God in his heaven.
As precious good is granted us by God,
And him with the whole soul we must obey,
1665   His law is easy, asks but filial love,
From which will grow the fruits of sanctity
And blessings of an honest life. For this
The soul entire to God must turn, for this
Secure may reign today, and later hold
1670   Eternal joy. Though reverence to the Lord
Requires us to obey his laws without
Expecting anything, he wished that such
Obedience would bring us great good and make
Us give our gratitude to Jesus Christ.
1675   You shall love your God and in him alone
Place all your trust: this is the supreme law.
But to the saints and their images pray,
Ask them for God's assistance and his grace
Your supplications to him they present,
1680   Obtain for you forgiveness of your sins.
For great is the mercy of God for those
Who love him, but they who forget him will
Endure eternal sorrow and great pain.
      When we are called upon to make an oath
1685   Before the omnipotent, not to things
That He has made, as witness of our acts,
We should swear by God in all our judgments,
Promises, covenants, and with the truth
And justice as the elder prophets sang.
1690   On the day consecrated to the Lord,
Rest calmly and to him due adoration
Render, the worship worthy of his great
And sacred majesty, with deeds devout.
Saturday was kept in the ancient law,
1695   Symbol and memory of past events,
But now we sanctify the day that Christ
Rose glorious from the deepest dark of hell
That he might live in everlasting triumph.
The Church commands us to observe that day.

---

44. See Eph. 5:23–25.

45. That is, forced into marriage.

1700 No work must be done on that day, for it
Is dedicated to worship of God,
And helping one's neighbor, or what can not
Be done on other days, when it is our
Virtue and our duty still to shun
1705 All diversions unworthy and malign.
        The first three commandments refer to God
And to holy worship of him, as we
Have seen above. What follows now concerns
Those that unite us in fraternal love.
1710   To your parents or to those in their place
Give love, and aid, obedience and respect,
And teach your children, be a good example,
Care for their good in soul and body both.
        Thou shalt not kill. If you are angered by
1715 Your brother, forgive his wrong with kindness,
Deny him not your help, remembering
That no one can in truth harm you except
Yourself with your own deeds, and how we are
All in pressing need of forgiveness, and
1720 That we are all obliged to follow Christ.
        Do not commit adultery, and despoil
The conjugal law, not even in thought;
Remain clean, free of all such wicked stain,
Faithful in soul and body to your spouse,
1725 Ignoring the perfidious pleasures that
All faithless, dishonest delights afford;
Adultery is a sin against the flesh,
Profanes the temple of the Holy Spirit,
Deceives the faith of matrimony, breaks
1730 The holy laws, and in ignoble death
Adulterers will be wretched criminals—
witness the words of Christ, of the woman
In adultery taken, in St. John[46]—
And last, for pleasure shameful and short lived,
1735 Their souls fall headlong to hell's deep abyss.
To prevent such a terrifying fate,
Avoid excess at table, and avoid
Excess wine, idleness, and sensual verse,
Conversation obscene and writings lewd,
1740 Contact with loose women, also excess
Of embellishment in your daily dress,
Practice holy fasting, and above all,
Ask for God's aid, and take the sacraments
Frequently. Thus will you banish the dread

1745 Monster of the flesh back to its lair.
        Thou shalt not steal what belongs to your brother,
Without trying to return it to him
As quickly as you can, no matter how
You took it, even without theft in mind.
1750 Stealing is a serious sin, and not
Erased until the goods have been restored.
But you, so far from stealing, proffer aid
To the aggrieved with charity and love.
        Do not speak ill of anyone, nor bear
1755 False witness, nor presume to tell a lie;
Speak always true, and be wise to speak up
When you should say in public what you know.
        Do not covet your neighbor's servants, fields,
Or land; do not pursue your neighbor's wife
1760 With lust; avoid thus dreadful punishments;
Without them live in peace and full content.
        And once the soul is well disposed, in faith
And justice confirmed, you will have to praise
God omnipotent, and in your own name
1765 And those of all your neighbors give him thanks,
And beg him also for his assistance,
That you may live according to his law
And reap thus precious fruits, today of peace,
Tomorrow bliss, sure of what he will grant,
1770 For he who raises his prayers up to God
From the deeps of his heart knows that he is
Enveloped by his love divine, and that
Faith constant and firm hope protections are
Against the snares and springes of the Devil.
1775   And what more efficacious prayer could be
Than that which Christ himself taught unto us?
Pray thus, he told us: Our Father, by whose
Divine and sovereign will we are raised up
From nothingness to life, may the Lord keep
1780 And redeem us, and save us, sending us
Legions of spirits celestial who are
Our guardians and companions attentive
Throughout our lives, and show to us the path
To bliss. May you, who see us commit sin,
1785 Tolerated or sometimes punished, yet
Always be moved to have mercy upon us,
Allowing us poor wretches to return
To your amity and your love and grace,
As we your children are loved by our parent

46. The episode of the woman taken in adultery occurs in John 8:1–11. Hernández's emphasis seems to require that Jesus condemns the sin of adultery.

1790 And Jesus' brothers by the holy waters;
      Of whom men say that you dwell in the heavens,
      But whose sovereign power rules the stars and earth
      And the deep oceans, penetrating all
      Is your holy presence, sustainer and
1795 The life of all that is, and without whom
      The globe entire would all at once collapse
      Into the abysses of nothingness:
      To your blest name glory, eternal honor
      May all beings render! And the devout
1800 In you the source of life will recognize,
      Giver of good and grace and love divine,
      Revere you above all, as lord supreme.
          May your reign come to us, justice and peace
      Reign sovereign in the world, with those great joys
1805 That come to us from Christ, the certain faith,
      Unconquerable love, and hope. May your
      Divine will prevail in us and extend
      Your gentlest empire to all human souls,
      Until the universe falls at your feet
1810 And Satan flees, deceits and traps frustrated.
      Thus after this long exile may we be
      In your celestial kingdom and our home.
          According to your will we may have all,
      Not according to ours by Adam's sin
1815 Darkened and diminished. We beg you, for
      Of all good you are the sole, unique source,
      And without you we will not attain bliss,
      Beset we are so many times by sins,
      Our souls by disquiet and daily toil.
1820 Thy will be done on earth as 'tis in heaven.
      Let the flesh cede, the spirit obey, and
      May both rejoice in esteeming your laws.
          Give us this day our daily bread with which,
      The body fed, the soul fulfils its duty.
1825 Because of the first sin the earth now turns,
      Once propitious for us, now hostile, hard,
      And bitter, and we earn our bread with sweat

      From our brows in accordance with your doom
      And your word. And if you benevolent
1830 Do not see us, all our work would be vain
      And all our undertakings useless too.
      And we do not pray, Father, for choice dishes,
      Only the sustenance that may renew
      Our drained strengths, restore warmth to our
          bodies,
1835 Exhausted by fatigue of daily toil.
      But also we pray for the bread, your word,
      And bread of Christ in the most sacred host,
      Which—as the body daily must be fed—
      We receive daily to sustain the soul.
1840   Forgive us for those errors we committed
      Against you, as we forgive those who harm
      Or injure us, for we offend you so,
      That your son suffered death upon the cross.
          Although the enemy tempts ceaselessly,
1845 Into temptation let our souls not fall,
      But to emerge victorious in the fight,
      Inspire us with your divine strength, for ours
      Without you cannot resist his attacks;
      You are our aid, protection, and our hope,
1850 And if you leave us, we are unarmed prey
      To the first strike of enemy attack.
      With your assistance we may now repel
      Assaults launched by the Devil, until we
      Enjoy at last your eternal abode.
1855   Deliver us from all evil. May it
      Never stain our souls with sin. May you look
      Upon us with kindness, and give us strength,
      That we may be apart from such disgrace,
      Suffer with patience sorrows and fatigues,
1860 Repel the dangers which do us waylay.
          All this, our Father, we implore of you
      And that your sovereign piety grant it us,
      In the name of Christ, always heard by you
      With love, whose intercession reaches all.

FIVE SPECIAL TEXTS:
CACAO, CHILI, CORN, TOBACCO, AND TOMATO

The five plants whose descriptions we place together in this section appear, hors de combat so to speak, taken from Hernández's manuscript drafts (BN MSS 22,436–22,139) and so represented in their fullest form. We have given these five a special place because they are plants that had an obvious, major impact on the world once they were exported from the Americas and because Hernández devoted much more space to these plants than to any others, on account of their alimentary, cultural, practical, and historical importance in New Spain. Furthermore, the various selections and editions of Hernández in the seventeenth century did not do justice to his narrative in these five cases.

Cacao

To speak of cacao is to bring to mind the great phases of human history. In the Old World and in primitive times, when people lacked the necessaries of life, which conse-quently had to be paid for, they would ask their neighbors for them but never paid with money. Gold and silver coin did not circulate yet; there were no graven images of cattle, kings, or princes. They lived by means of the barter system, as Homer sang,[1] with people providing one another with freshly picked fruit, until the day that coins with those thou-sand different images began to be minted. But signs of avarice never penetrated the New World, nor did ambition take root, until the arrival of our countrymen in their ships, brought here by the winds. The native inhabitants put no such value on gold and silver, which were plentiful. The most beautiful birds' feathers, cotton cloths, and precious stones, which this land produces naturally in abundance, constituted their most precious riches. The people of the pueblo knew only necklaces, bracelets, and armbands made of flowers, and to them these things[2] had no value. They went almost naked and lived a happy life, not preoccupied

---

1. The allusion is purely rhetorical.

2. Metals or metal objects.

by the future, by accumulating enormous amounts of treasure, or by increasing inheritances. They lived from day to day, following their inclinations and desires, in a modest state but tranquil and contented, and enjoying with great pleasure the best things that nature has to offer.[3] The seed of the cacao tree served instead of money, and this is what they used to buy things, when necessary, a practice that still survives in quite a few places.

And what is so strange about this, considering that in the kampongs of the east shells or the leaves of various trees and other things are all used in place of money? The markets were filled with this cacao seed, with which they carried on their commerce, and by means of a simple seed, goods changed hands. They also made from it a drink, since they had never discovered a way of making wine, even though in their woods all sorts of wild vines (of which we will speak in their places) grew, twined around trees and shrubs with their tendrils and racemes of different colors, sometimes bowing under their own weight. This most famous seed, which even today is a substitute for wine as well as money, we shall describe now, beginning with the tree itself. The cacahoaquáhuitl is a tree about the size of a citron tree, and with similar leaves, except that these are larger and wider, with oblong fruit that looks like a large melon, but striped and red, called cacahoacentli, which contains the seed, cacáhoatl, which as we said, serves for money among the Mexicans and makes a very pleasant drink. It is made of a blackish substance divided into unequal particles but well accommodated, tender, nourishing, quite sharp, slightly sweet, moderate or somewhat cold and moist in nature. As far as I know there are four varieties of this tree: the first, called quauhcacáhoatl, is the biggest of them and has the largest fruit; the second, the mecacacáhoatl, is of medium size, spread out, and with

fruit that follows the first kind in size; the third, known as xochicacáhoatl, is small, with small fruit, whose seed is reddish on the outside and like the rest inside; the fourth, which is the smallest of the four and is thus called tlalcacáhoatl, or "little," gives the smallest fruit, but is still the same color as the others. All of these varieties have the same nature and can be used interchangeably, although the last one is used more for drinks, just as the others are more suitable and convenient as money. The quauhpatlachtli will also be considered a member of this genus of trees, but it is a larger tree, with bigger leaves, fruit, and seeds, which are sweeter than the others and can be eaten like almonds, roasted or with sugar, although they are less suitable for making a drink. That drink, made from the cacáhoatl seed with the addition of nothing else at all, is commonly administered to the seriously ill, to mitigate heat, just as it is also given to those suffering from a hot disorder of the liver or of any other part. Four grains mixed with one ounce of a gum called holli[4] and drunk, are an admirable cure for dysentery; but they should first be roasted, the gum as well as the seeds, which are so fatty that oil comes out of them, while the gum is sticky and extremely glutinous. Excessive drinking of cacao brings with it numerous illnesses and diseases, because it obstructs the intestines, damages and destroys the person's color, and among those who use it to excess, it usually causes cachexia and other very serious diseases. But because so many drinks, both simple and compound, are commonly made from cacao, and are not prepared in any one manner, nor with the same ingredients, except that they are mixed with the flowers or other parts of plants that have been ground into powder, it will not be out of place if we pause a moment to describe them.[5] The first drink that we shall describe is known as atextli, or thin paste; it is a simple made from about a hundred grains

3. This paragraph is as close as Hernández ever comes to the trope representing the New World as an image of paradise. A text such as this would almost certainly have been cause for censorship after 1577. Columbus thought in 1493 that he had found the earthly Paradise (see Elsa Malvido, "Illness, Epidemics, and Displaced Classes in Sixteenth-Century New Spain," n. 4, in *Searching for the Secrets of Nature*).

4. Holquáhuitl, or holli tree (*Castilloa elastica* Cervantes).

5. In the *Quatro libros* Ximénez added, "And record their existence in contrast to what has already been written by Doctor Barrios with

more style and elegance." The reference is to a treatise by Juan Barrios usually known as *Del chocolate,* published in Mexico City in 1609. No original copy of this work is known to have survived. What appears to be most of the text is reprinted in Antonio de León Pinelo's *Question moral si el chocolate quebranta el ayuno eclesiastico* (Madrid, 1636), fols. 116–22, which can be supplemented by further quotations from the treatise in Gaspar Caldera de Heredia, *Tribunal, Medicum, Magicum, et Politicum* (Leiden: Elsevier, 1658), 468–76.

of raw or roasted cacáhoatl, well ground and mixed with as much Indian grain,[6] softened in a way that we will explain elsewhere, as will fit in the space of two cupped hands. But if a compound is desired it can be made with the further addition of the fruits, mecaxóchitl, xochinacaztli, and tlilxóchitl (plants that are described in the appropriate places),[7] also ground, the mixture then being stirred for a suitable time. Before it is drunk it should be poured from a considerable height into another container, until it produces a foam and the fatty particles, much like oil, rise to the top. Then you can drink just the lighter and more pleasant portion, or taste both parts separately, and hence with more pleasure. The property of the compound is that it excites the sexual appetite; the simple refreshes and nourishes very much. Another kind of drink is made with twenty-five grains of cacahoapatlachtli, which will be discussed in its place, as much cacáhoatl, and a handful of Indian grain; no other ingredients are usually added, because they are hot, and cooling and nourishment are sought in this drink. The third kind of drink, called chocóllatl, is made with grains of póchotl and cacáhoatl in equal quantities, and they say that it puts on extraordinary amounts of weight if it is used frequently. Both grains are mixed together, put in a vessel, and stirred with a wooden whisk until the fatty part floats and is airy. That part is then skimmed off and set aside. Added to the mixture then is a handful of the aforesaid Indian grain that has been softened; when the drink is ready to be taken, return the fatty part to it, and, finally, drink it lukewarm. They administer this, with great success, to consumptives, the underweight, and the emaciated. Another drink called tzone is made from equal amounts of Indian grain and cacáhoatl both roasted, then boiled with a small amount of the same grain softened, to act as a thickener. This serves as a refreshing food, not as medicine. Planted next to the quauhcacáhoatl to give it shade is the tree called atlinan, which has, to my knowledge, no other use, a picture of which we shall also provide. The cacahoaquáhuitl grows in warm or hot areas, in marshy, wet, or humid places.

Chili

Chili, or Mexican pepper, is the plant that produces those pods that the Haitians call *ajies* and that were known, according to some, by the ancients as peppers. The Spanish call them peppers of the Indies. It was taken a long time ago to Spain, where it is highly esteemed and where it is cultivated in gardens and tubs as an ornamental and as a useful plant. However, since there are many varieties among the Indians and it is used every day as an appetizer and as a condiment, scarcely a table is without it and since its many properties are known from daily experience, I have decided not only to discuss the varieties that grow in New Spain, which I will soon treat below, but also all the species that have come into our hands. I will illustrate them in drawings, describe their structure and leave for posterity an account of their properties and nature.

I shall say, then, that the leaves of all of the species are similar and that they are the same as those of the solanum except for the quauhchilli, which has smaller leaves. The flowers of the chili plant are white and from these grow pods, which in the beginning are green and afterward become a reddish color for the most part and finally take on the color of a raisin. They are full of small seeds. These seeds are flat, whitish, smooth and round. They are of bitter taste and of a burning nature—all this comes from the seed. They can reach the fourth degree of heat and are also dry to the third degree. When they are fresh, they abound in a certain "excremental" humor, which later almost completely disappears. They encourage flatulence and stimulate the sexual appetite, and at the same time soften the belly, not without a certain difficulty in urinating and a sensation of pain, especially for those who are unaccustomed to this condiment. We may say with good reason that the burning sensation is also the cause of this pain.

The chili plant also causes urination and brings on menstruation in women. It strengthens the stomach that has suffered coldness and it helps digestion if that has been hindered by cold. It stimulates the appetite when prepared

---

6. Corn.

7. Xochinacaztli is known in Spanish as "flor de oreja" or "orejuela." Tlilxóchitl is vanilla.

in a salsa with so-called tomame, and purges phlegmatic humors from all parts, but especially those that adhere to the joints of the hips. Some say that it is an effective remedy for consumptives, if the abdomen and the sides of the body are pricked with sharp objects that have been rubbed with chili. Some also say that they provide considerable nutritional value, both hot and dry, but that they can irritate the kidneys and inflame the blood and liver, sometimes causing kidney disease, illness of the brain and the pleura, pneumonia and other internal inflammations, eruptions and other similar symptoms. This occurs when they are used without moderation or very frequently as food, as the Indians, for whom it is a condiment, use it.

Going on to describe the particular species, we can say that the first of these is called quauhchilli by the Mexicans, that is to say tree chili. For the Haitians, ⟨the fruit⟩ is smaller and rounder, and the plant is smaller as well. It is called among them, chili from the woods. This is the smallest of all the chilis and is very similar in shape and size to tribacas olives.[8] All of the types of chili reach almost the fourth degree of heat. However, this one is the hottest of all. It is therefore used both as condiment and not as a condiment. It is mixed with other sauces instead of pepper. It grows year-round.

The second type is called chiltecpin, named after the mosquito because of its small size and color. Others refer to it as totocuitlotl, that is to say, bird dung. Among the Haitians, it is called "huarahuao" which sometimes seems even more "hot" ⟨to me⟩ than the first. However, it loses its color sooner. But there are three varieties of this type, differing only by the location in which they are produced and the season when they are harvested. The first is most common. The second, similar to the first, but darker, is called tlilchilli or "black chili." The third and last type is the smallest of all and follows in size from the second type which is of medium size. It is planted in the month of September and is harvested from December until the beginning of April. The third type is called tonalchilli, or chili of the sun. It is

usually planted in those places that are watered when the rains have already ceased, that is to say in August and September. It produces fruit from November to March. The Haitians call this "white chili." It is green at first, then yellowish, then orange, and finally it turns red like all the other types. The fourth type is called chilcoztli because of its saffronlike color which gives its color to the other ingredients with which it is used.

It is also called saffron chili for the same reason among the Spaniards who occupy the island of Haiti. It is about six or seven fingers long. It is somewhat thin and reddish while turning at times to the color of a raisin. It is planted in December and harvested from August until the end of the year. The fifth type is called tzinquauhyo because it is from the woods. It is called coral by the Haitians because of its shape and color. It is thin and about five fingers long. It is planted in March and is harvested all year long. The sixth type is called texochilli or dough chili because of its softness. It is long and wide with a certain sweetness, bitterness of taste and red color. It has a light spiciness, and is usually eaten with corn or with tortillas, that is, pancakes made from Indian grain. This type is called pocchilli when it is dried and smoked in order to preserve it for all year long. If this is not done, it quickly rots because of its excessive excremental humor. It can be planted and will grow at any time of the year. There is yet another type of chili known as milchilli, not smaller than the previous type but it tapers to a thin sharp point. This one also turns red in its final stage. It has its name because it is usually planted and collected at the same time that corn is planted and harvested.

I do not want to spend more time on the other species of chili that can grow in Haiti, among them the Spanish, whose fruit is similar in shape, color, and size to the blackberry or to our sweet cherries. This grows on a medium-size bush. There are two other kinds that the natives call, because of their similarity, pineapple point and bird's beak. The same goes for the maboyamboniada, the corniculada, the cacica, the hortense and all those whose history is more complex

---

8. Unidentified. As José M. López Piñero, José Luis Fresquet Febrer, María Luz López Terrada, and José Pardo Tomás point out (*Medicinas, drogas y alimentos vegetales del Nuevo Mundo: Textos e imágenes españolas que los introdujeron en Europa* [Madrid: Ministerio de Sanidad y Consumo, 1992], 265 n. 454), tribaca is a learned word of Greek origin meaning "exhausted" or "ruined," and in Latin it signified an eardrop made of three pearls, but it has nothing to do with olives.

than useful and that I believe I need not bother my readers with. All of these types grow in warm areas as well as cold or mild ones, but they grow more abundantly in temperate or warm areas.

Corn, or Maize, and the Drinks and Varieties of Tortas That Are Prepared with It

How extraordinary it is that, in the origins of the world and the crude beginning of time, all the appropriate things for comfortable living had already been discovered. And lacking wheat, that wonderful find and a gift from mother nature as precious as health itself, people had to resort to acorns and barley, with which today we fatten hogs and the most wretched animals. But let us consider that even in our time some people feed themselves on rice and millet bread, others on the pods of certain trees, others on the more familiar yucca, others still on the ilianthus and guaiaris,[9] and finally—not to stretch this into an interminable list—others live on tlaolli, which our countrymen call Indian wheat, and the Haitians call maize. But I do not say this to denigrate tlaolli, for, so far from condemning it, I praise it highly, and I do not understand how the Spanish, always diligent imitators of all things foreign, who know so well how to exploit other people's inventions, have still neither adapted for their own use, nor attempted to plant and cultivate this species of grain. Used properly, it is exceedingly beneficial to the healthy and sick alike; it is easy to cultivate, it grows abundantly and without any risk almost anywhere it is planted, and is hardly susceptible to damage from drought and all the rest of the rigors of the climate; and by means of this grain it is possible to relieve hunger and all the ills that derive from hunger. And in case anyone is surprised that there are people who can live without ever using wheat, who can feed themselves and live healthy and pleasant lives with foreign and almost unknown foods such as tlaolli, we may safely say that in Mexico it is important and continues to be used not just among the Indians but also among the Spanish. We shall say then that tlaolli, which we call maize (the more familiar and more common word for it)—for some

people today a Turkish grain, for others more properly an Indian one, and whose form we shall not discuss because it is known almost all over the world—comes in many varieties, distinguished by color, size, and the sweetness of the grains that cover the ears. They are mostly found with white kernels, but they also come in yellow, black, purple, pink, blue, or multicolored; and finally there are others, which, although they have white grains like buds, grow much larger, more tender, and in spears three times the size. All these varieties can be seen in images taken from living specimens here in my books. It is planted in March, with four or five seeds sown in holes one pace apart, and it is turned back into the earth in November, December, and January, when the ground is worked again; but depending on the different regions, which among these Indians vary a great deal over a short distance, owing to the situation of the land and to the nearly equal length of day and night, the crop is harvested later or earlier and is then threshed and stored. It is mild, or inclining a little toward hot and moist, of moderate substance, easily digested by all who are used to it, not coarse, not obstructive or viscous (an opinion held by some), which is obvious if we recognize that the Indians themselves live on this grain in the form of tortillas, and that they do not experience any obstruction, nor do they appear pallid. These people affirm that they have no feeling of heaviness in the stomach after their meals, only that after a few hours they are hungry again, just as if they had ingested nothing at all, and given the chance, they avidly fall to eating again as if they had never eaten before, or nominally at least, before the arrival of the Spaniards. But besides this, there is not among the Mexicans any foodstuff more common or more convenient for treating those suffering from serious illnesses; the way they prefer it is as an infusion, whose efficacy has been tried and tested thousands of times.

They say that this tlaolli is rapidly digested, that it is sufficient nutrition in itself, that it produces no sensation of heaviness, that it calms the stomach and chest, that it reduces the heat of a fever, especially if taken in the form of powder dissolved in water, the way the chemists prepare it, to provoke urine and cleanse the passages—in short, to clean

---

9. Possibly *helianthes* (Pliny's term) and *Rajania cordata* L., respectively.

the whole system. As it is abundant then in so many different grades of quality if it is prepared properly, and does not occasion any damage (unless, as one may admit, to those who produce an excess of blood and bile), we cannot agree with those who say that it is more hot than wheat, difficult to digest and assimilate, and that it causes obstructions in the passages; I would rather commend the Mexican doctors who dismiss infusions of barley on the grounds that they taste unpleasant and repugnant to the sick, preferring a gruel made of maize, which they call atolli. As used by these people, atolli is agreeable, harmless, and provides a pleasant and healthy food.

Let me explain right away, and as succinctly as possible, all the different ways of preparing these gruels for the healthy and sick alike, and I will leave until the next chapter the method of preparing tortillas from this same grain. I begin with nequatolli or atolli with honey, to which they add lime, such that there are eight parts water to six parts of this Indian grain, and one of lime; it is all put in an earthenware pot and placed over a low flame until it is tender; then it is taken off the heat, covered with linen, and finally ground in the stone known as metlatl; it is cooked slowly in an earthenware vessel until it begins to condense or thicken, and at that moment they add a tenth part of honey of maguey (which will be discussed in its place), and at the end it is taken off the boil as long as necessary to achieve the consistency of porridge, or Spanish polenta. This is cooling and moistening for those suffering from a hot, dry fever; it calms the chest, is very nutritious, strengthens and fattens the emaciated, and restores lost strength; it also cleans the body and is suitable food for the sick. Even to those who suffer from consumption this can be administered in the same form as a barley tisane, and is a great aid for those who pick up very serious illnesses. Some add Indian pimento in small quantities, but only when the healthy have to take it, or those not suffering from a hot fever, and made this way it tastes better and stimulates the sexual appetite. The Indians use this food at any time of day or night, be they healthy or sick, but mainly in the morning, and accompanied by something to drink. The Spanish have also begun to savor it, but mainly those born of Spanish and Indian parents, or Indians and negroes, or negroes and Spanish. (To what depths of vileness have our customs sunk that such diverse races can unite in vice!) They prepare in the same way as described above another kind of atolli called iztac or white, but when already done and served in the pots from which it is to be taken, they put green chili on top, with the so-called tomame, and salt to taste, all mixed and diluted with water, although some people consider the natural juices sufficient. They are also in the habit of preparing the so-called atolli agrio, which the Mexicans call xoxoatolli, mixing a pound of yeast or sour dough with two pounds of maize softened and ground as described above; the yeast is prepared with black maize, made into dough in the same way, which is then kept for four or five days until, eventually, the atolli has a suitable acidity. Once served, it has salt and chili added to it, and it is taken this way in the morning by the sick, so that it will clean the body, provoke urine, and purge the stomach. With the same yeast dissolved in fresh water and drunk, the body is cooled when it has become too hot, or tired from travel or work, or when the kidneys have been so irritated that the urine causes burning and ulcerates the urinary tracts.

White atolli, which the Mexicans call yollatolli, is made in the following way: the maize is cooked, as described above, but without lime or anything else; it is then formed into a mush, cooled, and diluted with water so that it can be drunk, the same as the agrio that I mentioned earlier. They say that this slakes the thirst—whatever the cause—and that it prevents the danger of having to swallow vast quantities of water. The chillatolli or atolli mixed with chili, as its name indicates, is made like the others, but with the addition—when it is cooked this way—of a quantity of chili diluted to the taste of the person who is going to take it. It is drunk mostly in the morning as protection against cold, tones up the stomach, aids digestion, gets rid of lingering phlegm, and clears the kidneys of all their imperfections. They also prepare nechillatolli, or atolli mixed with chili and honey, the same way as the others, but adding to it when it is half cooked these said ingredients, again according to taste. It augments thus the natural vigor and excites the sexual appetite. There is another species of atolli called ayocomollatolli, which is an atolli with beans and small pieces of dough. This one is made by adding chillatolli, epazotli, and the pieces of dough when it is all half cooked, and finally, when it is nearly done, whole cooked beans. It constitutes a splendid and most pleasant food, and by virtue of the epazotli, it purges the blood and raw humors. Chianatolli is described in the chapter on chia, but its name persuades me to include it here among the varieties of this drink. It is prepared from chia seeds, which are toasted lightly in a pan or a so-called comalli, then reduced to a powder and kept in this form all the year round. This powder is mixed with water and stirred until it acquires the necessary intensity to please the palate. Some people take it in this, the simplest style; others add chili to it before drinking it. Without chili, it soothes heat caused by fever or some other cause; it relieves walkers, especially in warm areas, and it is useful to all who take it as a most agreeable food. There is another kind of drink called chiantzotzolatolli, from a larger seed, of which we will talk in its place; it is prepared in a similar manner and serves the same uses, but this seed does not keep, and for this reason is only rarely used.

They also prepare michuauhatolli, that is, atolli with seeds of the michihoauhtli (of which, also, I will speak at the appropriate moment) by toasting the seeds, grinding them to a powder, mixing them with enough water so that the consistency is not too thick, and sprinkling it all with cooked maguey honey (they make three different kinds of honey from maguey, of which more in its place). It cleans the kidneys and the urinary tract, cures scabies in children, thanks to its purifying quality, and is a food among these people. There is likewise the tlatonialtolli, which mixes a small quantity of maize and a larger amount of dried, pulverized pimento, added to epazotli, and all put on the fire until this herb is cooked, which happens quickly; and it is drunk hot; it excites the sexual appetite, provokes urine and menstruation, and warms and fortifies the whole body. Neither must we omit the tlaxcalatolli, prepared from ground maize, and made in the comalli into tortillas as thick as three fingers; when these are well cooked, the skin is taken off, it is mashed into crumbs, blended with cold water and returned to the heat, stirred until it begins to thicken, taken out, served in bowls and eaten with a spoon; it revives and increases the strength admirably.

Even the cob, stripped of all its grains, charred and reduced to ashes, is commonly used to make olloatolli. This is ground, mixed in the proportion of one part to three parts corn, ground again all together, and put on the fire until the atolli is well cooked and has the consistency of polenta; it is served in bowls and chili put on it. It is of use to those with an excess of blood or heat. There is also, from corn cooked in common lye, the so-called quauhnexatolli; the corn is left in the lye long enough to soften it; it is purified thus and acquires a special flavor quite distinct from all the others; it is then ground, and cooked like the rest until it acquires the right consistency. Taken thus, they say, it purifies the blood although it has no other function, either medicinal or alimentary. There follows the izquiatolli, which is prepared from corn that is roasted and ground, but with a little bit of boiled corn added to it before it is all cooked again, and stirred all together until it is thick enough; with a little chili added to it first, people drink it who have weak hearts or such an excess of atrabilious humor that they are almost always melancholy. There are also hoauhatolli, which is made with strawberry blite and is drunk sprinkled with honey, and the michihozuatolli, which is prepared with michihouahtli mixed with a kind of blite that some people call a symphony on account of the harmony of its various colors. Of the diverse kinds of polenta and mush used in antiquity, others have already said enough; and having surveyed them all, I decided to write only about the things that are familiar to the New World, but are still not sufficiently known in ours.

How Bread Is Made from Corn

They soften corn in the manner I have described above, then grind it, and in their hands they form thin, medium-sized round tortillas, which they cook straight away in a comalli over hot coals. This is the most common method of preparing bread from corn. Some people make tortillas that are three or four times as large, and thicker. They make balls of dough about the size of a melon and cook them in a pot over the fire, sometimes adding beans. They eat these with great pleasure, for they are easy to digest and taste very good. Some make these breads one span long and four inches thick, mixed with beans and put in the comalli. Socially important Indians use corn to prepare tortillas, so smooth and paper-thin that they are nearly transparent, and small corn cakes that, despite their density are in fact translucent; but these things are only for the rich and powerful. But the bread that is cooked on a barbecue is unpleasant. Not far north of Mexico City live the Chichimeca, a fierce, barbarous and indomitable people. They roam through the hills and woods, partially covered with animals skins, feeding themselves by hunting and gathering, picking the fruits of wild trees as if they were animals. When these people want to eat meat, they hollow out a hole in the ground and fill it with red hot stones, and they wrap the meat in cornmeal, then put another layer of hot stones on top of that, and cover everything with earth; they leave it like that for as long as necessary to cook the meat perfectly. It is cooked when they take it out, and they love their bread cooked this way. This method began to catch on among the Spanish residents of Mexico, so I was able to experiment a bit myself; it is no secret that it is delicious. Let us say, finally, that toasted corn on the cob, or cooked with meat, either way is really good to eat.

Tobacco

The yetl is a plant with a short, thin and fibrous root, whose thin stems are five or more spans in length. The stems are villous, disordered, elongate and straight. The leaves are wide, oblong, and to a certain degree similar to henbane. Its flowers are like those of the henbane; when they fall, they leave berries or capsules full of seeds.

The Haitians call this plant tobacco—the same name that was transmitted not only to the Indians but also the Spanish—because the aromatic smoke of incense with this plant added to it is also called tobacco. Some among us call this "the holy weed"; others, nicotiana. But there is not just one species of this plant: there is another, called quáuhyetl, which has small white flowers. The stem is round and the leaves are straight and long. Both taste bitter and are hot and dry in the fourth degree, from which arises the error that these plants are cold, and that they belong to the varieties of henbane. Because even though they are not in form or shape very different from dark henbane, they are nonetheless opposite in properties. While they do cause sleepiness or drowsiness, this does not come from the cold or moistness

which of course they do not have, but rather from the heat, which excites the vapors that go to the head and induce sleep.

Let us turn now to the properties that are well known from daily experience. The leaves are put out to dry, and then they are rolled in the shape of a cylinder, wrapped with paper and shaped into tubes and lit. They are then smoked through the mouth or the nose. The smoke is inhaled through the mouth or the nose, closed so that the smoke may penetrate all the way to the chest. This causes expectoration and is good for asthma, a most miraculous cure. It is also good for respiration problems and related difficulties. But this smoke is not only good for these sicknesses but is also a good remedy for prolapse of the uterus. It gives strength to the head; it induces sleep; it relieves pains and rejuvenates the stomach. It cures headaches; it relieves sorrows and difficulties, and relaxes the spirit so much that one could say it is almost inebriating. Fresh leaves softened with oil are heated and applied to the top of the stomach and on the corresponding part of the back, but not to the level of the lungs, which they might irritate and inflame. This plant helps indigestion and cures surfeits to a notable degree. With each application it reduces inflammation of the spleen and the colon, together with pains caused by cold. It also cleans cancerous and chronic wounds, which can be cauterized with a few drops of the juice of the crushed leaves of this plant. One can also sprinkle wounds with the powder, which is obtained from the dried leaves of the plants. It can also be used on head wounds, provided the nerves and bones have not been injured. It is good for toothache. A small amount of tobacco is used to wrap the tooth, thus relieving the pains of the damaged tooth. The powder of the leaves is inhaled and taken through the nose, and this allows one not to feel the pain of whipping, and other afflictions of this type. It augments vigor and rejuvenates the spirit, to enable people to carry out work and other tasks. Those who take an amount about the size of a nut from the bark of the plant become intoxicated to the point that they lose consciousness and are almost half dead.

Those who use it too frequently, that is to say more than they should, suffer from discoloration. Their tongues become dirty and they suffer from palpitations in the throat, and from a burning sensation in the lungs, and finally die from cachexia and dropsy. However, those who use it moderately rid themselves of many maladies. Besides being very good for curing the French disease, it is also a good antidote for wounds from poisoned arrows. The wound is covered with tobacco powder, and left there until the powder and the wound unite and coagulate like a plug. This remedy comes from the cannibals of the islands near Haiti, who, when they receive poisoned arrow wounds from their enemies, use this herb. This is the only herb they had—and this is confirmed by the inhabitants of San Juan, in Puerto Rico, who, when they fought with these Indians and had received many arrow wounds, were able to escape death only because of this antidote to poison, in all those cases in which the arrows had not penetrated the guts. And I also learned from the Spaniards that this plant calms pains in the limbs and reduces inflammations, and that it takes away flatulence, disperses chronic and seemingly incurable pains, and that it is good for the various problems caused by fleas. What one has to do is sprinkle the house with a decoction of the leaves. It is cultivated in the same way as lettuce, and likewise is transplanted and cultivated in any land that is mild and humid. Prepared with dry leaves that have been mixed in the proportion of ten parts to one of lime, it is a highly praised medicament among the Indians, to the degree that their markets are full of this medicinal herb. Wrapped in a corn husk and placed between the mouth and cheeks, it produces a sweet sleep and tranquil repose of the senses and of the mind. It relieves men of their problems and readies them for whatever work they have to do, especially for walking. It is a good treatment for the stomach as well as for toothaches. It is also useful in other ways that we have not mentioned but that we can infer. Among those worthy of mention is the oil that the leaves have been fried in, as a cure for colic. Its juice mixed with tlilzápotl pits and wine, applied to the anus, is good for quartan fevers and for all feverish shivers.

Tobaccos That Are Used on the Island of Hispaniola, Which the Mexicans Call Picietl

On the island of Hispaniola they call "tobaccos" certain hollow pieces of cane, a span and a half in length, which on the outside are smeared with charcoal dust and on the inside are filled with tobacco and liquidambar (or xochiocotzotl), and also with other hot and aromatic things. These, when they are lit at the end where they are full, discharge smoke at the other; when the smoke is drawn in through the mouth, it gently induces mild euphoria, getting rid of the stress of travail and fatigue. In addition to this, by means of this benefit it gets rid of all pains, primarily those of the head; and helps one spit out the phlegm that usually runs down [inside] the chest, which is what usually engenders asthma. It comforts the stomach, but one should avoid its excessive use because often it greatly distempers the liver, burdening it with excessive heat, which is the cause of cachexia, poor condition of the body, and other incurable ills.

Tomato or, the Plant of Acid Fruit

Apart from the other species of solanum, which we will discuss among the plants of Europe, there are in this world other fruits called tomato because they are round and enclosed in a skin. They are dry and cold in the first degree and they contain a certain degree of acidity. The biggest of these are called xitomame, that is to say, tomame with the shape of a rough squash. The smallest are the miltomame which is to say the planting type—the type used for cultivation because they are usually planted at the same time as corn. Some of the first type are beautiful, a little bit bigger than nuts; they are green and later they turn yellow. They are called coatomame or "snake tomatoes." Others are of the same shape and size but in their later stages turn red. Still others turn yellowish to green to red and they are about the size of the eggplant, with each side slightly compressed and irregularly rough from the part that adheres to the stalk toward halfway down the middle. Others turn red when they are completely ripe. First, they turn green, then yellow, and then red. They are almost the same size and shape as the former. But in addition to being rough, they also have some irregular protuberances. Among the smaller varieties are those the size of nuts that are encased in a skin like a bladder, from which comes their name.

Among the smaller varieties, there are some about the same size as nuts and of a green color. Others are called yzhoatomatl which are larger than almonds, but smaller than walnuts and are encased in a skin like a bladder. They go through various stages from green to yellow or purple. Then there are those called miltomame, which are the size of almonds and the same color as the previous ones. Among these, we have the coztomatl and the tomatl, which are called xalatlacence in reference to the place where they grow. These are full of small seeds and they are counted among the principal medicaments with the character of heat.

There are other species that we will treat separately. They have proper names and a special nature. From the ones that we have seen above, they all seem similar to those of the solanum and even more to their species. But those that give the largest fruit also have larger and serrate leaves and the smaller ones have smaller fruit. In summary, the shape of the plant and its membranes all correspond respectively to the species Solanum. With respect to food, one can use them either in ground form or mixed with chili to make a very agreeable sauce that improves the flavor of many dishes and at the same time stimulates the appetite. By its nature, it is cold and dry and somewhat piquant.

Both its leaves as well as the fruit of the plant are effective when they are rubbed on the body. It can be used against St. Anthony's Fire.[10] It can cure blocked tear ducts and headaches. It is also good for stomachaches and heartburn and when used with salt, it is good for reducing mumps. The juice of this fruit is good for throat inflammation and it is also good for curing spreading sores when it is used with white lead, rose oil and lead oxide. For sinuses one mixes it with bread. As a remedy for the children's irritation called psoriasis,[11] it is mixed with rose water; it is added bit by bit to eye drops; it is mixed with egg to cure acute fluxes and, instilled in the ear, it cures earache. When applied with a bandage, it controls excessive menstrual flow and when it is mixed with chicken dung and applied with a wick, it is an excellent remedy for sinusitis. It grows anywhere—but especially in hot terrain where it grows either wild or cultivated.

Coztómatl, or Yellow Tomato

The coztómatl, or yellow tomato, has a thick, long, white root filled with shoots. It has tawny stalks and leaves like a nightshade's, to which species [it belongs], and a yellow flower, from which the name comes. Its fruit is covered by certain small bladders. The root is bitter and hot; it cures surfeit, dissipates wind, provokes urine; applied to the chest it relieves asthma [and] gets rid of pain in the belly, when it has been mixed with chili pods. When a decoction of it is drunk, or the root itself [taken] in the quantity of two oboli, it restrains fluxes of the bowels born of a hot cause; and when it is applied to the nipples [of a woman], it dries up milk. Moreover, it is usual to drink it a day after having taken tlalcuitlaxcolli, which we shall deal with in its own place [in this book], in order to strengthen and comfort. It grows in temperate lands such as Mexico in cultivated, moist places.

Huitztomatzin or Spiny Tomato

The huitztomatzin which some call huitztómatl and others neixpopoaloni meaning "that which cleans the eyes" is a bush with thick ramified roots, from which spiny stems grow four palms long. Its leaves are similar, up to a point, to spinach leaves. They are velvety and whitish on their undersides. The flower is purple with certain yellow filaments. It is there that they produce their fruit, which is similar to white cherries. The root is bitter, sharp and hot, almost in the third degree. Its bark, when mashed and drunk in a dose of half an ounce with water, evacuates all the humors by the inferior route. It is good for fevers, difficulty in breathing, and dropsy. It grows in the cold and humid regions of Témuac and Amaquemeca in level areas. There is another plant that is called, properly speaking, neixpopoaloni and is very similar to this same kind but it is taller, and has no spines or flowers. It is not bitter, and is astringent and cold. It takes its name from its virtue of cleaning the eyes.

---

10. Any one of a number of skin diseases, such as erysipelas.

11. Or any rash on a child's scalp.

QUATRO LIBROS DE LA NATURALEZA

The first substantial selection of the writings of Hernández to appear in print was the *Quatro libros* (Mexico City, 1615). Copies of this book are relatively scarce. We have collated copies at the Henry E. Huntington Library, British Library, and the Biblioteca Nacional and have found no sign of variant printings. Comparison of this Spanish text with the corresponding Latin of the Hernández manuscripts in Madrid demonstrates the obvious: the text of the *Quatro libros* is evidently corrupt, with frequently distorted syntax, omitted words, erratic punctuation, and eccentric spellings of the names of plants. Rival editions of the book were published in 1888, one edited by Nicolas León and published in Morelia, the other more lavishly printed but less reliably transcribed, by Antonio Peñafiel, and published in Mexico City.

Coapatli, Also Called Clamacazquipapan

(1.1.1)

Coapatli is the name given to an herb that has leaves similar to those of the peach tree, [but] somewhat broader, which from the beginning of their growth are attached to the stalk on its front side, leaving the other side bare. It produces round, cylindrical stalks. The small flowers [are] in umbels, and at their tips white shading to yellow. The root is fibrous; it smells like musk, [and] is bitter and glutinous. Because it is sharp and bitter, it has a hot and dry nature almost in the fourth degree. It grows in Yyauhtépec, [in] the Marquesado del Valle.[1]

Because it has this quality [the root] gets rid of the chills of calentures, expels wind, eases and joins together broken bones, provokes urine, purifies gross and viscous humors, [and] calms any pain whatsoever [that is] born from a cold cause. The natives say that its decoction cures bloody flux,[2] by evacuating [it]. The root's bark heals quartan fevers [and] gets rid of the pains of buboes[3] when one takes the root, ground into a powder, for nine days, in the amount of half an

---

1. A vast territory incorporating part or all of Coaxtla, Coyoacán, Cuernavaca, Oaxaca, the isthmus of Tehuantépec, and Tuxtla.

2. Dysentery.
3. Syphilis.

ounce each time. It does the same, with greater ease and certainty, when one takes a double dose of the medicine because on the first day it evacuates all the humors just as they say, but on the other days not so much. With nature lending support, it particularly cures this illness completely.

Atepocapatli

(1.1.9)

The herb called atepocapatli produces rough leaves similar to those of the almond tree. It has slender, cylindrical, purplish stalks sixteen inches long. The color of the flowers is somewhere between yellow and red. The root [is] transverse, from which come forth many others similar to the roots of the asphodel or the ranunculus; they leave an aftertaste of resin. They are viscous, not without a certain bitterness, apart from which they are mild in their scent. [This plant] grows in temperate lands and is found very easily in wooded places and in plains and flat fields. It blooms in the month of September, but the roots—which are what is used in medicine—are gathered from November to January and kept for the whole year. They are hot and dry almost in the third degree.

Drunk in the quantity of six oboli, which is a dram's weight, they cure any cold distemper, [and] cure sterility when it proceeds from such a cause. Some of the Indian doctors assert that drinking the decoction of this root instead of ordinary water gets rid of calentures completely—which does not seem a thing based upon reason, but perhaps I do not know [what] is meant by this—for with this remedy the shivers and chills of intermittent fevers are expelled; or, by being evacuated in some other way, the cause of the calentures ceases. It cannot be denied, however, that some cold qualities are hidden in this plant, with whose help what [those Indian doctors] say could happen.

Cassia Lignea, Cinnamon Bark, and Cinnamon

(1.1.11)

The cinnamon tree is a tree of medium size, whose leaves much resemble in shape those of the laurel or citron; they have many longitudinal veins, with three small ribs. The fruit [is] black [and] the flower white. The leaves have the same flavor as the bark, albeit less sharp and biting, but it quickly goes away.

The bark is stripped from the tree every three months: first the outer bark is scraped from the top [down]; even though some people say that [only] within three years does it grow new bark. When [the bark] is fresh, it is so slippery and sticky that it sticks to one's teeth if one chews on it. When it is added to pottages, it turns in a certain sense spongy; but afterward it hardens and turns into the substance and form in which we see it—about which it seems unnecessary to say anything, since it is so widely known. We will point out only that experience clearly has shown already that cassia lignea, cinnamon bark, and cinnamon consistently grow from a single tree and not from different ones, let people say what they will. The old herbals gave cinnamon different names in the olden days, so on account of the excessive value and price it commanded, avaricious merchants not only used to adulterate aromatic medicines, but also often used to give [the variously adulterated grades] different names, even though they came from one species, in order to raise them higher in esteem and price.

It grows abundantly on the islands of Mindanao (one of the Philippines), from where I have seen quite a large branch, and in other regions of the East Indies, and the most and best on the island of Ceylon.

Coapatli of Cuernavaca

(1.1.12)

The coapatli has somewhat long, rough, stiff leaves. The stalks [are] smooth and purplish, and their tallest are six palms high; on them are round, white, pilose flowers. The root is full of fibers. Coapatli grows in hot places. The root is sharp and biting, bitter and fragrant, hot and dry in the third degree, and of subtle parts. When taken orally in the amount of half an ounce, it expels wind, mitigates pains and stomach cramps, cures a cold, provokes urine, and heals colic admirably.

Yoloxóchitl, or Flower of the Heart

(1.1.20)

The yoloxóchitl is a tall tree with leaves like the citron, but twice as large and umbilical; the flowers are heart shaped with an abundance of white petals, reddish on the inside, thick, smooth, firm, glutinous, astringent, pleasant to taste, hot and dry, and if they are mixed with cacao shells or with a draft made from cacao, they strengthen the heart and the stomach and, if needed, they have a notable effect on looseness of the bowels. The pith, cooked together with mecaxóchitl, mexóchitl, xochinacaztli, tlilxóchitl, collopatli, and the tail of the opossum, introduced into the uterus, is an excellent remedy for sterility. This tree is valued very highly by the natives, as much for its medicinal applications as for the beauty and aroma of its flowers. These trees grow, amazingly, from a colorful pod, which dehisces when it ripens, so that seeds are scattered; wherever they fall, they grow; and when they are a span away they shrivel on the ground and stay dry for two months; some escape drying and are said not to flower. Some do not bear fruit: these are all over New Spain, planted frequently with all due care, and so they are sold more than twelve leagues from their place of origin, which is Yzauhtlan on the way to Veracruz.

Hoitzilóchitl, or Balsam Tree of the Indies

(1.2.11)

The tree that the people of Pánuco province call chucte, our people call balsam of the Indies, and the Mexicans [call] hoitzilóchitl, which means "tree that exudes resin," because it emits a liquid very much like Syrian balsam and is not a whit inferior [to it] in aroma and virtues. It is a tree the size of the citron, with leaves [like those] of the almond tree, although somewhat larger, rounder and broader. The flowers [are] yellow ⟨and⟩ on the ends of the branches. At first [they are] shaped like a large pouch, and as time passes certain [of their] petals ⟨become⟩ longer and broader than the rest; when they fall at the end, there is found enclosed in them a certain white seed that shades into a yellow color.

When the trunk or the bark of this tree is cut, at any time of year whatsoever ⟨but⟩ mainly once the rainy season has finished, this most precious liquid—celebrated throughout the world, which we commonly call balsam—oozes

forth, a deep yellow color shading to black, sharp and somewhat bitter to the taste. ⟨It has⟩ a vehemently strong odor, but a most pleasing one. It grows ⟨naturally⟩ in hot lands, such as the province of Pánuco, and many other areas; but it was brought to the gardens of Oaxtepec at the command of the Mexican kings, no less for the pleasure ⟨it provides⟩ than for its magnificence and grandeur. I[4] saw it every time I attended at that hospital [in Oaxtepec], while I was serving the poor for some years [there]. This same liquid also is extracted in another fashion, namely by boiling the finely chopped shoots and tender twigs in water and gathering in a glass vessel the liquid that floats upon the water; but this [kind] is inferior in its powers to that mentioned above.

Nevertheless, in whatever manner this liquid is extracted, it is hot and dry almost in the fourth degree and has subtle parts, not without some astringency and invigorating quality. It is useful for curing an infinite number of ailments; for, when it is taken on the tongue in a lick of three or four drops in the morning, while fasting, it strengthens a stomach weakened by a cold cause. It provokes urination and expels from the body wastes and superfluities from the kidneys and the bladder. It opens up the vessels [of the body] and cures difficulty in breathing. It gets rid of pains in the stomach and belly and puts good color in one's face. Some drops of balsam, beaten into an eggwhite and put on the face, get rid of blemishes and clean [the face] particularly [well], without risk. It preserves youthful vigor and a good state of health. In the form of suppositories placed inside the womb it attracts the afterbirth or a stillborn fetus. It makes labor shorter and easier; and it cures barrenness when it proceeds from cold humors. Anointing the exterior parts mitigates whatever pains may befall them from the same causes, in any part of the body whatsoever. It resolves tumors and expels wind; it comforts the brain; and when it is applied at the origins of the nerves, it cures all cold indispositions and palsy. It is a great remedy for the ailments of colic and pain in the side, and extremely useful for the ills of gout and viscous humors. It heals fresh wounds most quickly, and it does the same for old ones. When one anoints

---

4. Ximénez appears to have blended his own voice with that of Hernández. This sentence ("I saw it . . . years [there]") does not appear in two surviving MSS (JCB and BN).

the neck and shoulders with it, it gets rid of the chills of calentures.

The oil extracted by squeezing the seeds does the same, although it also is sharp and has an agreeable mild scent. It is fragrant to the taste and hot in the third degree. The protomédico of New Spain Dr. Francisco Hernández extracted it first, before anyone else; from whom those who have extracted it since learned ⟨how to do it⟩. It is very similar in scent and taste to the oil that is extracted from bitter almonds or peach pits, but [is] much more fragrant and vehemently strong and has more sharpness and acridness. All the rest of the Indies balsams have the same effect.

Balsam of Tolu

(1.2.14)

They tell me that in the province of Tolu, going from the city known as Nombre de Dios toward Cartagena, one may find some trees of medium size that resemble pines, with leaves like those of the carob, perennial foliage, and a soft, thin cortex. I am told that they grow in cultivated areas and that they exude from incisions a liquid called balsam, as efficacious as or better than the balsam of the Indies, described above, for everything that that one is used for.[5]

Molle

(1.2.15)

The tree known as molle[6] among the Indians and tree of Peru among the Spanish is a tall tree, beautiful in appearance, and most appropriate as an ornamental plant in the courtyards of private houses or in public spaces. It is leafy, and its branches grow green and purple on all sides, with leaves like the olive, but much narrower and thinner and disposed in one row on each side of the branch, angled toward the tip of the branches; it has clusters of small white flowers that then turn into green fruit, like a hawthorn seed or a little bigger, and when they mature they are mostly white

with a bit of red, enclosing a hard stone sheathed with a membrane of the same color. This tree exudes a teardrop from the trunk and the leaves, and the rest of the plant has the aroma of fennel and mastic. It is often classified as a species of mastic, as if it could be considered a plant *sui generis*. The leaves and the fruit last all year, some beginning to sprout as others are growing and yet others are maturing. It is a wild tree and does not require any special attention, although it has recently begun to be highly regarded and takes quite well to cultivation. It grows everywhere, propagated by sowing, cutting, or planting, but it flourishes best in warm places. Its flavor is tart, suggests bitterness with a slightly sweet edge, and astringency; and in nature it is hot and dry in the third degree. The pulp of the fruit is sweet, but the stone tastes as we have described. It strengthens and gives heat to the upper intestine, binds the lower one, and, some say, takes the place of turpentine, just as the seed can replace cardamom. It moves the urine, heals old or recent wounds, stops bloody fluxes, cures hemorrhoids, alleviates arthritis, makes films disappear from the eyes, clears flatulence and strengthens the limbs; it dries moist humors; mixed with lotions it resolves phlegmatic swellings. It also makes the teeth and gums firm and cures mouth ulcers. All of this can be achieved most efficaciously with the fruit, whether it is applied externally or taken internally.

Tecomahaca

(1.2.16)

The plant that produces the gum that we call tecomahaca, which the Indians call copal yhyac, [or] memeyalquáhuitl, is also called tecomahiyac, but [this is a] corrupt [form of] the name tecomahaca. This is a large tree that has round, serrate leaves. It produces a small, round, red fruit at the ends of its shoots, filled with seeds resembling a peach's pits. It grows in Mixteca and also in the province of Michoacán. It is a sharp, biting plant, odoriferous, with a certain astringency, hot and dry in the third degree.

---

5. BN MS adds: "I have spoken already of the other kinds of balsam, and when the pressure of time permits, I intend to treat the Haitian varieties."

6. Georg Marcgraf gives lentiscus as an alternative name for molle (1648 ed., p. 90); and the corresponding chapter to this one in the Rome edition (3.15) is headed "De Molle Lentisco Peruana," where the text veers off radically toward the end into something quite different.

When it is cut or incised—or sometimes spontaneously—this tree emits beads of gum well known throughout the world, in which is found the same virtue and temperament as the others we have described. Thus, there are some people who use it in place of myrrh. It cures wind pains, disperses sluggish and viscous humors, and corrects cold distempers when it is applied in the form of a poultice. It is such a good friend to a mother that when it has been thrown upon the coals and [afterward] put to her nostrils, it then frees up and heals those who are suffering from maladies of the womb. When applied to the navel, it stops menstrual flow, fortifies the womb and makes it stay in its place, [and] arrests menstruation and fluxes. When applied to toothaches and put in the cavities that [teeth] often have, it sedates them and arrests the decay. It cures and heals injuries of the nerves, [and] heals sciatica and gout when they proceed from a cold cause. When it is applied in the form of a poultice, it comforts the brain, the nerves, and the stomach. In sum, it is an extremely important remedy for all maladies born of a cold cause, as many people in Mexico have proved through experience.[7]

The Tree from the Province of Florida That They Call Sassafras

(1.2.27)

The sassafras is a large tree that has leaves cut and divided into three sections. The trunks are smooth, shading to a red color, and smell like anise. It grows in the province of San Agustín in Florida and in [the province] of Michoacán.

It has a hot and dry nature, almost in the third degree, and subtle qualities, by means of which it helps colic and pains of the side. It is a great remedy for difficulty in urinating and disorders of the kidneys, provided that they proceed from a cold cause. It expels flatulence, opens obstructions, and fortifies the internal organs. It cures asthma and other illnesses of the chest born of a cold cause; it prevents vomiting; it aids the digestion; it relaxes the abdomen; it is greatly beneficial for sterility of the womb; it provokes menstruation; and it is a great remedy for buboes, just as other alexipharmics usually are. It eases toothache; and it clears colds by consuming the cause.[8]

Tocpatli

(1.2.28)

Tocpatli is the name given to a small tree that grows in hot, flat places. It produces a voluble root, from which the trunk grows. Its large, serrate leaves, like those of the wild radish, look something like the iron [points] of lances. The flowers are white. The root is sharp, biting, and fragrant, and somewhat astringent; [it is] hot and dry in the third degree.

The decoction of its leaves and roots, both drunk and applied to the scattered lumps of buboes, cures them. I used this root much more willingly than ⟨I used⟩ the other [roots] that the Indians and the Spaniards ordinarily prescribe for the above-mentioned purpose, inasmuch as its humors were cold and tenacious, as they for the most part tend to be in this illness. The same root, crushed and applied in the form of a poultice, diminishes and consumes splenetic humors and restores the spleen to its former health.

Hoayacan

(1.2.29)

The Indians call this plant[9] guayacan; others call it matlalcuahitl or "blue tree," because its heart or marrow is this

---

7. The remainder of the text in *QL* is certainly by Ximénez: "Certain waxed cloths are compounded from this and other gums, for pains in any part of the body whatsoever. For if [the illness] is from a cold cause, [this] is a most blessed remedy that those persons tell me about to whom Canon Salazar gives alms (he will receive his reward in Heaven for such good work!); and its composition is as follows:

They receive waxed cloths, tecomahaca, balsam, castor oil, chili oil, axin, white copal, [and] yellow wax—a pound of each. All these things are melted in a glue pot and cooked until [the mixture] becomes quite thick; and then, after it has cooled a bit, half a pound each of ground cloves, nutmeg, orejuelas, anise, ololiuhqui are added. When they have been stirred together with one another

very thoroughly, the cloths are infused [with this mixture, thus] making waxed cloths; from which they cut off [pieces of] the size that are necessary to take away the pain." For axin, see *T, Animals,* 9.5, in "Italy, c. 1580–1651," below.

8. The remainder of this long chapter is attributable to Ximénez, who adds an anecdote to show that "it is good for turning brackish water fresh in an emergency, as we found while sailing from Florida to Veracruz in 1605, when, near the cove that they call Carlos's [cove], we lacked water."

9. Hoayacan: *Guaiacum officinale* L. See "Afternote: Abraham Munting," in "The Low Countries, 1630–1648," below.

color. This tree is of medium height, with a woody trunk, lean and spiny. Its leaves are a little larger than those of the rue plant. The bark is sooty even though the substance that covers the trunk is thicker and red. The wood is yellow and the marrow or heart is blue—hence its name. The bark is very bitter and thus the bark and the leaves are said to be hot to the second degree with a noted dryness.

The heart is not bitter. Its effects are used to cure the French malady[10] and chronic diseases of the head, chest, stomach, gall bladder, kidneys, and pains in other parts of the body. The method of cure is a remedy that, according to my way of thinking, should be very well known to all who practice medicine. There are two species—the one that we have just described, properly called guayacan, and the other, which is thinner and whiter in color, inside and out. It is a lighter color altogether, an ash brown. The wood of this second species is sharper and more fragrant, and is more useful and effective, and thus it is called "Holy Wood" because of the illnesses that it can cure. It is here that another author was mistaken when he said that the leaves of this tree are like the plantain, which was a manifest error. The leaves are the way we have said they are, as we have seen them thousands of times, and as Dr. Francisco Hernández, our author, saw them.

Others state that the hoayacan is a species of box, and I am with them, because the two are very similar. In using this wood, it is advisable that the wood that is to be administered is freshly cut and of an ashy color in all parts. It should be whole, full, and "grave." It should not be cracked or corrupted like plantain, but rather resinous, biting to the tongue and somewhat bitter. The heart of this tree is preferable to other parts. The wood should be picked when it is green, and it should be saved. There are so many trees of this kind in all the Indies! And I believe that they surpass the pines in their shape. It is not risky to say that anyone who takes the sap of this wood should be purged three times. Once before he begins his penance. The second time after fifteen days, and the third, thirty days after the treatment, when the patient has received absolution. The best time to take this cure is in the fall and spring, because taking it in summer would inflame the body too much. And if it were taken in

winter, the effects of the cure would be weaker, even though this remedy is always useful and never harmful. However, if this is taken in the summer or winter the excesses of the wood should be tempered by mixing hot things with wood in winter and temperate things in summer. It is good for bad breath, and keeps the teeth white and beautiful.

Yohualxóchitl or Nocturnal Flower

(1.2.30)

The yohualxóchitl, which some call cozcaquáhuitl and others yahoalxóchitl, or round flower, is a small tree, which has leaves like the elder, which species it resembles, although it seems to be more like the types of wild vine, but with less serrate leaves; it has umbels like those of the elder, clusters of little round yellow flowers, closed during the day, as is said, and open at night. From these hang fruits in racemes at first green and then red, and after a while purple; the roots are sticky, have a resinous taste and smell, and are quite odoriferous. It grows in Chapultépec, not far from Mexico City, at high altitudes, and it flowers in June; it is hot and dry in the second degree, and tastes bitter; applied in the form of a plaster it resolves tumors, or matures and opens them; it provokes sweat in some who are drunk, and in others it moves the bowel; a powder made from it gives shape to incurable wounds and cleans them; it cures scabies and leprosy and is a great remedy for tetanus and for women seized with fits of the mother.[11] Some eat the cooked leaves as a medicine, having first squeezed out the juice, and they say that this cleans out the body and fattens it, and that in a similar way it restores flesh by helping it to grow back, and that thus it consumes growths without causing any pain; and without causing any harm its leaves, placed on the skin, get rid of fears, fearful imaginings, and the fainting fits that they may bring about.

Nanahuaquáhuitl, or Bubo Tree

(1.2.32)

The nanahuaquáhuitl is a large, spreading, tall tree that has leaves similar to [those of] the olive tree, somewhat fragrant

---

10. Syphilis; also called the "French disease."

11. Eclampsia.

and bitter. ⟨Their⟩ decoction, when drunk copiously in the morning, cures the French disease. It grows in temperate places around Cocotla.

Quauhtlepatli, or Fire Tree

(1.2.33)

The quauhtlepatli, which the people of Michoacán call chupíreni, or "fire plant," is the tree that Dioscorides calls the rhododendron.[12] Its milky sap is astringent; nevertheless, the Indians say that, taken in the amount of four oboli, it very easily evacuates the phlegmatic humors of those suffering from cachexia, the French disease, or dropsy, especially if the illness proceeds from a cold cause. I do not believe, however, that such a strong medicine can be taken without any harm; and I judge it safer (and the Indians who indeed have tested it by experiment have said this) if it be applied in a moderate amount upon the navel, and in this way it may purge the body. It is also a very efficacious remedy for skin ailments, such as impetigo, leprosy, scabies, alopecia, and rashes. The people of Huexotzinco usually use it in a dose of two drams, ⟨or⟩ a little more or less, against intermittent fevers. It grows in Michoacán and Ocopetlayuco, near moist and watery places, where Dr. Francisco Hernández was on the point of losing his life because he had rashly tasted its sap, which is poisonous: the entire plant is most pernicious to humans. We could counter this by saying that many things, if tasted by a healthy man, would kill him, which may yet be given for a poisonous bite or animal bite, or other contagious diseases, quite safely, and the same milky sap, applied to swellings, resolves them.

Quauhíyac, or Fetid Tree

(1.2.34)

The quauhíyac is a large tree that has leaves like those of the citron, but sharply pointed. The bark is astringent and gives off an unpleasant smell. It grows in Ocuila, in rugged and rocky places. It has a hot and dry temperament. It stops up diarrhea and provokes sweat. Its juice, instilled in the nostrils, causes one to sneeze violently; and in this way it purges the head, getting rid of pains, and heals calentures. They usually store it when it is in season to use it year-round.

Cacapolton

(1.2.36)

This is a small tree with leaves like the cherry or capolin, purple stems, and blue flowers at the ends of the branches, which produce succulent fruit almost the size of chickpeas, red at first, then purple, finally turning black. The leaves are cold and astringent. They resolve tumors, control diarrhea, combat fevers and cure wounds. The juice from the leaves or fruit cures inflammations of the eyes. It grows in Ocoituco and Quauhquechulla, that is, in mild or warm areas.

Tlalámatl

(1.2.38)

The tlalámatl is a tree that has leaves like those of the sage plant, but thick and softer. Its flowers are spiny, small, and red; from which, in season, berries sprout. It is found in cold places. It flowers in February. Those who live on the lower slopes of the volcano near Mexico [City] call it quauhtlan matlatl.

The leaves, when crushed in the quantity of a fistful and drunk in water, are said to purge all the humors gently, without any irritation, by means of vomiting. Despite all this, it seems that it has a cold and glutinous and astringent nature. They say as well that the root, ground and sprinkled upon wounds, heals [them]. Ordinarily it serves as a food for horses, upon which they are nourished and grow fat, even though in the beginning it sets on edge the teeth of those who are not used to it.

Chatálhuich

(1.2.39)

The chatálhuich, which other people call zacaócotl and [yet] others the canafistula,[13] is a large and branchy tree, which

---

12. A MS note (eighteenth century?) in the copy of the Rome edition of Hernández at the Museo de las Ciencias Naturales, Madrid (call no. FE 4.264) identifies the quauhtlepatli as "Plumeria."

13. The canafistula (*Cassia grandis* L.) or drumstick tree is described in *QL* 1.2.56, below.

is green year-round. The trunk and branches have a certain red hair [upon them], and upon [the branches] the leaves [are] separated at small intervals; they are similar to the leaves of the lemon tree or the canafistula, but longer and whitish on their undersides. The blossoms are yellow, and the fruit is no more or less than the most delicate and most sour. It grows near riverbanks in the fields of Xocotepec.

The bark is hot and dry in the fourth degree, and variegated black and white in color. Ground and taken with water, in the amount of two drams, in the morning, it evacuates choler and phlegm by means of the upper and lower passages. It expels worms and maggots if by chance there are any in the body. It is considered by the natives a singular purgative medicine because of these effects. Mixed with axin[14] and applied behind the ears, the bark also gets rid of earache.

The skin of the fruit is sweet; and it has a flavor resembling that of the pulp of the drumstick tree. When it is drunk in the same fashion and in the same amount, it purges choleric and phlegmatic humors and softens the abdomen and provokes diarrhea gently. The same substance, ground up and made into an infusion in water, heals and mends tetters.[15] It strengthens split hairs and makes them grow long. The seed inside the fruit, ground up and drunk in water, reduces and expels fevers. All of this has been seen and proved by experience and out of curiosity.

Huitzmamaxalli

(1.2.53)

The huitzmamaxalli is a tree that has leaves [like those] of the mesquite or the tamarind. The flowers [are] yellow, with some seed pods, which usually grow [to be] good to eat. The trunk and branches of the tree produce horns like a bull's.

When tasted, the leaves seem to have no flavor. They are said to resist poisons and cure the bites of poisonous animals after the wounds are first scarified, and then the crushed leaves are applied in the form of a poultice, which in the space of about six hours gets rid of every trace of the poison's potency and draws it out, making the leaves turn black. The horns engender certain slender ants, tending to black [in color], whose bite is very poisonous and causes excessive pain that lasts an entire day. The eggs of these ants look like little worms. When ⟨the leaves⟩ have been ground into powder and instilled in the ears, and afterward the juice of the same tree's leaves is squeezed into them, the pain is eased. The juice relieves toothache, too.

It grows in the hot lands of the coast, in places near the northern sea,[16] both flat and hilly ones.

Canafistula, Which They Call Quauhayohuachtli

(1.2.55)

The quauhayohuachtli is a big tree that my countrymen call the drumstick tree, which has an almost ash-gray trunk. The leaves [are] like a laurel's; the yellow stellate flowers hang in clusters, from which grow the very-well-known pods that often are made into a conserve with sugar when they are tender. With this, choleric and phlegmatic humors can be purged without any danger or trouble, when it is given in the weight of three ounces. To discuss the drumstick tree['s pods] and their powers and uses after [they are] mature would apparently be an excessive and superfluous thing to do, for there is no one who does not know about this medicament. It grows in hot areas such as Yyauhtépec and Hoaxtépec, in flat, cultivated terrain.

The Somniferous, or White Sapodilla, Which They Call Cochiztzápotl

(1.2.59)

The cochiztzápotl is a large, scrawny tree, whose leaves resemble those of a citron tree, [but] sparse and disposed in

---

14. An unguent, common in New Spain, made from worms. Hernández describes it in *T, Animals*, 9.5. See See Bernardino de Sahagún, *Florentine Codex: General History of the Things of New Spain*, trans. Arthur J. O. Anderson and Charles E. Dibble (Salt Lake City and Santa Fe: University of Utah Press and School of American Research, Santa Fe, 1950–82), pt. 11 (bk.10, chap. 24, p. 89).

15. This term covers such skin disorders as ringworm, herpes, and eczema. It is not clear if Hernández means any or all of these specifically.

16. The Atlantic. See *Antiquities* 1.1, above.

threes. It has a variegated trunk with white scars [on it]. The flowers are small and yellow. The fruit is the shape of a quince, and sometimes of their size. Spaniards call it white sapodilla. It is a good fruit to eat, and has an agreeable aroma and taste, but [it is] not a very healthy sustenance: the seed inside is deadly poison. It grows in [both] hot and cold lands. The tree's bark is dry and slightly sweet, [but] not without a certain bitterness.

The leaves, when crushed and placed upon the nipples of a woman who is giving suck, cure the loose bowels of the children who nurse [from her]. The pits [of the fruit], when they have been burned and made into powder, cure gangrenous wounds, consuming all the corrupted flesh and cleaning the wound, engendering sound flesh and growing new skin with admirable swiftness. The fruit, when eaten, provokes sleep, whence comes the tree's name.

Coacamachalli, or Snake's Cheek

(1.2.62)

This tree is called coacamachalli because of the shape of its leaves, which are similar to the cheeks of a snake and in a certain way look like the leaves of the coanenepilli, even though the latter plant is twining and like a liana. This is a large tree. The flower is small and grows in spikes near the ends of the branches. It has pods filled with seeds like lentils. It grows in the countryside of Hoaxtépec, on the tops of wooded hills. When the leaves are applied in the form of a poultice, they mitigate pains even though these may be born of buboes; and it is good for lockjaw. The taste is astringent and sweet, and a little bit viscous. The temperament [is] cold in a certain way, or moderately hot.

The Tree Called Quamóchitl

(1.2.69)

The quamóchitl is a thorny tree that bears leaves like those of the pomegranate, but ⟨with⟩ less pointed tips and some heads similar to [those of] the epithymon at the extremities of the twig, but somewhat larger. It produces some small pods, which shade from green to a purplish color, with black seeds. Even though the seeds can be eaten and have quite a

pleasant flavor, they usually leave the mouth with a bad odor. It grows in hot regions such as that of Cuernavaca, and in all those towns around [there], in any areas and places whatsoever.

The root's bark is cold and astringent. It cures bloody diarrhea and other fluxes; as, thanks to experience, we used it with great benefit to the sick persons in the hospital of Oaxtepec, where there is a great superabundance of these trees. Its decoction heals wounds, grows new flesh and generates new skin, when it is put hot upon the wound with a small cloth. When they have been pulped with salt and applied in the form of a poultice, the leaves and seed pods cure a surfeit; and together with palm leaves, the juice of the seeds, which is contained in the pods, stops vomiting. Instilled into the nostrils, it attracts and copiously casts out all the ill humors from the head. It does the same, and even more efficaciously, if the seed is dried and powdered, with some rue leaves added to it, and taken like tobacco; and in such a manner it acts as a purge, for it attracts all the worms from the internal parts and wounds—all of which is clear already from many and most certain experiences. Thus, it is a tree well known by all.

The Tree Called Cacaloxóchitl, Meaning Flower of Roasted Corn

(1.2.70)

The cacaloxóchitl is a tree of medium size that has leaves like those of the citron tree, but much broader, which have many small veins that run from the middle to the sides [of the leaf]. The fruit are large, fat, red pods. The flower is large and very beautiful, and has a very agreeable and mild scent; these flowers are often used in bouquets and in the collars and garlands that the Indians usually use—for they hold these things in such esteem that they never dare to visit a person of any rank without first offering him some things of this sort. The juice of this flower is cold and viscous; when it is applied to the breast, it gets rid of pain. Two drams of the pulp of the fruit or the pod, taken, cleans out the stomach and intestines.

Many trees of this kind are found, which differ only in that their flowers are of different colors. Some are pure crimson, which they call tlapalticacaloxochitl. White ones are called iztaccacaloxochitl. There are plenty of others that, due to the differences of their flowers, have different names, such as tlauhquechulxochitl, huiloxochitl, ayotectli, and various other names that we omit to state, so as not to weary ⟨the reader⟩.

The thing that is most important is its marvelous virtues. A decoction is made from the bark of this tree thus. They take two pounds of the bark, which they pound in a stone mortar, to which they add seventeen pints of water; and they continue to cook it over a gentle fire until only one fourth part remains. From this they take ⟨a dose of⟩ six to eight ounces, lukewarm, every afternoon and morning: this is beneficial against thick and phlegmatic humors. It gets rid of pains in the abdomen and stomach; dissolves wind; loosens obstructions in the stomach, spleen, and liver at the beginning of ⟨an attack of⟩ dropsy; and gets rid of chronic headache. In particular it serves for those persons who have had serious illnesses and cannot finish convalescing. From the same, they make a syrup that is very useful for the same [purpose], by adding three pounds of sugar to the four pounds of decoction ⟨and⟩ cooking it until it assumes the consistency of syrup.

Capolin, Which Bears Indies Cherries

(1.2.71)

The capolin is a tree of medium size, which has leaves like [those of] our almond tree or cherry tree, slightly serrate. The blossoms are pendant from little stalks, from which develop fruit similar in every respect to our cherries—in shape, color, and size; in their seeds or pits, and in taste (except that they tend to the taste of mulberries) for which reason I believe that this tree should be comprehended as a species of cherry unknown in our hemisphere, even though it seems to some people that it ought to be comprehended as a species of the metzi. The fruit is a tiny bit sour and astringent, although when it reaches perfect ripeness it becomes sweet, losing a great part of its sharpness. It tastes pleasant, so much so that it seems certain persons who have sampled it vow that it is just as good as our own cherries.

[The fruit] is of a hot and moderately dry nature, with a certain astringency. From this fruit they make bread and wine, when there is a lack of one or the other; these give a sustenance that is atrabilious and somewhat harmful to the heart. They stain the teeth of people who eat them often; the stains can be cleaned off easily. In sum, there is no lack of persons who may dare to prefer this fruit to all the other fruits of summer, even though they be those of Spain; for Madame Gluttony is not content with less.

It flowers in the spring and bears fruit almost all summer. It is found in temperate regions, such as that of Mexico, where it is grown in orchards and fields, with care being taken to cultivate it.

The decoction of its bark, after it has been put out in the sun for fifteen days, drunk in the amount of an ounce, cures bloody diarrhea. Ground to powder, the bark removes cloudiness from the eyes, makes sight clear, and cures inflammations. It softens and moistens the tongue when it dries out due to lack of much ⟨moisture⟩ and violent heat; the juice, or the liquid of its shoots and tender stalks, does the same.

Zoconan

(1.2.74)

The tree called zoconan has a black trunk variegated with many spots, and leaves larger than those of the senna. The blossoms are white, [but] shade from white to red, and are shaped like a flywhisk. Crushed and mixed with resin and applied, the leaves cure ringworm or tetters. The leaves are bitter and astringent, hot and dry in the second degree. It grows in the mountains of Iztoluca. It is a famous tree and highly esteemed for these two kinds of illnesses that it cures, which are ⟨otherwise⟩ almost incurable.

Tepeizquixóchitl

(1.2.76)

The tepeizquixóchitl is a tall tree with flowers like the izquixóchitl, white, large like a fly swatter, with a pleasant aroma like the izquixóchitl, and just the same in shape. It is similarly cold and dry with some astringency, and not without a touch of sweetness; the bark of this tree, ground and placed on the gums, relieves pain and burning sensation, comforts and strengthens the teeth, and two drams of the bark, taken as a powder, detain belly fluxes. It grows in Chietla in the province of Oaxaca in warm places.

Ihuixóchitl, Which Means Flower That Resembles a Bird's Feather

(1.2.77)

This is a large tree that has large drooping leaves that grow in groups of five and that are very similar to those of the pinahuiztli. It has a red flower that looks like a bird's [feather], from which the name comes. There are other varieties of this tree, among them one that bears white flowers and another, white ones shading to green, but which are in all other respects the same.

The native Indians say that the person who carries a sprig of this tree will be agreeable; all those who have dealings with him will love him and be fond of him. He will rise to grace and favor with monarchs and great lords, in such a way that he will receive from them whatever is asked of them.[17]

As far as concerns its temperament, its leaves are cold and astringent. They correct and stop up fluxes. It blooms in the spring. It grows in hot and humid places.

Tlatzcan

(1.2.80)

The Mexicans give the name tlatzcan, or "fragile and glassy wood," to the tree that the ancients, Pliny among them, called the cypress.[18] Therefore I wanted to depict this tree, mentioned by very respectable authors but not seen by anyone that I know of in the Old World, as much for the above reason as because it is very common and frequent in all places here in New Spain where we are studying and describing plants, ⟨but⟩ principally in the temperate or cold ones. It has the same shape as the common cypress, but with the boughs extended sideways and almost inclining downward, from which its name comes. It is also of the same nature,

but its wood is more fragrant and just as good for carving. It grows upon hilltops and on their lower slopes, and its beautiful foliage embellishes mountain ranges and high hills. All year long it bears fruit like the common cypress's, but small, the size of hazelnuts. Its decoction, when taken, alleviates the chills of fevers; and its powder, taken in water, cures those same fevers. It is propagated by means of the root. Cuitlahoatzin, the prince of Iztapalapa, propagated these trees and with his determination caused them to be cultivated and valued in his realm. The uses and properties of this tree are the same as ⟨those⟩ of its fellows.

The Elder Tree, Which the Indians Call Xúmetl

(1.2.81)

The Mexicans call our elder tree xúmetl, and the people of Michoacán [call it] cundemba. It is of moderate size for a tree. Its leaves, when applied to the head, are said to get rid of the pain born of a hot cause. Placed upon the face and nostrils, it stanches nosebleeds. Taken by mouth, the ⟨leaves⟩ are said to cure intermittent fevers by expelling the cause of the harm, by means of both vomiting and diarrhea. Crushed and applied to the part [of the body] that hurts, it gets rid of the pains caused by the French disease and heals cramps and uterine pains in women who have just given birth. When the leaves and blossoms are boiled, and all is thrown into an enema, and its vapor is taken, it is extremely beneficial for hemorrhoids. They say also that the water in which its roots have been infused, when strained, purges the body and in this way stops up diarrhea and expels fevers, and heals other ills of the abdomen and stomach; and that the juice, when applied as a medicine, purifies and cleans out the passages.

The Tree Known as Guayabara, Which the Spaniards Who Inhabit Hispaniola Call Hubero

(1.2.84)

This is a large tree that has single leaves, which are round, thick, and a palm in diameter, with a vein across the middle from which other veins lead to the edge of the leaf itself and

---

17. In the margin is printed "A thing without foundation. It is not a natural power, and this cannot be believed."

18. Presumably meaning Pliny's cupressus cretica (*Juniperus sabina* L.) mentioned at 24.11.61.

make a very graceful arch. The fruit [is] good to eat [and] hangs in bunches, each berry the size of [one of] our grapes. The wood [is] solid and somewhat reddish. In a certain way [it] resembles [that of] Spain's kermes oaks.

At the time of the conquest, the leaf of this tree was the sole substitute for paper when there was a shortage of it and of ink. People communicated with one another with this leaf alone, writing [upon it] with the end of a wire or with a pin. One writes from one edge to another in [such] a way that it can be read with great ease; because after it is ruled, one puts [on it] white letters when the leaf has been recently picked. So far, it has not come to my attention that it serves any medical use at all; unless it is to make charcoal, for which it is an appropriate wood, or to extract very thick chunks of wood for butchers' chopping blocks and bellows of all sorts.

It grows on Hispaniola and throughout the Indies and mainland of the Ocean Sea,[19] where it is well known by everyone. Another tree grows [there], scarcely different from this one: slightly larger, but [with] a leaf of the same shape, except that it is more slender and without the small veins; the people of Hispaniola call it "star-of-night." From its leaf the Spanish used to make cards with which they played for high stakes at the time of the conquest. On these same leaves they drew the queens, jacks, and kings, along with all the rest, until [they could] place a deck of cards on the table.

The Soap-Bead Tree

(1.2.85)

In the province of Oaxaca and in Upper Mixteca and on the islands of Santo Domingo and Puerto Rico, very common large trees grow, whose leaves are somewhat similar to those of small ferns, and at their tips resemble [them] closely. They produce a fruit the size of a hazelnut, [or] a bit smaller, but it is not good to eat. But when its pit has been removed—which is a little larger than a chickpea, round [and] black like a musket ball—they throw this fruit into hot water (having removed the pit that I mentioned), and with that they soap their clothing as with real soap. It foams—as much and

as plentifully—the same as the choicest Spanish soap; and if necessary, one can easily wash clothes continuously with it. When the pits have been put out in the sun, they turn a very fine jet black; and after they have been turned on a lathe and pierced with little holes, they are made into very valued rosaries, almost as good as those that they call coyol—used ordinarily [for this purpose] in New Spain, where there are so many of such good quality that they can supply Spain— because they are very light but never break, like those of jet and bone. Each pit has a seed or pit inside [that is] very bitter to the taste, [like] peach stones, which the lathe turners remove with ease, and the beads are left hollow. These they make to the size they want, because when picking the fruit in the way they may wish, they make them as tiny as people request when [the seed] is put in the sun to dry.

Chillapatli

(1.3.2)

The chillapatli is a shrub with a fibrous root. The leaves are the shape of [those] of roses. The flowers [are] scarlet, two of which grow at the base of each of the leaves along the entire length of the stalk. It grows in the hot lands of Hoax-tépec and Yacapichtla, where we have investigated its powers. It is hot and dry in the third degree.

Taken by mouth, it mitigates pain in the abdomen. When a fistful of the leaves is taken with chilatolli,[20] they say it has admirable effects if it is given to people suffering from quartan fevers, ⟨for⟩ it gets rid of them right away.

Tlatlacótic of Tepoztlan

(1.3.8)

This has roots like new shoots, black on the outside and white inside, many cylindrical stems, somewhat purple, uneven, very long; leaves like the lemon but larger, somewhat crenellated, with longitudinal veins, and round, yellow flowers. It grows in the hills of Tepoztlan, Yauhtepec and Yacapichtla. The root is sharp, fragrant, of subtle parts, and its nature is hot and dry in the third degree; it is very good

---

19. The Americas. For the distinction between the "Indies" and "New Spain," see *Antiquities* 1.1, n.1, above.

20. See chili, in "Five Special Texts," above.

for those suffering from pain and swelling in the belly. It dissipates wind, purges the belly, and it is said thus to cure dysentery.

Aquílotl, or Voluble Plant That Grows Next to Water

(1.3.10)

Aquílotl is a voluble plant that grows next to water, so for that reason the Mexicans give it this name. It normally grows in humid and watery places, and it trails along the ground or twines around neighboring trees. There are two species of this tree, distinguished only by their names, the color of the flowers, and the relative size of the leaves. The first kind has white flowers, fairly small leaves, and is called aquílotl, whereas the flowers of the other kind are pale yellow, the leaves are larger, and it is called cóztic aquílotl after the yellow color of the flowers. Both kinds have rounded stems that are purple, woody, brittle, thin, and full of soft pith; the flowers are like those of the izquixóchitl, white, as we have said above, or yellow, no different in form and fragrance from those of that rose that is known among people today as the musk rose, from which this shrub, all in all, does not differ all that much. The leaves are like the blackberry, but whole, with longitudinal veins, and have an aroma like cucumber; the flowers are used for perfumes, and in coronets and bouquets, which are very common and familiar among the Indians; they extract from the flowers, by exposing them to heat, a very aromatic and pleasant essence. It grows in moderate or slightly cool climates. The leaves are bitter, and warm and dry almost in the third degree, so that a handful drunk with wine gets rid of flatulence; mashed and applied as a plaster, it loosens stiff limbs, and resolves tumors and abscesses.

Nacázcul, Also Called Toloatzin

(1.3.18)

The plant called nacázcul, which some people call toloatzin, is a kind of tlapatl that grows in the province of Hoaxocingo. It is a shrub that produces stalks like [those of the] fig. The roots are white and single-stemmed, the leaves like [those of

the] stinking vine: soft, thick, and hirsute. It has spiny fruit; and after the spines fall off, it is round and divided into four parts, like a melon. Its seeds are red and very similar to those of the radish's seed. It grows anywhere—on rubbish heaps and in the enclosures and ditches of Pahuatlan—and it is held in great esteem by the natives for repairing many kinds of harm.

The seed, dried, ground and mixed together with glutinous resin, heals broken bones admirably and restores dislocated bones to their proper places. For this reason, the Indians put some feathers on top ⟨of the mixture upon the injured limb⟩ and support it with splints; when this has been done, they place the sick persons in steam baths that they call temaxcalli, repeating this medical treatment as many times as seems necessary.

They drink the crushed leaves in water against pains anywhere in the body that are born of the French disease; and for the same [effect], [the leaves] are applied in the form of a poultice, together with yellow chili pepper. It needs only to be noted that one must not exceed the dosage, which has been stated already, because it could cause a certain insanity and encourage certain vain and inconstant fancies.

Iztaccoanenepilli

(1.3.24)

The plant called iztaccoanenepilli has leaves in the shape of a heart. It is a voluble shrub with a long, yellowish root from which sprout slender shoots that are rounded and green, and on those are the heart-shaped leaves that we have mentioned. The flowers go from white to pale yellow. One ounce of the mashed root, drunk, is said to bring down fevers, and if it is mixed with the yztauhyatl, or taken instead of it, it provokes urine, expels retained semen and blood clots, and induces sweat. It tastes sweet and is in nature cold or moderate.

Quauhtlepatli

(1.3.29)

The quauhtlepatli is a shrub with a thick, woody, red, fibrous root, from which grow woody stalks full of branches; serrate leaves like basil; and white flowers with red [in them], clustered on the ends of the branches almost in the manner of verticils. It grows in rural places in Xoxotla. It is of a slightly cold or temperate nature, dry and astringent. Its decoction cures all pains whatever, much like guaiacum, china root, or sarsaparilla. When taken in the morning for two weeks—or more, if necessary—it greatly benefits those who have dysentery and serves to stop up any other fluxes whatsoever.

Quauhtlepatli 2

(1.3.30)

This is a shrub with a branched and tawny-colored root, long and thick, from which grow twining and tawny-colored stalks, leaves like a lemon tree's, and a white and medium-sized flower. The root's cortex—which is cold, slightly sweet, and of an astringent nature—when it has been reduced to powder and applied, cures the rash that usually proceeds from the French disease. They say that it produces the same effect when it is taken and that in the same manner it gets rid of all skin infections. It grows in the hot areas of Texacahoaca, where it is greatly esteemed by the Indians for combating the said illnesses.

Xiuhcocolin, or Twisted Herb

(1.3.31)

This shrub from Hoitzoco has sparse leaves, almost with one cavity on one edge, oblong, pilose, and whitish, especially near the bottom. The round stems are thin, pale green and hispid with nodes spaced well apart. The flowers are like the bean's, and the large white root fades to red. It grows in warm hills and wooded places. The root tastes somewhat cold and astringent; its pulp, ground and taken with water in a dose of two drams twice a day, is antiemetic, especially among children; its juice cures mouth ulcers and sores in the genital area, and is very good for the eyes. The flowers mixed with milk provide the same remedies.

Mexóchitl

(1.3.33)

This shrub is the height of a man, has fibrous roots, leaves like those of the peach tree but a little bigger; small flowers

in dense clusters, yellow with a little red, and pods like the chili but with longitudinal lines on them. It emits a strong, acrid smell. It grows in humid valleys or in the hills of Hoeitlalpa. The leaves, crushed, are taken for poisonous animal bites, because by causing the patient to vomit they return him to health. The same, applied to wounds or sores in which there are worms, dispel and kill them.

Atlinan

(1.3.34)

The atlinan is a shrub with a thick and ramified root, stems with elongate, narrow, whitish, serrate, pilose leaves, almost like the willow, and flowers that are large and white. The root tastes of old chestnuts; the fragrant leaves taste resinous. It grows in the warm region of Cuernavaca, near streams and rivers, or in wild, flat places. The whole herb is warm and dry. A handful of mashed leaves taken in the morning reduces fevers, purging phlegmatic humors and bile, either upward or downward, without any harm. Introduced in a slightly larger quantity, this will purge those humors by way of the lower channels.

The Wild Grapevines of New Spain, Which They Call [Those] of Huachichiltic or Totoloctli

(1.3.39)

In many parts of New Spain there grow wild grapevines, but until our time the [native] people never cultivated or planted them carefully or methodically; for indeed they did not know the art of Bacchus, even though they drank too much of many other kinds of wines. Even today they do not neglect our [wine], but use it with the greatest excess and lack of temperance.

The fruit ⟨of the native vines⟩ is somewhat thick, with the flesh or pulp shading to a red color. It is wild but agreeable and sweet; and it seems to me that if it were to be cultivated, it would come to be soft and gentle in all its other qualities. These plants are very similar to our grapevines. The leaves and the tendrils have a cold and dry nature. They awaken the desire to eat; cure tetters; prevent swellings; reduce excessive heat; heal the inflammations of the eyes;

and mitigate the fever and pain of wounds, and dry the matter that is engendered in them.

Some people call them xocomecatl, which means "disagreeable rope." [This is] so because of the flavor, for the tendrils or running shoots wrap themselves around neighboring trees.[21]

Huapahualizpatli, or Medicine for Convulsions

(1.3.40)

Huapahualizpatli is the name given to a shrub that is as tall as a man, which has a rough trunk and branches, and [is] ugly to look at because ⟨these are⟩ for the most part bare of leaves, which are somewhat long and narrow. The supple yellow flowers grow in calyxes. It grows in Hueytlalpan, in high and flat places.

The decoction of any part whatsoever of the entire plant is given, lukewarm, in the morning and in the afternoon for a period of two weeks, or more if necessary, to restore lost movement. It seems to be cold and dry because it lacks taste and scent; and thus we are to understand that it creates these effects by means of some hidden property or by means of its dryness and astringency, which we have observed in many other medicinal substances of the New World.

Itlantli, or Old Woman's Teeth

(1.3.41)

The itlantli is a shrub to which this name was given because of the resemblance that its thorns have to the teeth of old women. It produces round, villous branches with a certain roughness, which tend to a yellow color, especially where they are most tender. It has leaves like a grapevine's, crossed by some veins that shade from yellow to reddish, but more pilose [than a grapevine's]. The flowers [are] white, and also tend to a yellow color. It produces fruit in bunches that are pendant from racemes all along the length of the stalk: green at first and afterward yellow, and full of many white little pits. [The fruit's] taste is bitter, viscous and astringent. It grows in hot and cold lands, in valleys and in flat and moist places.

A single leaf, cast into water and drunk, cures surfeit and also cures calentures by evacuating the cause; which it does, no more and no less, when it is tossed into water in an infusion. The liquor of a fistful of the leaves is given to be drunk against the inflammations of children's heads in order to cool them, for its heat is very moderate.

The Shrub Called Tenamaznanapaloa

(1.3.44)

Tenamaznanapaloa is the name of a shrub that some people call tenamazton and others tlalamatl. It has a big and single-stemmed root; leaves like those of the sage, large, whitish, and rough; white flowers that tend to purple, arranged in bunches and the shape of hazelnuts. It grows in any places whatsoever, both hot and cold. It has a cold, dry, and astringent nature. Thus, the liquid that runs from the tenderest stalks and shoots, when squeezed into the eyes, cures them if they suffer from any inflammations. It is applied also to tumors, inflammations, and swellings, and it cures calentures.

Tlacotequilizpatli, or Medicine of a Chopped Branch

(1.3.45)

Tlacotequilizpatli is the name given to a shrub that has many branches or "feet," two feet in length, woody, and round. Upon them it has serrated leaves [like those] of the oregano. The flowers [are] small ⟨and⟩ white. The root [is] long and slender, like a [man's] little finger, and woody. It grows at the summits of wooded hills in cold places in Upper Mixteca. It is hot and dry in the fourth degree; sharp, resinous, and glutinous to the taste; and very fragrant. It tastes something like coriander. Its decoction cures ills of the chest, expels wind, and mitigates pains of the stomach and belly.

Mintzitzin

(1.3.47)

Mintzitzin is the name given to a shrub that has red stalks four cubits tall, leaves like those of the peach tree, and white

---

21. Ximénez added: "In the province of Florida there are so many of them that the woods are full of them, in such a way that one almost cannot find a tree that does not have one embracing and living off it parasitically."

flowers. It grows in the temperate hills of Uruapa in the province of Michoacán. It is bitter and fragrant, a bit sharp and biting to the taste, hot and dry in the third degree. The leaves, crushed and applied in the form of a poultice to the stomach, provoke defecation and clean gross humors out of the intestines.

Chilpantlazolli

(2.1.6)

The chilpantlazolli or flag of dung, which others call tozcuitlapilxóchitl, hoitzitziltentli, chilpanxóchitl, and panxóchitl, is a small herb with leaves like long willow leaves, serrate and narrow, thin purple stems and long red flowers that are yellow at the edges, and an elongate, fibrous root. This grows in warm places in Tototépec and Itzocan. The root is sharp, hot and dry almost in the fourth degree, and burns the throat. Crushed and applied, it cures pains in the joints and pains caused by the French disease, is extraordinarily good for the spleen, for contracted sinews and restricted movement. It cures wounds and bleary eyes, and causes eyelashes to grow again; it also reduces phlegmatic humors. Crushed and taken with water in a dose of three drams, or its decoction instilled in the ears, it dries up pus, relieves earache and restores hearing. There is another plant called chichilácotl that is like this one, but it is sweet and has absolutely no medicinal properties, as far as I know.

Poztecpatli of Oaxaca

(2.1.15)

The herb called the poztecpatli of Oaxaca bears white leaves like the rue's, small [and] disordered, similar to the buds that sprout from the trees; the leaves last all year. They have exactly the same flavor as cress. It has woody stalks, dark in color, tending toward black. The roots [are] slender, like threads. It grows in rocky places and in the rough areas of the wooded hills of Oaxaca province. The stalks and leaves are hot and dry in the fourth degree. Crushed and drunk in the quantity of a dram, the leaves help the nerves and tendons and the stiffness of lockjaw, with something that may prevent the damage [caused] by a moist and cold cause. It

restores impeded mobility, as many experiments have shown.

Tlalatóchietl, or Plant Resembling a Small Pennyroyal

(2.1.16)

The herb that is known as tlalatóchietl is a foreign species of the pennyroyal or tragorígano. It has serrate leaves very similar to those of oregano, although somewhat smaller, arranged in pairs at intervals ⟨along⟩ the slender stalks. The flowers shade from white to red and sprout two at a time from the same base as the leaves. The root [is] long, delicate, and fibrous. It grows in rugged places and plains in Xalatlauhco, where they usually keep it in bunches in order to use it year-round upon the thousand occasions that present themselves. It is hot and dry in the fourth degree, and it burns more than the other varieties of its type. After one takes it in the mouth, it scalds the tongue; and then a little later it chills it notably, like a species of atochietl. Its decoction expels wind, gets rid of pain in the belly and the sides, expels cold, and provokes urine and sweating.

Tepecuitlázotl, or Mountain Cuitlázotl

(2.1.17)

This is a small herb with leaves like those of the pear tree, but larger, whitish stems a span and a half long, and a ramified root. It grows in Anenecuilco. The root is hot and dry in the fourth degree, with a sharp, burning taste; crushed and smeared on the back it relieves the shivers that accompany fevers, expels wind, purges gross and viscous humors, eases pains from a cold cause or from flatulence, provokes urine and menstruation, induces sweat, helps those suffering from convulsions or whose movement is impaired, strengthens the debilitated, and serves many other purposes appropriate to such a temperament.

Ichcatlepatli

(2.1.22)

The ichcatlepatli is an herb with medium-sized leaves almost in the shape of hearts, pilose and whitish underneath and green on top. Its many stalks shade into red. The greenish flowers [are] arranged in racemes. The fruit [is] round, somewhat hirsute, ⟨and grows⟩ near the base of the leaves. It grows in hot lands, in high and steep ravines and the gorges of wooded hills.

It is sharp and biting, hot and dry in the fourth degree, and has an astringent power. Its leaves at their tips smell like quince. Its decoction mitigates pain in the stomach. The powder of the root, placed upon wounds of the lower limbs, cures them remarkably [well]. The skin of the roots, when drunk, is said to heal dropsy admirably and with very great success, when taken in the amount of three drams or less.

Ixcuícuil, Which Means Painted Eye

(2.1.23)

This herb that they call ixcuícuil produces slender, nodular stalks filled with leaves like those of the rue, but longer; small white flowers near the bases of the leaves, and a root resembling that of the peony, dark-colored [and] shading to black on the outside, white inside. The root is what is used principally in medicine. At first it seems sweet to the taste, but then it burns and parches the throat. Its powder, drunk with water or added into a medicine, gets rid of pain in the belly; but it must be ⟨taken⟩ only in the weight of one dram. It is hot and dry in the fourth degree, and it has a burning power. They keep the root for the entire year.

Cempoalxóchitl, or Dianthus of the Indies

(2.1.29)

The plant that produces the flower that the Mexicans call cempoalxóchitl because of its great number of petals—is called dianthus of the Indies by the Spanish. The ancients, it is erroneously said, [called] it otona, or "Jupiter's flower." Seven major varieties of this herb are found in New Spain. There are others, differentiated and distinguished from one another by name and size, all of which have tough leaves, yellow or pale-colored flowers, and fragrant and subtle parts, not without a certain heaviness. Thus, they have a solvent and apparent virtue.

When the juice of the leaves is drunk, or the leaves are crushed and drunk in water or wine, they correct and moderate a cold stomach and provoke urine, menstruation and sweating. They get rid of the chills of intermittent fevers when they are applied externally before ⟨this stage⟩ ends. It expels wind, excites sexual appetite, and cures the debility of the body called cachexia by doctors, when such an illness comes from a cold cause or from vice and a bad disposition of the liver. It clears obstructions of the body's vessels, relaxes shrunken sinews, cures dropsy, and provokes vomiting when it is taken in lukewarm water. Finally, it is an admirable remedy for all cold ailments, evacuating the cause of the illness by means of urination and sweating.

The flower of the first variety is yellow, broader and with more petals than all the other kinds. This one properly is called cempoalxóchitl among the Mexicans, on account of the abundance and wonderful quantity of its petals (as has been stated), whose arrangement and shape resemble our own white rose in a certain way. This variety of the plant is the largest of all and has the largest petals. From this one is made a balm for wounds. ⟨The flowers are⟩ fried in ordinary [olive] oil, with a little of the juice extracted from this same flower thrown in until it is absorbed, and the rest is left; it is ladled out, strained, and kept for injuries. It is marvelous; and when it has coagulated with a little wax, it is a most famous cure for wounds and hemorrhoids.

The second [variety of the] flower they call oquichtli, which means "male flower," so called for the largeness of its petals and duct, in such a way that just as the first variety of all these plants has a notable advantage over the others in the largeness of its flower and petals, so—no more and no less—does this second variety surpass the rest, except in the size of its petals and in their number, in which the others exceed it.

The third variety of the flower they call tlapaltecacayatli because of the variousness of its colors. It is smaller than the second variety; but as we have said, it has more petals, which shade from yellow to green. The plant belonging to this flower is smaller than the other ones and has smaller leaves. The fourth variety is called macuilxochitl; it is almost the same as the third, but its color is pale. The fifth variety is called coaxochitl; it is smaller than all the above-mentioned ones and has as many petals, and in color it resembles the third variety. The sixth variety is called zacaxochitl amacoztl, which is yellow and smaller than the preceding one. The seventh variety is somewhat larger and is called tepecempoalxochitl; but it has the most delicate and yellowest flowers, just as the leaves of this same plant likewise are the smallest of all the varieties that I have mentioned.

I have seen ⟨that⟩ they grow wherever they may be planted, at any time of year, but best in hot places. They have been found in Spain for quite some time now. They beautify and adorn orchards and gardens with their blossoms, and not only in Spain; rather, people delight in this most noble plant in as many other nations as there are, but not one of them knows of the powers of which we have spoken.

Pelonxóchitl, or the Nasturtium of Peru

(2.1.35)

The plant known as the nasturtium of Peru may have been brought ⟨from there⟩ to Mexico, where Mexican ladies use it to beautify not only gardens but also pergolas, porches and windows. The Indians call this herb pelonmexixquílitl or pelonchili.

It produces almost round, slender leaves with some spines, which are pendant from certain small stems that do not grow directly from the middle of the leaves, but rather from one side of the circumference, almost at a slant. ⟨The leaves⟩ are green on their upper surface and somewhat pale underneath. ⟨This plant⟩ has a round, slender, twining stalk, which stretches out upon the ground and wraps itself around espaliers in gardens and arcades, where it is planted for decoration. It is very pretty and has a soft scent. The flowers are of an extraordinary, showy yellow color shading to red, as are those of the columbine or linaria, or those of the osiris. On their undersides these have a twisted little stem, which terminates on the upper side in seven sepals, of which two are bigger than the rest and two others [are] smaller than the remaining three. All have certain visible red lines, very similar to the wounds of Our Lord Christ as they are usually painted upon cruci-

fixes. The other three remain in the middle of the afore-mentioned ones. These have three markings in the shape of a crown of thorns.

⟨This herb⟩ is hot and dry almost in the fourth degree; and it so resembles our nasturtium in taste and power that there is no difference between them, such that even though they are very different in shape, ⟨this herb⟩ can be accepted comfortably in the species of nasturtium. It should be used in its place in medicines that call for nasturtium.

As we have said, it adorns and beautifies the gardens, espaliers, windows, and courtyards of houses, being planted in clay flowerpots. It is green and produces its flowers year-round, except when frost burns it too much and destroys it. They use its flowers in a salad, for they are very appetizing, so that afterward the main dishes taste even better; and it seems to be very useful ⟨for⟩ the maintenance of the stomach when it is weak due to cold or has wind pain. Crushed and applied, it benefits a cough; and when mixed up with alum and placed on the teeth, it rids them of pain. If one takes the leaves and flowers and crushes them together, and this mixture then is distilled in an alembic with some grains of alum, it is a singular wash for mouth ulcers and sores everywhere else in the body, as efficacious as the one they call "luminous water." Although it is somewhat hot, it heals the tumors and swellings born of a hot cause; which it does, even though it is hot [itself], by dissolving [them]. When [the swellings] stay gross and cold medicines are of no benefit, it cures inflamed wounds. They use this flower as ⟨we do⟩ our nasturtium, against pains from a cold cause.

It grows anywhere, but better and principally in hot places. It stays fresh and blossoms year-round; and vehemently cold weather does not impede it.

There is also another kind of nasturtium, which the Indians call mexixquílitl, which means "Mexican nasturtium," which they used to use when they did not have the one from Peru. It is a small herb that has very tiny leaves almost like those of the flax plant, but shorter. The stalks [are] woody, and its height from the ground is about a span. The seed has the shape and appearance of that of our own nasturtium; and even the plant itself seems, and is, of its species, since in scent and taste it is all one. It grows where it wants, without requiring cultivation. A friend has made known to me that he made an oil from this herb—which is not the point of what he meant to tell me, but rather that it had had many very good results against all illnesses from a cold cause.[22]

Purgative Root of Michoacán

(2.1.38)

The purgative root of Michoacán is known as tachuache, and the Mexicans [call it] tlalantlaquacuitlapille; some other peoples call it pusqua.[23] Three varieties of it are found. There are the male and the female, each of which in form and virtue is very similar to the other. ⟨This plant⟩ produces a long, thick root that exudes milky sap, and from the [root] emerge some twining, slender stalks that have leaves shaped like hearts, albeit small ones. The flowers [are] long and red. The fruit [is] similar to the cucumber in shape and size, covered with a certain white down ⟨and⟩ filled with a small, white, rather broad seed, with a few threads like silvery cotton that are hard to break.

The root is hot and dry in the fourth degree. When it is taken orally, it burns. If I had had it on an everyday basis, I would have had enough to censure other persons who have written thoughtlessly about it, things about which they knew not what they said; and there is no reason to marvel, since they saw it in their own lifetimes. It purges all the humors, but especially the phlegmatic, by means of the lower passage. In the amount of a dram and a half to two drams in water or wine, or in chicken broth or with a fresh soft ⟨cooked⟩ egg, it is easy to take, no trouble at all. Some people use its milk or the juice obtained by squeezing ⟨the root⟩ in place of scammony; and they even affirm that this same plant belongs to the same genus as scammony. They make tablets of it with sugar, and they swear that these pro-

duce admirable results. Moreover, some people usually leave the ground root overnight in an infusion, six drams of the root to six ounces of water; and in the morning they strain it and squeeze it, and give it to be drunk in water. I usually sweeten it with an ounce or so of matlalitztic or syrup or sarsaparilla or senna leaf, and in this way the purge is taken without any trouble. When there is a great dearth of scammony, it is usual to substitute the milk obtained from this plant's root in electuaries that require [scammony]. Some people use the root, after it has been squeezed, like ointment or in the form of a poultice; and with this they cure ailments of the eyes.

The third variety grows for the most part in black soil in rocky places. It has a more slender root. Taking two drams of this, one compounds a laxative electuary most conveniently, with an appropriate quantity of sugar, tzauctli, or tragacanth; which can be used with much satisfaction to evacuate choleric and phlegmatic humors gently. I doubt very much that ⟨any⟩ medicinal substance can be found in the Indies that should have an advantage over it. There are other people who make a syrup from its decoction that, when taken in the amount of three ounces, admirably purges the aforesaid humors with ease. It grows in many hot places in New Spain, even though that of the province of Michoacán—where it first was found and where its power was recognized—has a better name and reputation. It is also very common and familiar in Temimiltzingo, where they affirm that when this root is mixed together with the tail of an animal called the tlaquatzin (the possum), in equal proportions, it produces admirable results in provoking urine. The said root should be dried and stored properly year-round, care being taken upon gathering it ⟨to distinguish it from⟩ a certain root, which—being a very harmful, pernicious, and mortal poison—is very similar in appearance.[24]

22. This last paragraph is probably attributable to Ximénez.

23. To the title of this section Ximénez added: "and its differences and varieties, xalapa and matlalitztic."

24. Ximénez added: "When our author whom we are translating wrote his books, he did not have as complete information about the varieties of ⟨the purgative root⟩ of Michoacán as [is to be had] now, considering that the land of New Spain was not so frequented and well known as it seems ⟨to be today⟩. For since then

other varieties of the same root have been found, more benign in their operation and effect; even though it cannot be denied that the three varieties of it that our author mentions have been the most celebrated for their recognized effect because they are esteemed, for the purpose of purging, without counting many others that are not ⟨currently⟩ in use as these [are]." Ximénez expanded the chapter considerably, challenging readers to consider his description before accepting Monardes or López de Hinojosos.

Mountain Yyauhtli

(2.1.41)

They call this herb mountain yyauhtli or tepeyauhtli, for some people call it yyauhtli, without any other name. It is an herb that produces leaves like those of the other yyauhtli, or of the willow, but serrate and larger. The stalks grow as high as three cubits. The blossoms are reddish and rather large, in calyxes. It has many fibrous roots. It grows in hot and cold regions in the hills and valleys. It blossoms in the month of September. It is sharp to the taste and fragrant, and is hot in the fourth degree.

They say that when its juice is instilled into one's eyes, it cures [their] indispositions; and when it is applied to the head, it provokes menstruation and urine and expels from the tract of the kidneys and bladder all that might be able to impede good and free issue and operation. It expels wind, fortifies the stomach and all the other interior members that might be weakened because of coldness, corrects poor color, [and] stops up diarrhea. One takes its powder in the cocoa drink against coughing and against coldness in the chest. They often fumigate lodgings with this herb, throwing it onto braziers to perfume bad air and stench, especially that which the corrupt breath of sick persons usually causes. It cures surfeit and stomach cramp, together with the cold distemper of the stomach.

Chili, or Ginger, of the East Indies

(2.1.46)

That which the Mexicans call "eastern chili," the Arabs, Turks, and Persians call ginzibil; and in the apothecary's shops they call it ginziberis. Two kinds of it are found, one male and the other female. We dealt with the female in the previous chapter under the name of ancoa, ⟨which⟩ is common ginger, as it is called in Spain. It is an herb about two feet long, which has transverse roots full of knots and bumps, from which it produces stalks like canes. Upon them are long, narrow leaves exactly like those of the iris of Spain; and on the ends of the stalks [are] some flower heads resembling in a certain way those of the French lavender. It grows in all the provinces of the Indies where it is cultivated and planted, either from seed or from root cuttings. The one

that grows wild is very little esteemed. It also grows in the Philippines, whence it was brought ⟨and⟩ transplanted onto Hispaniola; where it [was] approved as well, for only it is tasted in all Europe and a great part of Africa. Even here in New Spain it has been found to be very good.

They plant this plant here in coarse, well-manured, very thoroughly plowed soils beneath the shade of some small trees, and in hot areas. In the month of March the root is divided into pieces the size of a [man's] thumb, ⟨which are planted⟩ at intervals five or six fingers' lengths apart from one another and as many [lengths] deep. ⟨Each piece⟩ is covered with earth, and then is watered as it is being planted and twice a week from then on, or only once [a week] if the soil is [still] visibly moist. It is to be cleaned and weeded in such a way that the plants [themselves] may not be pulled up or damaged, and the soil is dug ⟨to loosen it⟩ three or four times.

It yields a crop every year when the leaves fall from it, which usually happens at the beginning of January. The root must be pulled up, so that it can be kept easily. One has to scrape off the outer bark and then throw [the root] into a pickling vat, where they let it sit for an hour or an hour and a half. Then it will be put in the sun for the same length of time. Then it is laid out on mats or matting under a roof, until all the moisture has been consumed and the humor is exhaled. If it should appear that the roots thus [treated] are still damp, they have to be put in the sun ⟨again⟩.

If they are to be transplanted, it is necessary to keep them covered with earth in flowerpots, watering them with fresh water or rainwater as many times as has been stated ⟨above⟩, covering them up at night and exposing them to air and sunlight during the day.

To deal with the virtues and powers of ginger would be superfluous, since already so much is known already about these things throughout the world. The natives of Eastern India relate that when the roots are cut into small pieces when [the plant] is fresh, and mixed with other herbs, they often are eaten in a salad: with oil and vinegar so that it is smooth, not sharp or biting.

This root ⟨is grown⟩ in all parts of the Indies, just as it is among us, principally in flat, moist, low-lying places. With sugar, they make a preserve from this root, first chopping it very fine and infusing it with a lot of water so that it may be sweeter; this is gathered in season and well cured and prepared before they boil it in sugar. It is very good and tasty and tender to eat; but that which leaves threads in the mouth [is] bitter, is bad.

Tétzmitl of Tonalla

(2.1.49)

The herb called the tétzmitl of Tonalla appears without doubt [to be] a species of that herb we call sempervivum, for it has long, narrow, sparse leaves [that are] broad near the ends; round stalks; [and] roots resembling hairs. It cures pains in all parts of the body; it stimulates the desire to eat; it gets rid of pimples on the face; it provokes vomiting; and it cures burns. To provoke vomiting, one has to drink the juice; and in this manner it heals chronic and incurable illnesses. It is mucilaginous and has no notable flavor, even though on first contact with the tongue it tastes slightly sharp. It grows in warm terrain in lower Mixteca and on riverbanks.

Tlanoquiloni of Oaxaca

(2.1.53)

This is an herb with small, short, hairy, white roots. The pilose leaves are white underneath and resemble those of the common mouse-ear, only smaller. It has buds at the tip like the large plantain. It grows in the hills and in mild, wooded places in Oaxaca. The root, taken in a dose of two drams, is said to evacuate choleric humors; it opens obstructions of the spleen and cures itching and restores the whole body of one who has been adversely affected by bile. It seems sweet at first, but soon after, it burns the throat.

Nextalpa from the Town of Nexpa

(2.1.54)

The nextalpa, which is ⟨also⟩ called tlanoquizpatli, is an herb that has leaves like the olive tree's, but smaller. The stalks [are] round and like wood. The fruit [is] similar to that of the chickpea. There is a single root. By taking the weight of one

dram, one evacuates all the humors. It is a proven medicament with a very healthful effect. It is sharp and odoriferous, and hot and dry in the fourth degree; and it burns the throat.

Mecatozquitl or "Made of Cord"

(2.1.56)

Mecatozquitl is the name of this herb that grows leaves like lettuces, serrate, with stalks with round ends, a cubit in height; on the ends of which grow small yellow flowers that form fringes at the tips. The seed is soft and red, like that of the second sisymbrium, and gives off a very agreeable aroma. The root is like a radish, white and red, hot almost in the fourth degree and dry; and when its soft parts are applied in the form of a poultice, it relaxes and softens contracted and hardened members, provokes urine, dissolves wind and cures the pains that spring from it, and causes menstruation in women, comforts the stomach that has been weakened by cold, and cures wounds on the lower limbs.

Miahoapatli or Corncob Medicine

(2.1.57)

This is a small herb like the alsine that grows on the trunks of trees and feeds on them, with thin, short shoots, leaves like rue or a little smaller, and small white flowers. It is bitter, aromatic and hot in temperament. It dissipates flatulence and removes pains from a cold cause, when ground in the quantity of a handful and taken with wine. It restores and strengthens those who have given birth in the same way as the types of herb called cihoapatli; it stimulates the appetite and cures indigestion; it is also used as an ointment and applied in poultices to the head. Some people group it with ahoyacpatli, tancápaz, tezontequani, iceoalloyúhatl, and ichipinca.

Ayotectli

(2.2.1)

Some call this plant chichicayotli, that is, bitter squash, for it is a species of colcynthis or wild squash unknown in Spain. It has a round root with seven or more others, small and also round, hanging from it, yellow and purple inside and gray outside. The voluble branches bear leaves and flowers like the garden squash but smaller. The root and the hanging balls are very bitter. It grows in cool climates such as the mountains of Mexico, Tetzcoco and Oaxtepec. The root is hot and dry in the fourth degree. One dram of the root taken with water, or slightly more if introduced, is diuretic, and purges all humors by the upper or lower passages, but mainly the gross and phlegmatic, and is considered an infallible remedy. The Indians do not use the fruit for any medicinal purpose, however much it might be like our colcynthis in size, shape, and properties, although those are a little sweeter; I kept them dry for a year but they were useless because they were so bland, and could not even be ground.

Tzocuilpátli

(2.2.2)

The herb called tzocuilpátli has leaves resembling those of the basil, only much smaller and serrate, but profoundly rough. On one side they [are] whitish and not very different from those that the [herb] called cihuapatli produces. The stalks [are] round, hirsute, and whitish, yellow on their upper parts. The flowers [are] round and pilose. The root [is] full of fibers. It grows in the wooded hills of a hot land, such as the province of Pánuco. The root is odoriferous, resinous, and hot and dry in the fourth degree. When a decoction has been made of the root, and reduced by one third and [it is] drunk, once only, in a moderate amount, they say that it restores lost mobility. Instilled into the nostrils, it cures migraine by evacuating phlegm from the head by this route.

Ayótic Poxáhoac

(2.2.5)

The ayótic, which some call poxáhoac, meaning swollen and mild medicine, and others call olóltic, or round and circular, has a root much like a walnut in shape and size, white, solid, and lactiferous. From the root grow stems one and a half spans long, thin, reedy and nodular in parts; the minute white flowers produce three tiny white granules covered by a green membrane and arranged in a triangular pattern. It grows in temperate or hot places, such as Cuernavaca or Tepoztlan, while the chichimécatl grows in cold and wild places and has more pronounced properties. It flowers when other plants do. The thin elongate leaves look like blades of grass or leaves of chichimecapatli, to whose species this one belongs. It is a bitter herb with a slight touch of sweetness, and is hot and dry in the third degree. Two or three drams of the root, crushed and taken with water, or somewhat more if it is introduced, make a very effective purge by the lower passages of all humors, especially the bilious, and it may be used dried or fresh, although it is a light emetic.

Zazanaca, Which Others Call Coapatli

(2.2.6)

The zazanaca is so called for the down on the roots, which are thus very good for fueling a fire; these fibers are red, except that if you bite into them they show yellow. They have many long, round stems, and on them are oblong, serrate leaves, spiny at the edge, but strangulate when they start to sprout, and with lobes extending to each side of it, which gives them an unusual appearance; at the tip of the stems, pilose flowers that are pink inside and yellow and white outside, which separate into woolly strands. The root is sharp and bitter, and hot and dry in the third degree. It expels flatulence and, introduced, it relieves pains from wind or from cold causes by evacuating the intestines, expels worms, and cures diarrhea. Its powder, taken in a dose of two drams with water or wine brings the same relief, and cures surfeits too; it loosens the belly gently and eases sharp pains there, provokes urine and reduces fevers. The Michoacanese call this herb xararo, and say that the juice of its root cures pains from the French disease, restores free movement, gradually aids the recovery of people who are fading away because of obstruction or lack of digestion, it releases retained semen, strengthens the kidneys in women who have just given birth, and they say that the down that adheres to the root cures wounds and is highly inflammable. There are two other species of zazanaca, one of which is called xiuhtotonqui, of which we shall speak in due course. Zazanaca grows in humid, cold, or mild areas, such as Tetzcoco, near the mountains.

Hemionitic Cihuapatli

(2.2.8)

Because this herb cures the indispositions of women, and resembles the hemionitidis—for it is a species of satinwood ⟨to judge by⟩ by the shape of its leaves—they call it the hemionitic cihuapatli; but the Spanish women of New Spain call it "mother's herb." It produces many slender, round, straight, villous stalks from its one fibrous root. The leaves [are] long and soft, and in a certain way resemble those of the hemionitidis, whence comes its name. The flowers are white and in calyxes. It grows in all areas, both temperate and hot. It is dry in the third degree. For this reason three or four ounces of its decoction are generally prescribed for women who are giving birth, so that they may deliver [their babies] more easily with a good outcome. The decoction or juice is very useful for the breast. When a handful of the leaves has been crushed and given to be drunk in water or some appropriate liquid, they relieve stomach cramps, cure dropsy, and provoke menstruation. They plant it from root cuttings and from seed. They usually cultivate it as a pleasing and nice-looking thing, not only in gardens and orchards, but also in flowerpots and clay receptacles. Ladies and gentlewomen are in the habit of beautifying their halls and windows with it, and [also] their private pleasure gardens.

Cocozxochipatli, or Yellow-Colored Medicine

(2.2.12)

The cocozxochipatli is an herb that has leaves like [those] of the common bugloss. The flowers [are] yellow like those of the yellow chamomile, that is the buphthalmum, from which its name comes. The roots [are] similar to those of the peony. It grows in high places and plains of the province of Acatlan, [and] in temperate land in Lower Mixteca. The root is hot in the third degree and viscous. Taken by mouth, in the amount of an ounce, it cures bloody diarrhea, stops vomiting, and restrains blood wherever it is running too much.

Pezo

(2.2.15)

The herb known as pezo has serrate leaves, which are renowned and worthy of consideration, for others that grow next to their base become narrower until they end in a point; finally, these leaves are very notable because they have a peculiar shape, for nothing comparable grows in their manner. It must be conceded that they are similar to those of the sow thistle; the leaves of the pezo have stems longer than a palm, which grow from a thick, long root. The flowers are pinkish, hanging from a small stem and attached to the same root. It grows in temperate lands in the province of Michoacán. The root's taste at first seems informed by a certain sharpness; it is hot and dry in the third degree. This root is useful for the chest; it comforts the stomach that has been made weak by a cold distemper; and they say that when it is placed upon the pit of the stomach, it eases its pains.

Tecpatli

(2.2.16)

That which is called tecpatli is an herb five cubits tall, which has long rough leaves with folds [in them]; thin, straight, cylindrical, and twining stalks; flowers that are yellow near the center but white around [that], shading to reddish, placed in scarious little bases. The root is thick, full of fibers, and tastes like a carrot; but it is resinous and bitter and glutinous, for which reason they have given it this name. It is of a hot disposition and dry in the third degree; it has an agreeable odor. The juice of the root gets rid of harshness in the chest and is a singular remedy for palpitations and for blood in the bowels; and from this same root is made a very good lime for catching silly little birds.

The Herb Called Tuzpatli

(2.2.18)

The herb called tuzpatli has a round root the size of a hazelnut, with some slender fibrous tendrils, of a blue color; from the [root] grow delicate little stems, and upon them bending leaves almost like those of the sweet fern, but smaller and greener. It has small round flowers at the tip. It grows in warm and humid places in Tepuztlan. It is aromatic, and hot and dry in the third degree. They say it rids pain in the stomach and belly, dissolves wind, and that, drunk or made into a medicine, it cures surfeit and constipation by purging the belly.

Tepetlachichicxíhuitl, or Bitter Herb That Grows in Wooded Hills

(2.2.19)

The tepetlachichicxíhuitl, which other people call chichixíhuitl, is an herb with fragrant, serrate, rough, whitish leaves like a wall germander's. The slender, dark, round, smooth stalks grow three spans in length; on the ends of the stalks are hirsute white blossoms with yellow [in them], shaped like little stars, from which grows an oblong small fruit. The root is white and fibrous. It grows in hot hills. The root is fragrant, hot and dry in the third degree, with subtle parts that have a certain bitterness, from which it takes its name. It is an herb of great importance, whose juice greatly alleviates indigestion and afflictions of the chest when it is administered every day in the morning, since it purges phlegmatic and bilious humors by means of the upper channel as well as the lower.

Tlacopatli of Malinalco

(2.2.21)

Tlacopatli of Malinalco is the name given to an herb that has leaves in the shape of a heart or small shields; slender, nodular, twisted, twining stalks; fruit a little larger than hazelnuts; [and] a root full of fibers. It grows in Malinalco or Ytzoco, and in Tlalmalca, and in other similarly hot places. It is hot in the third degree, bitter and fragrant, and has a strengthening power and a sharp taste.

The root cures deafness; and when it has been mixed with turpentine, it cures the cold and the pains that usually proceed from it; resolves swellings and abscesses; [and] clarifies the vision. Made into small wheels and strung together like beads, and placed around the neck, it cures rheum and gets rid of the cold and bad humors of intermittent fevers and cures wounds by evacuating and dissolving the humors. When it has been mixed with turpentine, it eases broken or

dislocated bones and restores them to their original vigor and strength. It cures deafness on its own and benefits ⟨those suffering from⟩ eye troubles. It expels wind, and generally helps almost all the cold illnesses.

Totoncaxoxocoyollin

(2.2.23)

The herb called totoncaxoxocoyollin—which some people call atehuapatli, which means "medicine which grows by streams," and other people call texoxocoyolin—produces only one red, hollow stalk, full of bright red leaves, like those of the grapevine, to which [this herb] is very similar, with tendrils that also tend to red. The flowers are reddish, round, and grow on long peduncles on some of the longest stems. The seed [is] very small and from a yellow color shades to red, collected in capsules almost shaped like banners put together as if they were joined with a membrane, with another circle of the same color and same material in such a way that it forms a right angle. It has a white, round root almost covered in hairs. It grows in the mountains and rocky places of temperate lands such as those of Mexico and Tetzcoco. The root tastes bitter, with some degree of sharpness; it is hot in the third degree. When it has been crushed and infused in some liquor that is suitable for its intended purpose, it cleans out the intestines. It releases detained semen, and when it has been kept, it benefits inflamed eyes [and] provokes urine. When it is drunk in the amount of a dram and a half, it evacuates all humors by means of the lower passage.

Tragorígano of Cuernavaca

(2.2.24)

Although many of the Spaniards who live in the Indies call this plant pennyroyal, it seems closer in form and nature to tragorígano, which is known in Spain as oregano. It is much more rational to give it the name of tragorígano, so that is what we will do. It is a large herb with leaves like marjoram, purple stems, fibrous roots, oblong flowers that are white and pink and grow in calyxes, and the flavor of oregano and pennyroyal. It grows in mountainous, humid places in warm areas, such as Cuernavaca. It is known from experience that its decoction is extremely good for inducing menstruation, it cures cachexia and dropsy, it opens obstructions, restores lost color, expels wind, provokes sweat, restores full movement, reduces spleen, draws out the most deep-seated humors, purges viscous and thick humors, stimulates a weak appetite, and cures chronic, stubborn illnesses that have not responded to any other treatment. The leaves, chewed and kept in the mouth like tobacco, give extra speed to hunters and quench the thirst. Its nature seems to be the same as oregano or pennyroyal.

Nanahuapatli, or Medicine for the French Disease

(2.2.33)

The nanahuapatli—which others call the palancapatli because it cures sores—has a long, slender, and fibrous root; faded, lengthy leaves resembling those of the common mouse-ear; a flower like an apple's on the end of the stalk; and a bitter seed. It is hot and dry in the second degree, with a bitter flavor and aromatic smell. Made into flour and ground into powder, it cures putrid sores; for which reason, as we have said already, it is called palancapatli by some people. It eases those who are sick with biliousness and those who have suffered the bite of the Panucese viper that they call the mahuaquitli. Crushed, dissolved in water, and taken in the amount of a handful with some suitable drink, as often as needed, it completely extirpates the contagion called the French or the Neapolitan disease, drying up and also getting rid of the little sores and little swellings all over the body—which clears up with a dazzling light something that preoccupies and disturbs many people: to know that this illness had its origin in these West Indies and was spread to other regions of the Old World, since it has among this people a native, proper, and ancient name. It grows in temperate places, such as Tepoztlan.

Temécatl of Yyauhtepec

(2.2.34)

Temécatl of Yyauhtepec has rounded, wavy, soft leaves with a strong odor—fetid to put it bluntly. The twining runner-

like stalks full of tendrils; and succulent fruit hanging in racemes almost all along the stalk's length. It has a large root. Its nature is hot in the third degree and it has a bitter taste, so some people call it chichicpatli, or "bitter medicine." Crushed and applied, the leaves cure sores, indigestion, and pain in the belly, or any other ill that may come from the French disease. When taken, they provoke urine and get rid of flatulence.

Xiuhtotonqui, or Hot Herb from Tototepec

(2.2.35)

The [herb] that they call xiuhtotonqui is an herb that has serrate, rough leaves, almost in the shape of a lemon's, but bigger ⟨and⟩ whitish. The root [is] ramified and similar to that of the hellebore, covered with down. The whole plant is so similar to the zazanaca that it seems [to be] one of its species, as it has the same virtues, differing only in the shape of its leaves, which, although they are rough and somewhat long and serrate, suggest that their origin is not the same as zazanaca. It is very easily found in flat and hot places.

The root is bitter, hot and dry almost in the third degree, and has subtle parts. Its decoction usually is given to kill worms and to expel them from the body. It ⟨also⟩ expels wind; provokes menstruation and urine; cures dropsy; and thins and attenuates the humors, even if they may be born of the French disease—or Indies disease, since it is certain that it emerged from here, as we have stated. It comforts the stomach and is very healthful for the chest.

Chilpan, or Wasps' Nest Herb

(2.2.38)

The herb called chilpan produces leaves, not only from the roots—which are numerous, tawny-colored, and fibrous—but also from the stalks, which are two cubits in length and sometimes longer. The leaves are long, like those of the willow, thick, and narrow; in some parts they tend to scarlet color. It produces red flowers at the ends of the stalks, in striped calyxes, whence the Mexicans have given it this name, for they are a vermilion color, like the big wasps of a hot land. It grows in the month of September. It is raised in temperate places, such as the fields of Tetzcoco and Mexico, and in other flat lands and wooded hills.

When the root is drunk in some suitable liquid, in the amount of one dram, it usually evacuates choler by means of vomiting, but sometimes by means of diarrhea. Other people say that when these roots have been ground up and made into powder, they stop nosebleeds; or when drunk or infused in some appropriate or astringent liquid. It is bitter and hot, and it usually burns the throat a little bit when it is drunk.

Chipecua, or Firm Herb

(2.2.39)

The [herb] that they call chipecua is a little herb that produces many slender, somewhat purplish stalks from a root that is fibrous; and on [the stalks there are] leaves like [those] of the flax plant, long and delicate. The flowers [are] yellow, on each of the bases of the leaves. It grows in Tacambaro, in the province of Michoacán, in temperate lands or those inclining to cold. There it is held in much esteem by the natives. It has a bitter taste and [is] hot and dry. Thus, when it has been crushed and given to be drunk, it provokes sweating; relieves gout and pains in the joints, and any other pains whatsoever that may have their origin in a cold cause; and besides this, it restores lost mobility.

Nanacace

(2.2.43)

The nanacace, which means "angular plant," or "plant with corners," is an herb that has leaves like a grapevine's but somewhat longer, which are shaded a little bit to purple. It has a single red stalk, at the top of which grow yellow flowers covered with rather long scarious sacs. The root is thick and short, and in some way resembles an acorn: divided, fibrous, and covered with a sort of down. It grows in mountainous, temperate places, such as Xochimilco. The root is bitter; and it has just enough bite, when tasted, to suggest that it is hot and dry, and that it also cures fevers by evacuating the cause, and gets rid of all coldnesses. Moreover, the Indian doctors say that, raw, it provokes sweat and moves the bowels; and that, cooked, it stops up fluxes and cures blood in the bowels.

Teixmincapatli, or Medicine for the Eyes

(2.2.44)

The teixmincapatli is an herb with long narrow leaves, purple stalks, and small round yellow seeds; the root is ramified. It grows in hot terrain and at high altitude. It is a slightly bitter herb with a hot and astringent nature. It cures the sores of the eyes—hence its name—and those of women's and men's genitals, if the powder of its leaves or its root is sprinkled upon them after they have been washed and cleansed with water. It grows in hot, elevated places in Tepecuacuilco, and upon the tops of wooded hills.

Tlaltzilacayotli

(2.2.45)

The herb called tlaltzilacayotli has round leaves, mostly serrate on one side, narrow branches trailing on the ground, and a white flower. The fruit is like green chili, from which its name comes. The root is long, white, and almost an inch thick. It grows in rocky, dry hills in the province of Huexotzinco. The root has a bitter taste, and is hot in nature, so taking three drams gets rid of pains caused by the French disease, although it causes some terrible accidents, the Indians say, because it is customary one day after the purge to put the patients in the steam bath known as temaxcalli, in which they bathe with hot water.

Tlatlacizpatli

(2.2.46)

The tlatlacizpatli has leaves like oregano, minutely serrate, thin short stems, small white flowers, a delicate seed, and hairlike roots. It is bitter and somewhat mucilaginous, so they say that it is a very effective cure for coughing and for fluxes from the head, taken with water in a dose of one dram.

Iztáuhyatl, or Bitter Salt

(2.2.49)

The iztáuhyatl is an herb much like absinthe in form and properties and thus in New Spain it is commonly used as a substitute, which has led the Spanish to corrupt its name, calling it estafiate ⟨or absinthe of the Indies⟩. There are two varieties, one with narrow leaves, the other with much broader ones. It grows in mild or warm places, and it seems to me that it could be cultivated in Castile, from seeds taken from here. It removes pains from a cold cause, and relieves flatulence, it is useful for the chest, cures colic pains and helps the liver. Mixed with quauhiyetl or picietl, which we call tobacco, it strengthens the internal members, succors children who vomit their milk and are satiated. If the seed is taken orally, it clears obstructions. Mixed with the leaves of a certain tree, which smells and looks like the laurel and is called ecapatli, or Indian laurel, it cures perlesia, and its decoction is extremely useful for washing the legs when they are swollen. The leaves are mashed and formed into pellets like pills with honey and placed under the tongue that is swollen. It is a good cleanser and hence clears the head of phlegm.

Tlaelpatli of Acatlan

(2.2.50)

The tlaelpatli of Acatlan has narrow and elongate leaves like alsine, narrow, cylindrical stems one span long, ⟨seeds in flower spikes,⟩ and a long, narrow root. It grows in any climate in Acatlan, near hills. Ground and taken in a dose of half an ounce, the root cures dysentery, hence its name. It is very astringent with some bitterness and heat.

Tlanoquilonipatli

(2.2.51)

The herb known as tlanoquilonipatli produces leaves [like those] of the flax plant, long and narrow, whitish and villous. The stalks [are] round and also whitish; the flowers yellow, spiky and supple; the root long. It grows in the cold heights of Upper Mixteca. The root is somewhat sharp, mucilaginous, and not without some bitterness. When it has been ground up and taken in the amount of a dram and a half, it purges all the humors. As for its temperament, it is hot in the third degree.

Chilpanxóchitl

(2.2.52)

The chilpanxóchitl, also known as miccaxóchitl or medicine for the dead, is an herb with leaves like the leek, red

stems one cubit long, and on them flowers of the same color in calyxes. The small root is full of white fibers and tiny balls, which are somewhat bitter, and all of it we know from experience to be cold and to cure fevers. Three drams, or more if necessary, with water, given as a drink, will reduce inflammations of the breasts. Applied topically as an unguent it cures those suffering from epilepsy, from which it gets its name. ⟨Its nature is moderate and somewhat phlegmatic. It is native to wild and mild places, frequently found in the Mexican countryside, and could reasonably be classified among types of narcissus.⟩

Ahoaton, or Small Oak

(2.2.54)

The ahoaton or small oak, which others call tlalcapolin or small capolin, is an herb with serrate leaves like those of oregano, wall germander, or ilex, only smaller—hence its name—and the leaves are pale green on the underside, darker on the upper. The stalks are reddish; the flowers are scarlet, small, and slightly elongate; the berries are green at first, red later, and finally black, and contain a yellow-colored stone; the long, fibrous root is yellow and of average thickness. The root has an astringent taste and an equal balance of tart and sweet, it is odorless, and by nature it is cold and dry. If it is boiled in the proportion of three ounces to three pounds of water until it is reduced to one-third, and then administered like ordinary water, it comforts women in childbirth, helps prevent dysentery, fortifies loose bones in the ribs, and, like other medicines that provide relief, it eases the aches and pains of people who are tired from a long journey, from running, a fight, or some similar exertion. This plant is found in mild areas like Temichtitlan, or cool ones, and in rocky or mountainous terrain.

China Root of Michoacán

(2.2.56)

There is found in New Spain another species of china root, which we usually call [the china root] of Michoacán because it grows in that province. It is none other than an herb that has a root like [that] of a reed, but thick and heavy, from which its stalks grow like reeds. They are smooth, like those of the reed, and long as a thumb. It has big leaves at intervals, shaped like hearts, with certain veins that cross them lengthwise, which the other [species] also have. It is similar to [the others] in its virtues. It grows in the province of Michoacán, where they call it phaco.

Tlalayótic, or Tlatlalayotic, or Indian Veronica

(2.2.58)

The tlalayótic is an herb that produces small, round leaves resembling those of that plant they call numularia, or veronica. [The leaves are] arranged in pairs on both sides of the stem. It has voluble, slender stalks two spans high. The fruit is good to eat and very similar to the squashes from which its name comes. The root [is] long and smooth almost its entire length. It grows in flat places.

The root [is] viscous and exudes sap; although it has a certain bitterness, it seems to be predominantly cold and dry. It is drunk against the pain and burning sensation of calentures. It stops diarrheas, both those of humor and those of blood; it cures hiccups; it provokes urination; it relaxes shrunken sinews; it cures the wounds and blisters of the mouth. One should take note that if one is attempting to provoke urination, it ought to be given to be drunk in the cocoa beverage that we call chocolate; and if one wants to restrain it, it ought to be with cocoa, but it ought to be boiled. It is to be taken in the amount of two drams each time.

Tozancuitlaxcolli or Mole Guts, or Mole of the Indies

(2.2.59)

The herb called tozancuitlaxcolli has roots massed together like intestines, from which its name comes, stems with leaves like oregano, but rougher and entire, and at the tip, red, bell-shaped flowers. It grows in low-lying places or hilly ones in cold areas such as Chalco, Coatepec, and Xochimilco. It is a common herb, known to everyone as much for its notable astringency as for the unusual form of its roots, which few plants have. The root is cold, astringent, and

slightly bitter. It strengthens the stomach and moderates heat in it when ground and taken in a dose of six drams with water. It cures putrid and cancerous sores, fattens those suffering from consumption, and is commonly prescribed by Indian doctors to strengthen women after childbirth. Taken in a dose of one ounce, it controls fluxes of the belly and dysentery.

Quauhxócoc of Cholula

(2.2.61)

The quauhxócoc produces finely serrate leaves divided into three folds for the most part. The stalks [are] nodular and a span and a half in length. The succulent root [is] like a turnip that shades from white to soft red. It grows in moist places in the province of Cholula. The root is bitter and somewhat sour; the leaf is sour, but good to eat, in such a manner that it seems that this herb belongs to the varieties of xoxocoyolin, which in Spain we call sorrel, which it resembles very much. It produces fruit in berries quite like those we call tomatoes.

The root, when it is crushed and taken by mouth in the amount of two drams, gently purges the stomach and guts, and gets rid of heaviness and weight in those members. It also is given to children, in the amount of only one dram, in the morning, while [they are] fasting.

Purging Amamaxtla, Known as Friars' Rhubarb

(2.2.62)

The root of this plant reproduces and imitates the root of true rhubarb in flavor, color, aroma, substance, and properties in such a way that, if the leaves of this one, which come to a point (while those are narrow at the base and wider at the end), were not different, anyone examining both plants would say that this one is the same Alexandrine rhubarb. All in all, we think that this garden sorrel is a close relative of true rhubarb and can be substituted in its absence, and will serve the same purposes. So of course it purges bile gently and with certain tonicity, which comes from its coarse and astringent properties, in line with the experiments we have done with it among the Spanish many times,[25] and in Mexico too, where it is now found in abundance thanks to the care of Bernardino of Castillo,[26] a man whose notable work is worthy of a panegyric, skillful and valiant in his youth as he combated his enemies, and most careful in his maturity, up to his final days, in the sowing and cultivating of all manner of rare and exotic plants. But as it has subtle parts, which are purgative, and others coarse and astringent, the Indians are in the habit of using the sap, squeezed out in doses of a dram and a half as a purge, and that which is left, in the same dose, as medicine to bind the stomach. Two drams taken whole are sufficient to purge bile in those whose stomachs are on the delicate side, which we can certify from personal experience. One dram of its juice mixed with two drams of an electuary made with the softest sticks of black cinnamon clears bile first of all, and secondly, phlegmatic humors. It grows, cultivated, in all sorts of places, but principally in the warmest, such as Cuernavaca, in moist and fertile terrain. Four years after planting, the root can be used as medicine; it is pulled up at the beginning of summer, cleaned, broken into pieces called boletos, the same size as those of common rhubarb that are customarily brought to us from the East, then they are sorted on tables and turned at least once a day so that they do not lose the juice that they have in such abundance. Four days later they are threaded onto a tough string and hung in the shade, in suitable places where sunlight does not penetrate, and in this way, after two months they are completely dry, and then they can be collected and kept. I have said all this about the so-called friars' rhubarb, not because I am unaware that this plant is also cultivated by the Spanish in places near Madrid, but because in New Spain it is found in abundance in the garden of the above-mentioned gentleman, while many plants from our country are lacking, for the foreign medications brought across so many seas to these regions wind up shriveled and decomposing. I wanted, likewise, to remind the Spanish that with a little care they too could grow this plant in whatever quantities they like, and in the absence of better rhubarb this one could be accorded the prior authorization of the doc-

tors. Finally, the legend that identifies this friars' rhubarb with the Alexandrine: when King Francis[27] of France let the Turks occupy the port and city of Marseilles, they gave true rhubarb seeds to a number of friars—hence the name—from there it was taken to Spain and brought to the Indies, so those who have no faith are proved foolish.[28]

Neizotlalpatli of Tototépec

(3.1.1)

This herb takes its name from vomit, which it provokes. From its ramified roots grow voluble stems decorated with leaves like scammony distributed at long intervals, oblong, but wider at the bud, and white flowers. It grows in warm and flat places. The root is hot and dry in the second degree and is very fetid. They say that, taken in a dose of one ounce, it gently purges bile and phlegm by expulsion both above and below.

Ocopiaztli

(3.1.2)

The ocopiaztli, which other people call the hoitzcolotli, or "scorpion's sting," is a thorny herb that has leaves [like those] of the cirsium,[29] full of longish, narrow thorns. The stems are long, narrow, round, and smooth. On their ends are certain small heads full of thorns, very similar to those of the teasel, covered with purplish blossoms. It grows in flat and rugged places in Tenayuca. The root very much seems [to be] something sweet, and smells like the field eryngo or the chirivia. It is hot and dry in the second degree.

The Indian doctors often give its decoction, or the liquor in which it has been infused for a while, to people convalescing from calentures, in order to [make them] evacuate perfectly by means of urinating or sweating the remains of the humors that caused such fevers. With this, [the convalescents] finally get well and are left free of the illness in every respect. In addition to this, those suffering

---

25. BN MS reads: "for thirty years or so."
26. For some information on this man, see Somolinos, 197, 200–201 (quoting this passage).
27. In BN MS he is King Henry.

28. Ximénez added a long paragraph of his own, with details of where else this rhubarb grows and the case of a patient suffering from cholera who was cured with it.
29. Any of the prickly herbs of the Compositae.

arterial gout benefit in the same way. It is often used in the same way for other, similar things, with a good result.

Tepececentli

(3.1.4)

The herb called tepececentli has purple leaves that grow in the shape of those of the lemon, but larger, stems almost five palms long, cylindrical, purple, an inch thick and nodular at intervals, and a long, voluble white root with nodes on it. The fruit is like the chili, full of flat seeds, round, and surrounded by down. The root is soft outside and in, and has a strong but quite pleasant aroma, rather like a peony, and is hot and dry in the second degree and thick. It feels hot in the throat, but it is not burning. Crushed and taken in a dose of three drams with water, it is said to purge all kinds of humor by the upper and lower passages.

Tlaelpatli of Tonalla, or Medicine for Dysentery

(3.1.8)

The herb called tlaelpatli of Tonalla has narrow leaves like flax, delicate, long, cylindrical stems, and a long, thin, fibrous, white root. It grows in Tonalla, in lower Mixteca. The root is hot in the first degree, with a strong fetid odor, and is somewhat astringent. Taken in a dose of half an ounce, it cures dysentery.

Aphatzipuntzúmeti

(3.1.10)

The [plant] known as aphatzipuntzúmeti has leaves similar to those of basil: round, thin, and hanging from long stems. It has a green stalk, cylindrical and straight, at the end of which are round flowers similar to those of the yellow chamomile, of a tawny color shading to white. The seed much resembles that of anise. The root is single-stemmed, [and] is hot and dry. It grows in cold places in Michoacán, and smells like cilantro. When it has been dissolved in water and drunk, it cures blood in the bowels and those persons who suffer from quartan fevers; its decoction is most useful for washing one's legs.

Aphatzipuntzúmeti 2

(3.1.11)

The aphatzipuntzúmeti produces only one stem, six spans long, thin, cylindrical and striated, with two or three delicate roots like worms, and long, narrow, serrate leaves, thin like those of the almond. If they did not have a touch of gray in them and were not smaller and serrated, they would look like the willow. Its yellow flowers grow in lines and at the extremities, and the seed looks like that of fennel. The root has an aroma like coriander, but tastes like carrot and is hot. It grows on mountain peaks and in cold places, such as Pátzcuaro in the province of Michoacán. Mashed and taken with any suitable drink, it is used to cure, so they say, dysentery and quartan fevers.

Cacahoaxóchitl

(3.1.12)

The cacahoaxóchitl or cacaoatl flower is an herb that has heart-shaped leaves, stems a span long, purple flowers and thick, fibrous roots. The root is sweet, with a trace of bitterness, enough to make it hot. Half an ounce, powdered and taken, cures dysentery. ⟨It grows in Yancuitlan, in Upper Mixteca.⟩

Chichiántic of Coatlan

(3.1.14)

The chichiántic of Coatlan is an herb that has leaves like those of the nettle, but with their buds covered with [a substance] like feathers. The stalks [are] square and bare. The flowers [are] purple ⟨and⟩ very similar to those of the china root, to whose species it appears to belong. The roots are like hairs. It grows in hot regions, such as those of Yyauhtépec and Coatlan.

When the leaves have been crushed and given to be drunk in water, in the amount of half an ounce, they stop diarrhea. It has a hot, dry, astringent nature; and it has a strong smell. It usually restrains the flow of blood in pregnant women, however it may be applied.

Michcuitlaxcolli or Fish Guts

(3.1.17)

They call this herb michcuitlaxcolli, or "fish guts," due to the shape of its root, from which slender stalks sprout, and upon them delicate white flowers. It grows in Pánuco province. The root is hot. Ground and applied as a poultice, it cures wounds with admirable swiftness, even if they be cancerous and otherwise incurable, for which reason the native people hold this plant in great appreciation and esteem. Ground and drunk, the leaves cure jaundice and provoke urine. The root, sprinkled as a powder upon the superfluous growth in the eyes, gets rid of it and cleans it out. It is said as well that, when it has been made into an electuary, it purges the body, in such a way that it gives spirit to and enlivens languid, weary, lazy persons and makes them diligent and quick to endure any travails whatsoever.

Nextlácotl of Yacapichtla

(3.1.18)

The herb nextlazolli of Yacapichtla puts forth leaves like a lemon tree's, although larger and rough; stalks as tall as a man; blondish flowers covered in scarious calyxes; [and] single-stemmed roots. It grows in cold or hot terrain, in moist places and mountain passes. It is aromatic, hot, and dry. The decoction of the roots or the leaves, drunk in the quantity of two drams, provokes urine and is extremely useful for women who recently have given birth.

Tecopalli, or Stone Copal

(3.1.21)

The tecopalli, which is what we might call in Spain "incense of stone," is an herb that produces leaves like those of the acocotli, or Indian lovage. The stem [is] hollow, like that of the giant fennel, and nodular and white at intervals. The fruit grows in calyxes at the ends [of its stalks], in the fash-

ion of a fly swatter; and they [are] very delicate and downy. The flowers [are] villous. The roots [are] similar to threads. It has a hot and dry nature; and therefore, when its powder is mixed with the root that they call nanahuapatli, it usually heals the humors and swellings that are born from the French disease.

Tzonpotónic

(3.1.22)

The people of Cholula give the name tzonpotónic to a certain kind of foreign erica, which is a plant that has downy leaves like [those] of the willow or the coniza. The flowers [are like those] of the erica, which shade from white to reddish, with a small red center. The root [is] single with threads [in it]. It grows in hot terrain such as Huacachula. It has a hot and mucilaginous nature. Its decoction cures a cough and surfeit; it gets rid of pains in the belly; it relaxes and cures joints and articulations impeded by an abundance of humors; it provokes sweating; and it expels wind.

Icelacocotli of Cholula

(3.1.23)

The herb icelacocotli of Cholula has leaves [like those] of the fennel, but thicker and broader, which have a soft scent. The stalks [are] a cubit in length, with filaments and many leaves, and a calyx containing abundant white seeds resembling a vertebra: round and resinous, with sharp edges. This [seed], when chewed, burns the tongue. The root is thick and long and smells like incense. From this description, it clearly is the true rosemary that Dioscorides described under the name fructifero.[30]

Iztacxíhuitl

(3.1.24)

The herb iztacxíhuitl, which some call tecacapan, and others chichihua xíhuitl, is a variety of creeper that was brought

---

30. Ximénez added: "Before Doctor Francisco Hernández, no one had depicted it with a true image and drawing; for the one that Andrea Matiolo presents does not match completely Dioscorides' description. It grows in moist places and in the ravines of wooded hills. It has the same powers that Dioscorides attributes to the rose-

mary. It bears a fruit called cachiri; although the people of Cholula and Tlaxcalla, where it grows, affirm that when its decoction is drunk, it cures smallpox and the spots that usually break out during sanguineous fevers."

into Spain a long time ago, vulgarly known as nun's kiss. It is by nature hot and glutinous, cures eye trouble, provokes urine, and expels retained semen.

Axixpatli of Cuernavaca

(3.1.25)

The axixpatli, which can be called axixpatli of Cuernavaca after its place of origin, has oblong and serrate leaves like mint and tiny purple stellate flowers, quite long, which spring up from the base of the leaves around the tip of the stems. It grows in the warm regions of Xochitépec and Cuernavaca, in flat and wild places. It lacks any notable flavor or aroma and thus is excessively hot. The roots, mashed and taken in a dose of one dram with a decoction of licorice or something similar, make a notable diuretic, clearing obstructions in the urinary tract and anything else that impedes urination. I have seen another herb with the same name in Quauhquechulla, though this one is aromatic and hot in the third degree, with a ramified root, serrate leaves like willow, and medium-sized white flowers. A handful of the leaves of this one, taken with water, also provokes urine.

Cóltotl

(3.1.27)

The cóltotl is an herb that puts forth slender yellow stalks full of leaves like those of the herb cecuridaca, which in Spanish is called *encorbada;*[31] on the ends of which stalks grow flowers like cornflowers, which shade from yellow to reddish. The root is bright yellow, long, and single-stemmed. It grows in Mexico and other temperate and rugged places. It clearly has a moderate nature. It has the taste and smell almost of licorice, from which it happens that when it has been ground and mixed with axixtlácotl and with chichicxíhuitl, it is applied to any part that hurts as a result of passing wind, or cold, [and] thereby gets rid of the pain at once. Moreover, when it is applied to the spleen, this remedy decreases it when it is full of humors. When it is drunk in the amount of a half ounce, it relieves the chest and refreshes

the mouth, benefits [those who have] smallpox, stimulates the appetite, and provokes urine.

Tatacanáltic

(3.1.31)

The herb called tatacanáltic produces leaves [like those] of the willow. The flowers [are] small and purple. The root [is] long and tapers; from it are pendant little balls the size of walnuts. It grows in the heights of Yacapichtla and Ocoytuco. Some people call it teuhquilitl. The root is sweet and has little heat. It is prescribed as a diuretic and in order to temper the burning of calentures. It also cures old wounds when it has been ground up and sprinkled upon [them].

Tlatlauhquichichiántic

(3.1.32)

The herb called tlatlauhquichichiántic, which some people call coztic, or "light reddish," produces some longish serrate leaves. The roots from which the stalks grow [are] like threads, numerous, round, and yellow, and resemble those of the hellebore. It has white flowers in calyxes and fruit like rather elongated acorns. It is cultivated in the fields of Témuac, which is a somewhat hot land, and also in Tepuzcullula [and] in Lower Mixteca, where they call it tlatlahuipátli because of its color, which shades from light reddish to [darker] red. It is given in a drink against calentures; and, after it is mixed with chichimecapatli, so that it may ease heat, it is drunk against smallpox in the amount of two drams' weight. It is instilled into bloodshot eyes, for although it possesses some quality of heat, it also has a moist and bland nature.

Tlallantlacacuitlapilli, or Tail of the Small Possum

(3.1.34)

Two kinds of this herb that they call tlaquacuitlapilli are found—male and female. The male has leaves [like those] of

---

31. Meaning "leaning over."

the nightshade: sharp-pointed, and twisted near the points. The stalks [are] voluble; the root long, slender, fibrous, and white. The female, also voluble, has an ash-gray, nodular stalk and broader leaves. It produces large white flowers in the winter [and] long fruit, longer than the flower, filled with yellow seed and covered with white down. Both have the same nature. It grows in the hot lands of Tlaxmalaca and Cuernavaca, in moist places and mountain passes. The root has no notable scent, and a certain sweetness resembling that of the licorice is found in it, but it leaves a rather bitter aftertaste. Both are of a hot and moist temperament. When it is taken in water in the amount of half an ounce, by itself or with the addition of a little chili, it expels stopped-up urine and cleans out the ducts of the kidneys and the bladder. The decoction of the roots gets rid of calentures by provoking sweat, and alleviates pains of the body.

Xochipalli

(3.1.36)

The xochipalli is an herb six cubits long with sinuous leaves somewhat like those of the mugwort. The stalks [are] as thick as a finger. The flowers [are like those] of the cempoalxóchitl, but smaller, and shade from a yellow color to red. The roots [are] slender and long. It grows everywhere you step in hot areas, and it is an herb that everybody knows. It is used only for its flower, which is moderately hot and has an agreeable scent and flavor. It comforts the heart; [and] heals eclampsia and [also] ulcers, especially those of the mouth. The flowers are particularly useful for dyeing—I say, for [dyeing] gray hair—and for painting images and [other] things of a yellow color or that tend in a certain way to red. For this they are boiled in water, together with saltpeter, and at the end the juice is squeezed out and strained. Painters and dyers use it as we have stated.

Zacanélhuatl of Cholula

(3.1.37)

The herb called zacanélhuatl produces single roots, with some stalks a span in length, and upon those leaves and fruit like those of the anagallis. It grows in the dry lands of the territory of Cholula and in Lower Mixteca. The root is sweet and has a temperate heat. When it has been crushed and thrown into water, and dropped onto a tetter or blister, it is said to cure them. It provokes urination and opens and cleans out its tract, moreover expelling [kidney] stones.

Tonalxóchitl of Ocoituco

(3.1.47)

The tonalxóchitl of Ocoituco, which some people call tonacxóchitl—which means "flower that grows with the sun"—is an herb, of which two varieties can be found. The first produces leaves [like those] of the basil, but larger and not serrate; stalks that twine at intervals, two spans long; big, long flowers [that are] yellow on the inside, and somewhat whitish on the outside, and in the vicinity of certain labia that it has, cloven and purple. From [the flowers'] interiors emerge some hairlike yellow ⟨filaments⟩. The flowers smell like capers and have a sweet flavor. The root [is] single-stemmed. It grows in all hilly regions and places whatsoever, close to trees, even though sometimes they may be found in flat places and orchards, with care [being taken] for its cultivation. It is moderate or slightly inclining to cold; for which [reason], when it is drunk in the quantity of a handful [mixed] in barley water or chicory water, it cures fevers completely. When applied externally, it alleviates erysipelas because it is also moist and glutinous in nature. The second variety of tonalxóchitl, because it has white flowers, they call yztac tonalxóchitl. It differs from the previous one only in this; but in its virtue and shape and all the rest, it is similar.

Matlaliztic of Tetzcoco

(3.1.50)

The herb called matlaliztic produces leaves shaped like those of the plantain, serrate and sparse, not dissimilar to the sprouting of the cane's leaves, but smaller and whitish. The stalks [are] full of knots at intervals of three fingers, ⟨and are⟩ round and hirsute, as thick as a finger and two spans long. The flowers [are] blue and grow in umbels, principally on the ends of the stalks. The roots are like those of the *triorquis,* the difference from which seems minor, but they are small and numerous. It grows in the wooded hills of Mexico.

The root resolves tumors and swellings born of a hot cause when they are crushed and applied in the form of a poultice. When given as a drink in the quantity of two drams, it stops up the impetus of the humors, represses the abundance of the blood, and cools off heat. It is covered with a thick bark. It is sweet without any bitterness, which causes it to provoke lust by increasing wind.

Totoncaxíhuitl, or Totonicxíhuitl

(3.1.54)

This herb is called totoncaxíhuitl, or totonicxíhuitl,[32] because it produces leaves similar to birds' feet—that is to say, sinuous and divided into five or more angles, like the cinquefoil. The people of Atotonilco call this plant caxtlat-lapan because, like the rest of the herbs of this name, it twines itself around and climbs by means of the limbs or neighboring trees. It puts forth a root shaped, and sized, like a hen's egg or a pear, which exudes milky sap. From this root grows a round, viscid stalk that goes crawling along the ground; and upon it [are] some leaves such as we have mentioned. The flower [is] purple like that of the mallow, but smaller. It is readily found in temperate and cold lands. It blooms in the month of August or September. The root has a hot power and an agreeable flavor. When it is crushed and drunk in the amount of one ounce in water, it evacuates all the humors by means of the lower passage, without any sort of trouble.

Ichcacalótic

(3.1.58)

The so-called ichcacalótic—which is also called tlapan-quipatli, which means "cracked medicine"—is an herb that produces round leaves in circular groups, with six in a round, with some other, smaller, whitish, slender, short

ones; and at the end of them some small flowers. The roots are similar to hairs, with which it affixes itself to stones. It grows on the slopes of moist places in hot lands, such as is [the land] of Pahuatla. It is, without doubt, a variety of that herb that the Greeks call lichen, which is similarly hot and moist; but it is good to eat, and it is useful for repulsing swellings and abscesses.

Yexóchitl, or Yetl Flower

(3.1.59)

The yexóchitl—which some people call eloxóchitl, or corn-cob flower; and others [call] zauquixóchitl, or reddish yexó-chitl—is an herb with a large root, which is white on the inside. There are pendant from it, as if from a small rope, another five or six longish roots, very similar to pigs' kidneys but somewhat longer and fibrous. This main root sends out some squared and nodular tendril-like branches marked with four striations. The small branches grow from the knots themselves, filled with twigs resembling those of goosefoot. The flower is longish and yellow, and from it comes the name. This flower usually grows in the summer and smells smoky. It grows in cold lands and rugged places, such as the countryside of Xochitépec.

The root is sweet and good to eat; it has a temperate nature, somewhat inclining to coldness. They say that the juice benefits inflamed eyes, and its decoction [helps] bloody diarrhea. Its powder cures lesions of the mouth and the other members, when they are specially sprinkled with it, if the person who has them is suffering from some hot distemper.

Quamiáhoatl, or Tree-Spike

(3.1.60)

The quamiáhoatl,[33] which other people call tlamacazipa-pan, or (as it were) "priest's-hair," has a hairy, reddish-colored root, from which stalks grow like those of the everlasting flower that modern people call vermicular, to

---

32. A late-eighteenth-century MS note to the equivalent text in the Rome edition identifies this plant as "ipomoea heterophylla Ort. Decad" (copy in Madrid, Museo de las Ciencias Naturales, call number FE 4-262).

33. Identified as Lycopodium, MS note to Rome edition, Madrid, Museo de las Ciencias Naturales, FE 4-262.

which it would be entirely similar if it did not have slender leaves. When these [leaves] have been crushed and applied to the head, they preserve an abundance of hair, and they produce the same effect when they are applied to the other hairy parts of the body. They say that when this plant is taken in water in a dose of two drams, it evacuates all the humors, but especially the phlegm, thus curing people who suffer from cachexia, dropsy, the French disease or pains in their joints, and those who are impeded in their movement. It lacks a noticeable flavor, even though it emits a certain fetidness that reveals heat. It also is similar to the spurge and should be classified, as I believe, among its varieties even though its stalks are branchy, which does not occur in the spurge. For that reason, I have elected to describe it and paint it, even though I do not doubt that it is the same [spurge], distinguished only by the soil in which it grows; or at least it is related to it. It grows in craggy and hilly places of Tepoztlan; and usually it also is sown in kitchen gardens for medicine.

Teuhxóchitl, or God's Herb

(3.2.1)

The herb called teuhxóchitl produces many slender, round, viscid, green—and occasionally reddish—stems full of leaves like those of the wild basil: downy, purplish, and delicate, which sprout before summer. The root [is] tender and double, longer than the entire plant; it exudes milky sap, and is white inside and tawny-colored outside. It grows in cold lands and has a cold nature, in the second degree. For this reason, when it has been crushed and drunk, in the weight of four scruples, it quenches thirst and moistens the tongue, and softens and mitigates excessive heat. It is a great remedy for restoring the heated liver; and in addition to this, it has a particular power against poisons. It softens them and gets rid of their force.

Atlanchane

(3.2.5)

The atlanchane has leaves like the willow, long round stems that are thin, smooth, yellowish, and hollow, which trail along the ground, and are no thicker than goose feathers. The flowers, which grow at the tips of the branches, are oblong and are like yellow capsules. The roots are ramified. The roots are cold and dry, astringent, and control dysentery and almost all other fluxes.

Cicimátic

(3.2.6)

The herb called cicimátic is similar to the turnip. It has a fibrous root, from which grow the leaves in groups of three in the shape of a heart and similar to beans, a variety of which it seems to be. It produces some small pods, and they grow red flowers that hang from the stems in racemes. It grows in hot lands and also in temperate ones, such as Mexico. Its nature is cold and viscous.

When it has been made into powder and put on wounds, the root cleans them and causes new skin to grow. Because of this, many people call this herb palancapatli, or "medicine for wounds." It is an admirable remedy for eyes that suffer from lesions and inflammations; it dissolves the cloudiness and superfluous flesh that grows in them. It stops up the flow from the womb and comforts women who have just given birth. The decoction of the root cures bloody diarrhea.

Cutiriqui, or Matlacaza

(3.2.10)

This herb, which the people of Michoacán call catiri, the Mexicans call matlacaza. It produces leaves resembling those of the domestic betony, smooth but smaller and more delicate. The stalks [are] smooth, purplish, round, and nodular at intervals. The flowers [are] yellow, and ⟨there are⟩ some rather long pods filled with triangular seeds not unlike mustard. The roots [are] small and almost round, white and fibrous, similar to small onions wrapped in a sort of black covering. It grows in cold terrain, such as that of Chimalhuacan and that of Chalco, in harsh and rocky places. The roots are cold and moist, and taste like jicama. They are good to eat, raw or cooked; and [the root] is said to cure fevers.

Nequámetl

(3.2.16)

The plant called nequámetl,[34] which means honey drinker, is a variety of the maguey similar in its properties to its fellows. The stalk and the fruit are of a rare shape: the stalk is as thick as an arm, and on its tip, covering it all over, are the fruit, ⟨which are⟩ oblong, shaped like small pears. The leaves are a little more than an inch thick, rough on the sides, and very sharp at the tip. It grows in hot regions. There are many other varieties of maguey, to whose depictions I have added only their names and the places in which they grow, since nearly all have the same virtues and are little different in form. The first is called mexoxoctli, or "green maguey." The second [is called] néxmetl because of its ashen color. The third [is called] quámetl, or maguey of the woods, and is discolored, with a fibrous root shaped like a thick, long sprout. The fourth is called hoitzitzímetl, whose long thorns and roots are purple. The fifth is the tapayáxmetl, or Tapayaxin maguey, almost the same as the previous one. The sixth is called acámetl, or "reedy maguey"; its leaves are whiter near the root, and its thorns and roots red. The seventh is called black maguey because of its dark color, even though its thorns and roots are a mixture of black and tan. The eighth is the xilómetl, or "hairy metl," with red thorns and roots, slightly sparser than in the preceding varieties.

Tlacámetl, or Great Maguey

(3.2.18)

This is a variety of metl, almost of the same shape and properties as the others, and with the same applications; but it especially gives vigor and strength to weak women or those who suffer from fainting spells. It has been given its name because of its [large] size.

Quetzalichtli, or Maguey Resembling the Quetzalli, or Feathers of the Quetzaltótotl

(3.2.21)

The quetzalichtli, which is also call the pita metl, seems to belong to the metl species. It reaches the height of a tree; it

has a thick, fibrous root that gradually becomes slender, and spiny leaves similar to those of a metl. Everything that is usually made from the metl is made from it, although textiles more delicate and more greatly esteemed [i.e., than those made from the metl] are made with its thread. It grows in hot places in Quauhquechulla and Mecatlan.

Omimetztli

(3.2.24)

The [plant] that they call omimetztli is an herb whose leaves are shaped almost [like those] of the basil, ⟨but⟩ somewhat deeper, shading from green to purplish. The stalks [are] red and slender and twining. The flowers, at the tips ⟨of the⟩ branches, shade from white to reddish and [are] small. From these come round pods filled with seed. The root is tender, thick, long, white, and fibrous; it has no scent or taste. It is glutinous, with a cold and moist temperament. Some people call this plant omitotonqui; and other people [call it] poztec-patli, and others still [call it] tlalticcopatli. It grows in high and rugged lands in Tememeltzingo and Ocopayuca and Tototepec, its shape showing some variations in some ⟨of these⟩ places.

The root restores broken and dislocated bones to their proper places. When it is applied in the form of a poultice to the parts of the body that have been traumatized in a fall or from a blow, it undoes [the displacement] with notable success. It also helps people who pass blood in their urine. It gets rid of pains ⟨and⟩ prevents abscesses.

Tepizticxíhuitl or Robust Herb

(3.2.27)

This has thin purple stems, small, serrate, round leaves somewhat like maidenhair but smaller, yellow flowers tinged with red, oblong, contained in a calyx almost like a rose's. It grows in hilly or wild places in the Mexican region. The root is usually cut in September and kept for future use. Its root, which is the principal part used in medicine, evacuates (when taken) urine retained for any reason; its nature is cold and moist, which also helps it reduce fevers.

---

34. Metl, in this and the two following descriptions, is the Náhuatl name for maguey.

Tlápatl

(3.2.28)

This plant has white ramified roots. Its fruit is round and similar to the prickly pear. Its stems are green and the leaves are like those of the wild vine, wide and divided by deep recesses. Its flowers are white and large and in the form of a calyx. This plant grows in many places but primarily in Tepecuacuilco and Mexico. Its temperament is cold and it has no discernible taste or smell. A decoction of the leaves is rubbed on the body for fevers, especially the quartan fever, or it can be applied in the form of a small suppository or pellet. The fruit and the leaves are good for pains in the chest. When these leaves are instilled with water and placed in the ears, they are good for deafness. Placed on a pillow, they bring sleep to insomniacs, but taken in large amounts they induce madness.

Tzauhtli

(3.2.33)

The herb that they call tzauhtli produces leaves [like those] of the leek, with certain lines that run the length of them. The stalks [are] straight and knotted; and upon them are some flowers that shade from yellow to red, resembling in some way those of the iris, although [they are] much smaller. The root ⟨resembles⟩ those of the asphodel: white and fibrous. It is found everywhere, high or low, but mainly in hot lands. It is cold, moist and glutinous.

A consummate and very tenacious paste is made from it: painters use it because it makes the colors adhere strongly. The images that they paint ⟨with it⟩ do not darken or wear away so quickly. The root is cut into small pieces and put to dry in the sun. It is ground up, and thus they make the paste with water. The Indians also say that when it is taken by mouth, in the amount of one ounce, this root cures bloody diarrhea, and moreover benefits ⟨those who are suffering from⟩ the rest of the illnesses that proceed from diarrhea and looseness ⟨of the bowels⟩.

Iztaczazálic, or Viscous Herb

(3.2.34)

This herb known as iztaczazálic is a type of voluble plant that takes its name from its extreme viscosity. It is white inside, red outside, and has virtually no taste. It produces long, rounded stems that twine around one another, and on them are leaves like garlic or those of the herb called colt's foot, slightly serrate. They say that it bears neither flowers nor fruit. It produces racemes similar in shape and size to wild grapes with many tendrils and berries everywhere, as we saw in the grapevines. It grows in rocky terrain and temperate mountainous places such as Mexico. The decoction of the root cures diarrhea. One ounce of the same root, drunk, is very good for tiredness after a long journey, mends fractures and if it is added to xochinacaztli, called orejuelas in Spanish, and drunk in the same quantity, they say that it provokes urine, it is usually given to people getting into a bath after a serious illness, and to women after childbirth for comfort. They say that, applied topically, it eases pains, repels inflammations, and reduces fevers, because it is cold, moist, and glutinous in nature.

Huemberequa

(3.2.40)

The herb called huemberequa produces round leaves in bunches of three, but the one in the middle is much larger and rounder than the others. The stalks [are] long. The fruit [is] small and in bunches; it grows all along the stalk, at the bases of the leaves. The somewhat woody root is long and tapering. This plant grows in the cold and rugged terrain of the province of Michoacán.

It has a cold and astringent nature, with which it usually gives benefit to those who have calentures. The decoction of the roots and the leaves, used as a mouthwash, heals and gets rid of pain in the teeth; it also gets rid of any other pain. The same decoction, squeezed and applied as a liniment on wounds, heals them admirably, even if they are born of the French disease. It raises any welts and itches on those persons who urinate on it and ⟨then⟩ pick them.

Quauhmecapatli

(3.2.43)

The quauhmecapatli is a variety of sarsaparilla whose roots are sent to Spain; with large heart-shaped leaves, twining and spiny stalks, a branched root, no fruit, and tendrils that sprout from every part [of the plant], and many berries. It grows in the fields of Tototépec, Metztitlan, and Quauhchinanco; but the best of them all grows in the region that is called, because of its depths, Honduras.[35]

Teuhquílitl, or Prince's Herb

(3.2.45)

The [plant] that they call teuhquílitl is an herb that has sharp leaves like those of the pomegranate, which grow in threes from every node in the stalk. It has many reddish, round, slender, woody stalks. It produces flowers at the tops of the branches, disposed in racemes, reddish, where small pods grow, enclosing a seed composed of tiny granules, which in the beginning are white but turn black after they mature. The root [is] slender and long, yellow on the outside and pale inside, shading into a whitish color.

When the root is drunk in water, in the amount of about three drams, it mitigates the heat of fevers because it has a cold and dry constitution and is astringent. Hence it stops diarrhea, and restores the stomach and comforts it when it is weak because of great heat.

Tlalmatzalin of Huexocinco

(3.2.49)

The tlalmatzalin is an herb that produces leaves [like those] of the almond tree—long, narrow, and serrate—hence its name. The stalks [are] delicate, square, and a little more than a span in length. The delicate purple flowers ⟨grow⟩ at intervals. The small roots [are] similar to turnips. It grows in moist places and in the ravines of the wooded hills of Huexocinco. It has fragrant leaves; they are somewhat hot, but the root is cold and dry in its nature and has almost no scent or taste. When [the root] is crushed and given to be drunk in water, together with four grains of cocoa, in the amount of three drams, it is said to be a gentle purge for the belly and all the body. It cleans out the urinary tract and is notable for moderating heat.

Alahoacapatli

(3.2.51)

The alahoacapatli has slender leaves like those of the flax, but smaller, and white flowers; the root is white, transparent, fibrous and twisted. It grows in the cold regions of Yalhualiuhcan, on the mountain slopes. The root, crushed and taken in a dose of an ounce and a half with water of bugloss and natural water, is said to evacuate all humors. There is also a spiny alahoacapatli, which seems to be a variety of tunas, which we will discuss in connection with those.

Cacamótic Tlanoquiloni

(3.2.53)

While some call this plant cacamótic tlanoquiloni, others customarily refer to it as caxtlatlapan and apitzalpatli. It has a rounded root, white and soft, from which sprout delicate, cylindrical, and voluble stems, leaves in the shape of an Amazon's pelta[36] or ivy, but more angular, and flowers that are mauvish purple, shaped like calyxes or cymbals. This one grows wild or cultivated, with robust vigor, in hot or temperate areas such as Pahuatlan and Mexico, and could be transplanted to various places in Spain. Two ounces of the roots taken at bedtime purge the stomach with wonderful gentleness and safety, and furthermore they remove bilious and other humors from the veins. What shall I say of their sweet and pleasant taste, not a whit inferior to the muscat nut or to our pears? Why proclaim eternal human discontent, and remain tormented by a thousand medications, when there is in nature such an abundance of mild and benign remedies?

Coapatli like Asphodel

(3.2.54)

The herb that they call the asphodel-like coapatli produces long, white roots like those of the asphodels, which explains

---

35. Honduras was given its name because the waters close to the coastline there are extremely deep. *Las honduras* means "the depths."

36. See Hernández's allusion to the Amazonian pelta—a shield—in *Antiquities*, 1.1, above. The context here suggests that "Amazon's shield" may be a vernacular name for a Mexican plant.

its name; or [like] those of the matlalitztic. From these roots come long leafy stems exactly the same as those of the leek. The flowers [are] in the shape of spikes on the ends of the stalks, similar to the little flower heads of the French lavender. It grows in Quauhtla. The root is soft and filled with juice. It has no noticeable scent or taste. They have a cold and moist temperament. When they have been crushed and applied, they are useful against snakebites; and they do the same when they are drunk in the water of ashes.[37]

Coapatli from Yancuitlan

(3.2.55)

The herb coapatli of Yancuitlan produces rough branches, with narrow, villous leaves [that are] whitish on their undersides. The flowers [are] yellow. The root [is] long and slender. It grows in the cold heights of Upper Mixteca. It seems [to be] of a cold and mucilaginous nature.

It cures ⟨the effects of⟩ poisoned drinks and snakebites, ⟨the latter⟩ when it is applied to the wound three or four times a day or given to be drunk, added to some appropriate liquid. ⟨This is⟩ as the clear and manifest experiment has shown upon a farrier—whose name I do not remember—who was living as the lover of an Indian woman, who gave him a snack of some tamales at six in the morning. At eight o'clock he started shouting like a madman, spewing froth at the mouth, all swollen and blue as an iris. When his trouble was seen to come near his legs, ⟨and he was⟩ like a man already breathing his last, an Indian came bearing this root. [The farrier] began to recover somewhat; and thanks to a ⟨potion to induce⟩ vomiting that we gave him, he threw up a great quantity of poison, so we gave him the drink immediately afterward. Thereupon he slept until four in the afternoon; and ⟨then⟩ he got up and walked around. By repeating this ⟨course of treatment⟩, after some days he was seen [to be] cured and well. But in the end, it happened that the same misadventure befell him four months after that.[38]

Huacuicua, or Dream of the Animal That Is Called Huacuiaya

(3.2.60)

The so-called huacuicua is a voluble herb that produces leaves shaped like those of the ivy, but narrow and long. The flowers [are] reddish. The stalks [are] slender, round, and downy. The roots [are] thin. It grows in flat, temperate, somewhat moist places, such as Uruapa. It lacks any notable flavor; but despite this, its decoction loosens the belly and its powder does the same. When drunk in the amount of two drams, it mitigates extreme pain in the belly, especially from a cold cause.

Purging Motinense Herb

(3.2.62)

This has small leaves shaped like ivy leaves, red flowers in calyxes, and rounded capsules that enclose the seed; the stalks are red and twining and the root is fibrous. It grows in Xiquilpa and in Tarímbaro, in the province of Michoacán. The seed, crushed and taken with water in a dose of a dram, purges all humors without any harm.

Tzaguángueni

(3.2.67)

The tzaguángueni—which other people call the zacualpa plant for the place where it grows, and others call totzinxitl, and some people also call comatlquilitl, and the people of Michoacán [call] xerotzi—is an herb that produces long, narrow leaves, for the most part in bunches of five, similar to those of the herb [called] iztafiatl or absinthe of the Indies. It has stalks six spans in length. The flower [is] reddish. The root [is] fibrous. It grows in the flat fields of Cuernavaca, in moist areas. When it is applied to hemorrhoids, or tied on the arm, it dries up and consumes them.

---

37. It is not clear what this means.

38. Unfortunately, the text ends here, so we do not know if he survived the second episode. The tone of the passage hints that he did not. Most of this paragraph is by Ximénez.

Yolopatli, or Irina

(3.2.75)

The yolopatli is an herb also known as irina, for the virtue that it has in comforting the heart and because the shape of the leaves resembles those of the iris. Two kinds of this herb are found. The first grows leaves like the iris's, but smaller and narrower; flowers resembling those of the omixochitl; roots like small vines, reddish, a bit long and stringy. It may belong to the narcissus species. It grows in Quauchinango, which is a hot land, in mountain passes.

The roots, when drunk in the amount of an ounce, are said to cure pain in the heart and its other indispositions. It cures fevers and is a particular remedy for wounded persons who have fallen from some high place, and for those who have been whipped. Some people say that it heals fainting spells, sadness, and other illnesses of the chest, when one takes it upon going to sleep. It is cold and moist in nature. It has no notable scent or taste.

The second kind is called yolopatlipitzahuac, which is an herb that has no stalk or flower or fruit. Its leaves are similar to those of the plantain, but thicker, more tenacious and narrower, and which grow only one or two to a root. It too grows in the same hot region, in rocky places. When it has been ground up and drunk, it heals calentures of any sort. When it is applied to the body, it refreshes it admirably.

AGUSTÍN VETANCOURT, TEATRO MEXICANO

Fray Agustín Vetancourt (1633–1700) incorporated some texts of Hernández, Agustín Farfán, and Gregorio López (who, he said, made use of the material that went into the *Quatro libros* [p. 54, 1.2, cap. 11, para. 194]) in his *Teatro mexicano: Descripcion breve de los sucessos exemplares, historicos, politicos, militares, y religiosos del nuevo mundo occidental de las indias* (Mexico City, 1698). Vetancourt was vicar of the chapel of San José de los Naturales in the Franciscan monastery in Mexico City. His own great work, the *Arte de lengua mexicana* (Mexico City, 1673), includes the comment that Nebrija's methods—methods that influenced Hernández—of studying European languages do not work very well in the New World.

Vetancourt's sole source for Hernández was the *Quatro libros,* from which he took about fifty chapters and abridged or paraphrased them, noting that the *Quatro libros* had been "well received" (1.2.11). Vetancourt seems to have been unaware of any European printings that included Hernández texts. His abridgments are terse, often dispensing with such luxuries as verbs. Until the new edition of the *Quatro libros* prepared by Antonio Peñafiel (Mexico City, 1888) and Maximino Martínez's *Plantas medicinales de Mexico* (Mexico City, 1933), Vetancourt's text was the last printing of a significant selection of Hernández to be published in Mexico.

Xaltomatl

Xaltomatl, sandy tomato, is a species of solanum, has a root like a small sweet potato, leaves smaller than the lemon, grows in cold lands, and sandy and mild; its root is cold and dry and has the same virtues as the solanum; broken in water, weight of one ounce, it expels wind, cleanses by the lower conduit, is good for bloody diarrhea, is prescribed to those suffering from tabardete,[1] and ground, and given to

---

1. This word covers a multitude of illnesses, including cocoliztli, tertian and quartan intermittent fevers, and even syphilis. It is discussed in the first chapter of Francisco Bravo, *Opera medicinalia* (Mexico City, 1570).

drink in pulque or honey water, it provokes sweat, and expels pockmarks. Mashed, it can be used in plain water in place of lentils, and from that enemas are frequently made, as many experiments have shown.

Cocoztomatl

Cocoztomatl, also called cocoztic and cocozton, is a voluble shrub, with thick leaves, divided in three points, white flowers, and small like those of the izquixochitl, from which grow white fruit, the root yellow, which has no aroma, nor any notable taste, its temperament is cold, and diuretic, made into powder and taken in any liquor, quantity of half an ounce, it provokes urine, expels gravel, purges phlegmatic humors that obstruct the conduits, suppresses fleshy growths there: also, mixed with oil of sweet almonds, with a cotton thread dipped in egg white, inserted in the urinary tract, like small candles, it has a wonderful effect; this root mixed with a purgative medicine, purges the belly. There is another herb called coztomatl, which is a yellow solanum with brownish stems, the fruit covered with certain sacs, the root thick and white, grows in cold and humid terrain, like Mexico, the root is bitter, and hot in nature. It cures indigestion, expels flatulence, gets rid of belly pain, controls diarrhea from a hot cause, and applied to a woman's breasts, it educes milk.

THE LOW COUNTRIES, 1630–1648

JOHANNES DE LAET

The first European publication to include significant portions of Hernández's descriptions of the plants of New Spain was *Beschrijving van West-Indien* (Description of the West Indies), by Johannes de Laet (Leiden, 1630). This was the second Dutch edition of de Laet's work, the first having appeared in 1625 with no mention of Hernández. De Laet acquired a Spanish text of Hernández between 1625 and 1630 and began to translate it. In the 1630 edition of de Laet's work, descriptions of plants by Hernández replaced those from Monardes and Oviedo that de Laet had used in the first edition. The 1633 edition, in Latin, contained many more selections, which were repeated when the Latin edition was translated into French in 1640. The section on Guatemala, which includes parts of the *Quatro libros* on cacao, corn, and passing comments on birds, has been translated into Spanish (*Mundo Nuevo o descripción de las Indias Occidentales: Libro VII, Guatimala,* translated by Marisa Vannini de Gerulewics [Guatemala City: Academia de Geografía e Historia de Guatemala, 1991]).

We have translated selections from de Laet's manuscript, British Library MS Sloane 1555, whose order we follow. De Laet's printed work, which paraphrased or abridged his manuscript, was not an edition of Hernández but a description of the Americas. The printed text does not create or maintain any special order that Hernández had given his descriptions. Much of de Laet's ordering of the chapters in his manuscript is the same as Recchi's, but in parts it is completely unlike that of any other surviving text; this ordering suggests that, even if he was translating the printed text of the *Quatro libros,* he did not respect its arrangement.

Copalquáhuitl, or Gum-Bearing Tree

(1.8)

The leaves of this tree are like the oak's in shape and size, but longer; the fruit is round, dark red, and tastes like the resin that comes from the tree. It exudes this resin spontaneously at times, and occasionally it can be induced with incisions; it is given the name of copal specifically, although the Indians really mean by this word all types of gum and resin, and restrict the name to trees that exude them. This resin, as is well known now almost throughout Europe, is colorless and clear, and hardens into broad chips. In Xicalan, in Uruapa, in the province of Michoacán, there are some trees no different from this one, which produce a golden resin, which species I have seen and of which I shall say more later. It grows in warm places, flat or hilly but damp, in Cuernavaca, Tlatzinco, Teotlalco, Copalla and Michoacán. But there is some difference between the wild and the cultivated, both in the shape of the tree and in the color of the resin, for which reason we give illustrations of both.[1] Its temperament is hot and dry almost in the third degree, somewhat astringent, solvent, and with a delightful aroma. The smoke from this resin, like that of the wood or the roots of this same tree, clears headaches from a cold cause, cures strangulation of the womb and, generally speaking, relieves all illnesses from a cold or moist cause. The same goes for other kinds of copal. Wax, as the Mexicans call it, is made from this resin, and others; used in this way it is good against all pains.[2]

Copalquáhuitl Patláhoac or Copal Tree with Broad Leaves

(1.9)

Although, as I said above,[3] the Indians normally give the name copalquáhuitl par excellence to the tree that we have described in the previous chapter, and copal to its resin, they give the same name indifferently to all the fragrant resins that come from any tree of this kind. But the Spanish use the name copal only for those trees that yield white resin, while those that produce blackish resin much like incense they usually call the incense tree of the Indies or moving spirit. But as there are many different varieties of this tree, we shall treat them separately.[4] The copalquáhuitl patláhoac is named for the breadth of its leaves, which are wider than those of all the others belonging to its genre. It is of medium size, grows untidily with serrate leaves that, at the tips, are similar to the plant known in Spain as sumac, in color, bitterness, and dryness, as well as shape and size. It has branches like wings, which produce a white resin quite different from that of the copalquáhuitl, but in smaller quantities, and said to have the same properties. It grows in warm places, especially in Cuernavaca, where it is very common.[5]

Tecopalquáhuitl or Wild Copal

(1.11)

This is a mid-sized tree with leaves like the strawberry tree, and fruit like acorns, containing a single nut covered with a kind of slimy resinous film, which encloses a white seed useful for many purposes. This tree exudes a gum like European incense in aroma, taste and virtues, which I judge is a relative thereof, because I have heard say that also in the Philippine Islands it grows everywhere. The people who live here in New Spain commonly call it ⟨incense⟩, though some call it spirit of the Indies. It grows in warm places in Papalotícpac.[6] All parts of this tree are hot almost in the third degree, and dry, with a pleasant

1. This is Hernández speaking: de Laet did not give illustrations of these plants.

2. It is interesting that de Laet (and his source) should omit Hernández's observation that the aroma can be smelled "once ⟨the resin⟩ is put to the fire; it is customary to worship the gods with this aroma or smoke (tecopalli is also used for this purpose) and the first conquerors of this land were received with this, whom this rude and ignorant people called teteuh, that is, gods."

3. In the previous chapter.

4. In the *Quatro libros* the equivalent of this sentence is "But as it is our intention always to proceed with clarity and discrimination, and many species of these trees yield similar liquors and resins—

some very similar but others very different from one another—we shall treat each species separately, explaining the differences among the resins, although to all appearances they have the same properties as the trees themselves."

5. The text from the BN MS reads: "It grows in warm places, principally in Cuernavaca, where we saw this tree frequently, even inside the very pueblo, and if I am not mistaken, it would be no difficult matter to have it shipped to Spain and planted in the warmer parts of the land there." De Laet's marginal note in the MS and in the 1633 editon of *Novus Orbis,* finishes with a brief reference to Monardes.

6. The BN MS adds that this plant could be transplanted to warmer regions of Spain.

odor. With the smoke ⟨from all parts⟩ it strengthens the stomach, heart, brain, and uterus; it removes rheums, consumes chills, warms cold parts of the body, restores a prolapsed womb to its proper place, and makes firm and fixed anything that is loose.

Copal de Tototépec

(1.12)

This is a large tree with dark green leaves like those of the golden apple tree. It exudes a gum that is very similar to the copal and is gathered in the same way, in small chips, and is kept for the same uses.

Cuitlacopalli, or Copal Dung

(1.13)

This tree (which is also called xioquáhuitl because the scabrous trunk looks as if it has suffered from leprosy) is medium sized, with small round leaves; it bears acidic fruit in spiny racemes, very fragrant and viscous. It produces a white gum that is somewhat fragrant, in nature hot in the third degree and moist. It grows in warm regions of Yyauhtépec, only in mountainous and rocky places.

Tecopalquáhuitl Pitzáhoac, or Narrow-Leaved Copal

(1.14)

When I was in Tepoztlan with the object of studying plants, and also in Hoaxtépec, I came across another medium-sized tree that exudes resin, or a type of incense that is virtually colorless, though it does tend slightly to gray, with the same rare properties and aroma of the preceding tree,[7] but with leaves arranged in a line from one side to the other of the branches, small but not serrate, and slightly larger than those of rue. The fruit is small, red, shaped like a round pepper, and adhering at more or less regular intervals to the branches. The resin of this tree mixed with the dung of ants and babies, and taken two to three times in a dose of one ounce, cures those who have delirium without a fever.

Xochicopalli, or Flowering Copalli

(1.15)

Xochicopalli is a medium-sized tree with leaves like mint, but more deeply divided and growing together in groups of three; the stems are very fragrant; it exudes a reddish liquid with an aroma much like lemon, and which has such similar properties to the ⟨other copals⟩ that it must belong to the same species. It grows in warm places in Colima and Michoacán. There is another tree of this name that exudes a similar gum, but its leaves are like the xocoxóchitl.[8]

Mizquixochicopalli

(1.16)

The mizquixochicopalli, also called xochicopalquáhuitl, is a large tree with leaves like the golden apple and a trunk marked with white spots, and small red flowers. It produces a gum the color of fire that is called spirit by some and copal by others, which is efficacious, for all the same purposes as the other kinds, but mainly as a perfume and to strengthen the head. It grows in very warm places in Copitlan and Colima.

Balsam Shrub (Tarascan maripenda)

(1.20)

This plant appears not to be a tree but a shrub, but it is to be recorded among the trees, on account of its similarity to the previous one [quauhconex 1.19], also a maripenda shrub, with a round trunk twenty spans tall, and blackish branches. Its leaves are similar to the spicula, thick and wide, green on top but purple underneath; fruit in racemes hangs from a red pedicel, six spans in length, like grapes but more sparse: these are green at first, then red, and finally turn deep purple. The natives use the leaves as pipes for smoking tobacco. They take the shoots and branches of this plant (however, not the seeds) and chop them minutely, and boil them in water until they have cooked down and acquired the consistency of syrup. This liquor is a wonderful cure for old wounds, and stanches blood in recent ones.

---

7. LMS 1.13.

8. Probably a transcription error: Hernández (BN MS) has "yoloxóchitl, which grows among the Teocaltzincans."

Copáltic, or Resin-Bearing Tree like the Copalli

(1.27)

This is a tall tree, smooth, covered with a skin or layer that it sheds spontaneously (which is why it is called xixio), with leaves like basil and fruit slightly larger than the hawthorn, green at first and then turning red. This tree produces a white resin that is quite fragrant, but in small quantities. It grows in warm and mountainous places in Texaxáhuac. The pulp is hot in the second degree, fragrant and pleasant to taste, with a certain bitterness. The resin is widespread among the Mexicans as a very effective cure for dysentery. Taken in a dose of one obolus with water, in which it dissolves at once making it milky (which they then call quauhcitlali), either on its own or mixed with copalli, cures dysentery and retards a bloody flux in any part of the body. Larger doses, however, should be avoided.

Tzinacancuitlaquáhuitl or Tree That Produces Resin like Bat Dung

(1.28)

Gums that are commonly known as lacca are not, as is commonly but falsely believed, produced by ants, but by drops that exude from this tree, which in the Indies is called tzinacancuitlaquáhuitl, which means tree that bears gum that resembles the excrement of bats. Small leaves grow at intervals on the branches. This tree grows in warm areas of Oastepec and Cuernavaca, where it is sometimes called xochipatli quauhxihuitl. It grows too in the east Indies, where it goes by several names. To find out about its uses, one must consult the Arab doctors. This gum is mixed with turpentine to make lacca, which is commonly used to seal letters; and if it is added to these other things it becomes quite thick, then ground and the whole lot cooked, it forms a paste that, subjected to heat, softens at once, but when it cools it hardens tougher than iron, stone, or diamonds, all of which it can break, which I know by observation.

Mesquite or Acacia

(1.31)

The mesquite is a very common tree in New Spain. It grows spontaneously in all kinds of places, though mainly in the hills, or any place that is mild or cool. It is scrubby and spiny, with tiny leaves like feathers disposed in a line on either side of the branches, a flower very similar to that of the tamarind and almost the same shape, and edible pods, oblong, sweet, and very pleasant tasting, full of seeds (hence its name), hanging everywhere. The Chichimeca make tortillas from the seeds, as a substitute for bread. This is the true acacia of the ancients, which produces real gum arabic, and it is found in great quantities in New Spain, though perhaps through negligence it remains unknown in Europe and is not yet imported there, but what is taken away from here is adulterated. There are many varieties of this tree. Its nature is cold, dry and astringent. The liquid it exudes, or which is extracted from the shoots of this tree, or better the water in which they are soaked for a while, admirably alleviates eye problems when it is applied. The decoction of the rind helps to control excessive menstrual flow; it cures scurf and impetigo. Some classify the axin, nacazcolotl and a few other trees that grow in New Spain among types of acacia.

Mesquite of Michoacán

(1.32)

The people of Michoacán give the name tzizítzequa to mesquite. It grows spines, and its leaves are more slender than the common mesquite. It is also a species of acacia, and produces an excellent gum arabic; it is found everywhere and has the same properties as the ⟨common mesquite⟩.

Íczotl

(2.4)

The íczotl, which the Spanish call mountain palm, and some of the Indians call quauhtepopatli, or medicinal wild brush, produces from one root two or three stems and white fragrant flowers in hanging racemes with six petals: from them grow fruits like pine nuts. It grows in mountainous places, whatever the climate. The fruit is cold and glutinous, so its seeds, roasted and crushed with chia, or with white lead in any astringent liquid, are a great cure for dysentery and prevent vomiting. A decoction of the leaves and the root cures syncope and calms fears if it is taken at the onset of an attack.

Some say that it also cures indigestion caused by some other illness, which I could not guess how to verify, whether or not it really strengthens the stomach. I must not omit mention of the way they make thread from the leaves of this tree, to weave cloths and mats, better finished and tougher than the ones they make from maguey.

Nopalnocheztli, or Cochineal of the Indies That Grows in Certain Tunas

(2.6)

In Mexico, in a certain genus of tunas called nopalnocheztli,[9] which grows in places sheltered by nature from possible damage by animals, some little red worms can be found. These are white on the outside and red inside; sometimes they grow naturally, sometimes by human cultivation, taking account of the previous year's seeds of the tunas. The Indians call them nocheztli and the Spanish cochineal, a name perhaps derived from coccum, or the insect of which this is a species. Some judge that these little worms are quite distinct; but although I am fully aware that the cochineal of the Old World does not adhere to tunas, which do not even exist there, but to the leaves of a certain ilex that the moderns call kermes oak; that it has astringent virtues, and that its internal part is called kermes on account of its excellence, while in its exterior part, which is more common, the Greek name is preserved, however, as these are worms, they serve equally to dye linens scarlet, and are indiscriminately used by painters and dyers, I am convinced that they should be classified in the genus of coccum or cochineal, from which, as we said, perhaps the Spanish name came, just as those that grow in Peru live in the roots of the plant called pampinula or teucrio. A purple dye can sometimes be extracted from the nocheztli, or a red one, according to the way it is prepared. A particularly exquisite color can be obtained if it is mixed with a decoction of the tree known as tezhoatl, of which we shall speak in its place, and alum, and stirring the sediment, which is kept in the form of tablets. Mixed with

vinegar and applied as a poultice, it binds, alleviates wounds, strengthens the heart, head, and stomach, and is very good for cleaning the teeth.[10]

Copalxócotl, or Resinous Plum Tree

(2.9)

Copalxócotl, which in Michoacán is known as popoaqua, is a tree with leaves like our plums, and fruit like small apples, sweet and very astringent, and which exude a supremely glutinous gum. It grows in warm regions, particularly in Michoacán. A salve or foam made from this cures fevers and is prescribed for dysentery and diarrhea. The wood is very good for carving, and better than the rest for making images, besides being soft enough that it does not split, rot, or decay easily. It tastes and smells like the resin of copal, from which it takes its name.

Copalxócotl

(2.10)

This is the other tree that has this name, but this one has larger round leaves terminating in a small point. It grows in Tlaquiltenango, in the part called Marquesado del Valle. The fruit of this tree is astringent and binding, and if it is cooked it has a pleasant flavor. It is wholly equivalent in properties to the other copalxócotl. The middle of the seed is sweet and is said to be very effective in curing scabies and leprosy.

Xalxócotl or Sandy Fruit

(2.11)

Xalxócotl is a tall tree, which the Haitians and Spanish call guayabo. There are three species of this; we will not deal with one; of the other two, the first has leaves like the golden apple, but smaller and more villous, white flowers, and round fruit full of seeds like those of the fig, from which it takes its name, which means sandy fruit. The leaves are

9. Opuntia. *Nopal* is the Náhuatl name for different kinds of *tuna,* and *nochtli* the name for the fruit of the opuntia. *Tunas* is an Arawak word.
10. Hernández added, in the BN MS, "Purple dye was used in antiq-

uity, contained in certain veins in the throat, to dye cloth, and give clothes Phoenician splendor. But after all this time this dye has fallen into disuse, which the world, never satisfied with new discoveries, always restless and changing, could once again gather."

acidic, astringent, and very fragrant; they cure skin diseases and are used in baths. The bark is cold, dry, and astringent; its decoction alleviates swollen legs and cures fistulous wounds. It is said also to help deafness, and to ease stomach pains because certain parts of it are warm. The fruit is hot and dry, mainly on the outside and the firm part, while the inside of the fruit is more bland and has moderate heat. It smells rather like bugs, yet it is not scorned at table; indeed it is considered by many to be pleasant to eat, and not entirely useless either, for more than a few maintain that it aids digestion and warms the stomach when it has been weakened by a cold cause. The second variety bears much larger fruit, almost without that strong, bitter aroma for which it is much esteemed. They grow in warm places, hilly or rural, but mainly in Cuernavaca and all of the Marquesado, where they are common. From the leaves of the other comes a most useful syrup used against belly flux, and as efficacious as dried roses. It is made thus: they take six pounds of the crushed leaves and leave them to macerate overnight in twelve *quartillis* of water; they put this to the fire until it is reduced by one-third, strain it, and add six pounds of best sugar, and cook it until it has the consistency of syrup. The dosage is as much as needed in proportion to the seriousness of the illness.

Quauhayohuachtli

(2.15)

This large tree, which the Spanish call canafístula,[11] has an ash-colored trunk, leaves like laurel, yellow flowers, star-shaped and in racemes, from which the famous sticks grow. These sticks are used a great deal: while still soft and fresh they are prepared with sugar and taken thus in a dose of three ounces to purge bilious and phlegmatic humors without any harm. There is no need to say anything about its practical uses because its virtues are so well known. It grows in warm areas such as Yyauhtépec and Hoaxtépec, in fields and gardens.

Quauhayohuachtli, or Pumpkin Seed Tree

(2.16)

This tree, which produces purgative pine nuts, is a tree of medium size, with large leaves like the burdock, rounded and angular, and fruit like common walnuts, containing three stones embedded in shells, the same as our pine nuts in shape, size, pulp, and stone, but with different virtues, for these have the property of purging all humors, and especially thick and viscous ones, by both conduits, but especially the upper; this is generally prescribed for chronic illnesses, in the number of five or seven, always an odd number—even nine—for what reason I do not know. Usually, it has been previously roasted, dissolved in water or wine and steeped for some time. It is by temperament hot and thick. This tree grows in fields in warm regions such as Tepecuacuilco and elsewhere.

Quauhtzápotl or Anona

(2.20)

Quauhtzápotl of the Indies (which the Spanish who live here in New Spain call anona, and other natives say texaltzápotl) is a large tree with leaves like the citron but narrower, white flowers with three points, in fragrance and delicacy of aroma like succulent pears. The fruit is variegated with reddish and green blotches; it is about the size of an American melon and looks like the altzápotl. Its pulp, full of small black seeds, looks like that famous dish called blancmange[12] on account of its color as well as its blandness, though it is less pleasant and less nutritious, encouraging wind and "off" humors. The seeds of the fruit cure diarrhea, and between Tzontzonate and the town of San Salvador a certain type of anona grows, whose seeds number ten or twelve, which purge bilious and phlegmatic humors gently and without side effects. It grows in warm places in New Spain and the island of Hispaniola.

---

11. See *QL* 2.1.56.

12. Denoting any number of dishes or sauces. See Constance B. Hieatt, "Sorting through the Titles of Medieval Dishes: What Is, or Is Not, a 'Blanc Manger,'" in *Food in the Middle Ages: A Book of Essays*, ed. Melitta Weiss Adamson, Garland Medieval Casebooks 12 (New York: Garland, 1995), 25–44.

Acueyo or Cihoaxóchitl or Omeliquitl

(3.5)

This herb has white leaves like the cumin plant, and stems like fennel, only it is usually four cubits high; the stems are sometimes pale green, occasionally dark green, the thickness of a thumb with nodes at intervals; it has a fibrous root. The stems are eaten raw and are used to season food, for they have a pleasant aroma as well as taste. It is hot and dry in the third degree, pungent, and of subtle parts. A decoction, taken or infused by a clyster, dispels flatulence and the pains that arise from it, corrects cold, clears obstructions, warms the interior parts, provokes urine, purges the kidneys and bladder, and does the same for the uterus; it excites venery,[13] provokes menstruation, opens the pores of the skin and elicits sweat and, finally, it attenuates and expels[14] gross and windy humors. It grows in warm places next to streams in Oaxtepec.

Tlilxóchitl, or Black Flower

(3.10)

This plant is voluble, with leaves like the plantain but fleshier and longer. They are dark green, sprouting at intervals along the stem. Long, narrow sheaths that are almost round grow from the stem. These sheaths, the vanilla beans, smell like musk or balsam of the Indies, and they are black—hence the name. It grows in hot, moist places. These are hot in the third degree and are usually mixed with cacao as well as with mecaxóchitl. Two vanilla beans dissolved in water and taken will provoke urine and menstruation, if mixed with mecaxóchitl. It hastens birth, expels afterbirth and a dead fetus. It strengthens the stomach, and expels flatulence. It heats and thins the humors. It invigorates the brain and heals fits of the mother. It is said that these vanilla beans are a similar remedy against cold poisons and against cold poisonous animals stings. It is also said to be one of the most aromatic plants in this region.

Hucuiro (Utzicuro)

(3.13)

This herb bears serrate leaves like sage, whitish on the underside and wider at the base, hanging from rather longer pedicels; the flowers are a color between blue and red. The root is long and narrow; its smell and taste are like lavender; it is hot and dry. It cures stomach and belly pains, and purges, by vomiting, bilious and phlegmatic humors, if the hot decoction is placed on the stomach and the treatment repeated the next day. It grows in the mild hills of the province of Michoacán.

Tzontollin, or Hairy Reed

(3.16)

This is a kind of round, sweet-smelling reed (and belongs perhaps to the esquinantum of Dioscorides). It has hairy roots, and from them round, smooth, hollow stems with yellow heads and oblong at the tip. The roots are sweet, fragrant and astringent. It alleviates cough, provokes urine, strengthens the stomach, heart, and head, firms weakened members, alleviates uterine afflictions, binds loose bowels, and ⟨cures⟩ rheums.[15] It grows in Nexpa in the province of Totonacapa in mountainous or flat places, provided they are dense and humid.

Chichimecapatli, or Medicine of the Chichimeca People

(3.21)

The chichimecapatli, which is also called yamancapatli because its root seems to be sweet, has long, thin leaves, a thin stem one cubit high, a root the shape and size of a nut, white inside, black outside, which exudes a sap that is very thick and glutinous. It grows in mild or slightly cool regions in Mexico and Tetzcoco, in places that are rugged and mountainous. The root, either fresh or dried (though dried is better) taken with some liquid in a dose of one scruple, purges

---

13. The opposite of the text in BN MS, which says it inhibits venery.

14. Literally, "cooks."

15. There is no verb governing "rheums" in de Laet's MS.

all bad humors by vomit or stool, though dried is better for purging below. It is hot in the fourth degree and very effective, hence it must not be given indiscriminately to just anyone, only to those who are strong enough to take it, and are not suffering from any acute illness, or to those who have not responded to gentler treatments. They say too that it rids flatulence and eases colic pains. With four ounces of the root and one ounce of cocoztic, a doctor from Cholula prepares this famous purgative throughout New Spain for a variety of diseases. It is a virtual panacea, as the two things are mixed together, with four ounces of best sugar and made into small balls; they are put in the sun to dry for thirty days. It is taken in the quantity of a dram; all of which is known from reliable accounts.

Purgative Cococxíhuitl

(3.26)

This is an herb with thin, heart-shaped leaves, pilose on the underside and green on top, growing at the tips of the stems, which are rounded and villous, and small yellow flowers; black seeds in groups of three, in size and shape like chickpeas, and enclosed in capsules that sprout from the same place as the leaves. It has a root full of fibers; the whole plant has the taste and aroma of thyme, and it is hot in the fourth degree. Taken in a dose of one dram it purges all humors, but mainly gross and phlegmatic ones, by the upper and lower passages, and can be administered also to children in a small quantity appropriate to their age and physical capacity.

Poztecpatli of Oaxaca

(3.32)

Poztecpatli of Oaxaca is an herb with leaves like rue, white, small, and rolled up like those of trees that are beginning to sprout; they last the whole year and smell like the nasturtium, without any difference; it has woody, gray, almost black stems; the soft roots are fibrous. It grows in rocky places and rough mountainous areas in Oaxaca. The roots and leaves are hot and dry in the fourth degree. Crushed and taken in

a dose of one dram, the leaves are good for sinews and tendons, if the trouble comes from a cold and moist cause; and they restore movement, as I know from observation.

Iztacpatli of Yohualapa

(3.42)

This has a fibrous root, thin stems with leaves like basil, entire, and round yellow flowers which like thistles separate into filaments. It grows in hot, flat, humid places in the region of Igualapa, hence its name. The root is sharp, slightly bitter, and hot and dry in the fourth degree. The leaves, chewed in a dose of one ounce, or a decoction of the roots, taken, ease pain in the belly and get rid of worms.

Iztacpatli of Atotonilco

(3.43)

This herb, which in Atotonilco they call iztacpatli, produces long, narrow leaves like those of flax; whitish, round stems one and a half spans long, and nodular roots. It grows in the said province in dry, flat, cold places, where Brother Juan[16] Zimbrón, religious, used it a great deal, so much so that the Spanish gave his name to it. It is an admirable purgative medicament, whose power is recognized everywhere. This same man would make an unguent from it that was a great remedy against all kinds of pains from a cold cause. The root is hot and dry almost in the fourth degree, and fragrant. The root in the quantity of half an ounce is ground and made into a tablet, dissolved in wine that has been strained two or three times, and drunk to purge the body abundantly and without harm.

Cihuapatli of Yacapichtla

(3.47)

This cihuapatli, which is also known as pitzahoac cihuapatli, has leaves like sage, glutinous like them, which stick to your hands if you touch them. Flowers at the tips of purple stems, disposed in corymbs. The root is fibrous: by nature it is warm

---

16. "Francisco" in BN MS.

and dry in the third degree, with a bitter and sharp taste; it seems much like coniza, which, if it were not distinct because of its flowers, would have to be classified among its species. A decoction, taken or applied, admirably resolves humors that have invaded the joints or nerves, and eases any pains, whatever their cause. It grows in warm land in Yacapichtla.

Eráhueni

(3.50)

Eráhueni is a herb with leaves like oregano and round stems, narrow, blue flowers; it has a twisted, glutinous, long root. It smells like cilantro but its taste is very much more bitter. It grows in mild places like Tancítaro. Its nature is hot and dry in the third degree and it is of subtle parts, so that its decoction, infused by clyster, cures acute intestinal pains, provokes urine, dissipates wind, clears obstructions, reduces body fat and is helpful in various similar ways.

Xoxonacátic

(3.60)

Xoxonacátic has leaves that are similar to those of the onion, only smaller and narrower, and small yellow flowers hanging from tiny pedicels; the round, succulent root is like a hazelnut covered with black filaments. This plant grows in cold, humid places, in the rainy season. A couple of roots, crushed and taken with water, will purge all humors by the lower passage without causing any harm. It is a light, safe remedy, with a gentle action, which can be given to the very young and the very old, to those with a fever and those without, those confined to bed and those working normally; it is used fresh or dried, but more frequently and more effectively dried. It keeps for two years—three if necessary. It is good against asthma, for its nature is hot in the second degree, phlegmatic, and it burns the throat a little.

Cococaquílitl, or Bitter Aquatic Plant

(3.62)

The cococaquílitl is an herb with leaves like basil, but more deeply serrate, sinuous and with yellow tips; and stems in groups of three; flowers like great betony or wild cempoalxóchitl, whose leaves are scarlet and produce calyxes, not unlike those of the cornflower; the roots are fibrous; the plant is three cubits high. The flower and leaves are fragrant and bitter to taste, rather like a nasturtium, which gives this its name. The natives eat these like vegetables. It provokes urine and the terms, gets rid of flatulence, warms the stomach, attenuates gross humors, helps the uterus, however it is applied. It belongs to the species of cempoalxóchitl.

Chichioalmemeya, or Milk-Bearing Plant

(3.64)

Chichioalmemeya takes its name from the milky sap it exudes, which is a very useful medicine; it is the only plant of its kind, belonging as it does to the tithymalus. It has serrate and rough leaves like the chestnut tree's, cylindrical purple stems, oblong red flowers in capsules, which become yellow toward the tips; the roots are long, soft and red. It grows in rocky places near hills in cool areas. The pulp promotes evacuation in those suffering from quartan or tertian fevers, with such good results that immediately after evacuation the patient recovers; it should be taken in doses of two drams dissolved in water. Some add to it, to improve its taste, four grains of cacao or Spanish hazelnuts or even almonds, and administer it thus every morning after the reduction of the fever, avoiding evenings when other medicines are being taken.

Cempoalxochític

(3.69)

The herb cempoalxochític produces spiny, serrate, bitter leaves like chicory, compressed and concentrated like hornets around their root; stems a few inches long, and yellow flowers that separate into filaments, from which it gets its name. The root is similar to the radish in shape and size. The decoction of the root, which is bitter, infused by clysters into the stomach, expels urine, and calms intestinal pain. It is bitter, of subtle parts and is hot and dry in the third degree: it alleviates the cough and, instilled in the nose, it induces sneezing and clears phlegm.

Cenanan of Tetzcoco

(4.7)

Cenanan of Tetzcoco (which is also known as cenantli or centliynan) is an herb that produces broad and somewhat elongate leaves [similar to the mullein in color, downiness, and size]. Its white flowers are arranged like a small fan, and its root is thick and long; the almost flat fruit looks like the chili, from which it gets its name. It grows in temperate or cold places. It is hot and dry in the third degree, and has a bitter taste. It kills worms in sores, and is useful against old wounds in animals; it eases toothache, applied as a plaster it resolves tumors and abscesses, and used in a clyster it brings out hardened feces, and it relieves colic pains.

Tezompatli, or Medicine like the Tezontle Stone

(4.20)

Tezompatli has a root the size and shape of the pear, only slightly larger and reddish, resembling the gemstone they call tezontli—hence its name. Hanging from it are thin long leaves;[17] there are two types of this ⟨plant⟩. The first produces a similar root, with three or four round, woody stems, nodular and full of leaves at long intervals, fleshy, entire, or crenellated in distinctive ways, with many veins and a red main dorsal vein. The fruit of this plant is very similar to the chili pod hanging from a pedicel, filled with small, round, flat seeds. It grows in the hills of Acolman. The root is bitter, with a strong aroma, hot and dry in the third degree. They say it clears obstructions and cleanses putrid wounds. Taken in a dose of two or three drams with wine, it relieves colic and coughing, purges the intestines and expels flatulence. The leaves exude a sap, which, applied, resolves abscesses. The other type of this herb has similar stems and root, but the leaves are more copious, wider, and with fewer veins, villous on the underside and soft on top; this one also gives off milky sap, tastes bitter, and has the same properties.

Coyolxóchitl

(6.9)

This is a voluble herb, with leaves like reeds, but shorter, and similar to the small plantain, with the same distinct longitudinal veins. The stem is round, purple, and broad, the size of a goose feather. The flowers grow in the form of calyxes at the end of the stems, very elegant in color, red verging into green and variegated with little spots; inside is a tiny, barely visible seed. The flowers are in nature cold and mucilaginous, although they do contain some hot and sharp parts. The liquor expressed from them stops rectal bleeding and nosebleeds. The juice of the root brings down the heat of fevers; it cleans pustules and stops the belly. The flowers are also used in garlands. It grows in mild climates, such as Mexico, in wild and cultivated places alike, and brings a touch of elegance to any garden.

Maguey

(6.12)

Of this tree, as Francisco Hernández writes,[18] there are several varieties;[19] the one that they call metl having large leaves like the sempervivum,[20] prickly on both sides, and very sharp at the tip; it bears an oblong yellow flower that is star-shaped in the upper part; called metl coztli, or coztic metl, has smaller leaves than the foregoing, and fewer thorns, which are black, and leaves that are yellow on the outside; its flower is sky blue tending to pink. The third Mexican metl has even smaller leaves, which are thornier and dark green. And there are others still, too many to mention here. One should also note that Francisco Hernández and Francisco Ximénez do not call these plants trees, but include them in the descriptions of herbs, although they do say that the first kind grows to the height of a domesticated tree.

---

17. MS has "root" for leaves.

18. This section was taken from *Beschrijving van West-Indien* 5.2, the first appearance of Hernández in the printed text.

19. José Ignacio Bartolache, *Mercurio volante* 8 (December 9, 1772), noted that European botanists use the term *áloe americana* too generally—even Hernández. But Bartolache repeated that Philip II had been a generous Alexander to his Aristotle, and added that the work of Hernández was, he had heard, worthy of its place of honor in the "cabinet of curiosities of our court."

20. MS has "aloes."

Mexócotl or Plum Maguey

(6.15)

This is a spiny plant belonging to the species of maguey, which bears sweet, acidic, round fruit like plums, from which it takes its name, which looks something like the fruit known in America as the pineapple; sometimes it is bigger. The fruit is edible, juicy and pleasant to taste. The leaves are like the maguey, or really more like the pineapple, spiny and brownish. The root is fibrous and thick, the stem round and thick; the plums are white (like acorns), tending to red; under the skin is a very soft pulp, sweet and sour as we said, with a flavor like pineapple and full of round, hard seeds that are white at first and later turn black. It grows in rocky places in warm areas in Tepecuacuilco. It is cold and dry; the fruit, mashed, chewed and kept in the mouth, cures fissures caused by heat.

Tepemexcallin, or Mountain Maguey

(6.17)

Tepemexcallin has the form of the metl, but with thin little spines. Crushed and eaten or rubbed on, it restores movement to stiff or paralyzed limbs, and cures any other muscular affliction. It is native to mountainous and rocky places in warm areas, such as Tepoztlan.

Poztecpatli of Mecatlan

(6.44)

This has leaves like those of the peach, opposite with two at each node, and red underneath; thick, round, nodular stems; rubicund flowers of five petals with a red pod in the center. It grows in the fields of Mecatlan. It is cold, dry, and astringent with some bitterness. The stems and leaves, crushed and applied to the affected areas, dissolve humors and abscesses; they have the same effect if they are taken; as the name indicates,[21] they cure dislocated or broken bones.

Tlatauhcapatli

(6.48)

This is a species of geranium, with a round, white root, leaves like the vine, and red flowers resembling a stork's bill.

There are two species of this root, differing only in color, one tending more to white, the other to red, but both similar and with the same virtues. Both of them grow in cold or warm areas, in hilly or wild places. The root, the part that is mainly used as medicine, is by nature cold, dry, and astringent, with quite an acidic taste. It cures dysentery and other fluxes, and inflammation of the eyes. Mixed with all cold and astringent medicines, it produces good results, and alleviates all laxity. It reduces fevers and combats excessive heat, especially if accompanied by moisture, it strengthens the teeth, makes the gums firmer and healthier, purges phlegmatic humors, relieves pain if the affected area is washed with water in which this has been dissolved, ripens tumors and opens abscesses, encourages fertility in women, and cures ulcers in the mouth and elsewhere. The natives swear that, mixed with chili, it alleviates coughing and expels urine, and that on its own it purges bilious humors, which I cannot verify, unless it has more astringent properties.

Mecapatli of Mecatlan

(6.61)

The leaves are heart-shaped, the stems voluble and yellow, from which it gets its name. It has a purple flower like the caxtlatlapan contained in yellow calyxes, and a long, narrow root. It grows in the warm region of Mecatlan, in wooded places. Its decoction purges gross and cold humors, and expels harmful animalcules from the belly. It must be taken in the mornings and cooked while it is still fresh, for once it is dry it is of no use.

Hoitzitzilxóchitl, like Oregano

(7.4)

This is a shrub which from just one root has many woody branches, and on them leaves like oregano, which is why I have given it its familiar name. The flowers are red, curved, and in the shape of the spear called a halberd. The aroma is like sage, the taste bitter, its temperament hot and dry in the third degree, and of subtle parts. Some say that it removes feverish spots, perhaps strengthening the heart,

---

21. The alternative name means "medicine for fractures."

and expelling the humor through the pores of the skin, or even by some arcane, occult property. It is the nature of this plant to expel flatulence, aid digestion, helps cold parts of the body, and expels excrement retained in the intestines.

Pinahuihuitztli

(7.32)

The pinahuihuitztli, also called cocochíatl because it is a soporific if applied to the head, and mere contact with it is seen to induce sleep (easier for the natives than for the Spanish), is a shrub four spans high. Its stems are thin and spiny; the leaves are grouped in bunches of six, not unlike those of the ihoixóchitl; the root is ramified, and the flowers and fruit are like those of the chestnut tree, green then red, hanging in racemes. It grows in warm places in Tepoztlan, Quauhtlan, and Hueitlalpa, and in the hills of Yacapichtla. They say that it encourages love between two people, but they cannot explain when or how this happens. The leaves taste somewhat like those of the radish; they are cold, dry, astringent, and very glutinous. The juice of the root cures tertian fevers as well as bloodshot eyes, induces sleep and cures belly fluxes. This is the shrub whose leaves, on the merest contact with a person, or with the wind, shrinks and droops, which makes me suspect that this is the same herb or a relative of the plant that, in the Philippines, the Spanish call the sensitive plant, about which various things are written (how accurately I do not know) which certainly are not true of the one that grows here: for it has upright stems the thickness of a goose quill, ten or twelve from a single root, each one with twelve leaves distributed in four series two inches apart; that the leaves are like those of the radish; blue flowers, which before they open look like larks' tongues, and divide, once opened, into three small leaves; that it happens that human touch offends it, even brushing the very tips of the leaves with the fingers will make it wilt, and all the leaves start to fall, that the stem collapses wherever it is touched, and the part that falls turns black, as if it had been charred; that any human touch will cause it to break down and fall; not that this happens when it touches a tree, a stick, or any other object—no, only human touch; that it is insipid and has no medicinal properties. They say too that in Malabar a plant grows that shrinks just the same way on contact with the human hand, that it has leaves like the polypody,[22] and yellow flowers. Others tell of one that grows in Peru, which also dries up when it is touched, like those that grow in Spain, especially in Cádiz. But what we have written about the pinahui⟨huit⟩ztli, we have proved from experience, having tested it on numerous occasions.

---

22. A fern of the genus *Polypodium*.

JUAN EUSEBIO NIEREMBERG

In the early 1630s in the library of the Imperial College in Madrid, the Jesuit scholar Juan Eusebio Nieremberg consulted the Hernández manuscripts that are preserved today in the Biblioteca Nacional in Madrid. Nieremberg also used the Escorial copy that Hernández had presented to Philip II. Some of Nieremberg's transcriptions from the Escorial manuscripts provide us with unique texts, simply because nobody else ever wrote them down before the fire destroyed the originals in 1671. Several of these are descriptions of plants that, in the surviving drafts, Hernández had placed in appendixes to particular books. As Hernández himself wrote, "Although in these books of ours on the history of plants there is nothing that I have not seen with my own eyes and tested for aroma and flavor, either by personal experience or that of others, I have added here, in these five chapters, plants native to the Philippines, based on the firsthand evidence of very reliable witnesses. I have added other Indian plants, taking them from Diego García de la Huerta, who has been to Goa." Because our texts focus on Mexico, we have excluded such chapters, except for the odd case in which Hernández says that a plant native to India or the Philippines also grows in New Spain. Nieremberg's text, his only work that was not theological, was published as *Historia naturae, maxime peregrine* (Antwerp, 1635).

Hernández did not include his brief description of the tiburon in his book on fish or aquatic animals. It is part of a separate essay, preserved now in Madrid, Ministerio de Hacienda, MS 931, fol. 57v. This Latin text was translated into Spanish and published in *OC* 6:492. Rafael Martín del Campo's concise introduction to the Spanish text argues, convincingly, that Hernández conflated information about several different kinds of tiburon, which in any case is not a fish but a species of shark.

The Fish Called Tiburon

(11.20)

This is a saltwater fish of the elongated cetaceous order, up to fifteen spans long, and the width of two human bodies. It is voracious, fast, and quite intelligent. Its crescent-shaped mouth, two spans wide, is about a foot below the face, with three rows of teeth on top and four beneath, which fit into one another like the teeth of two saws. It has five gills on each side; the face is round like a frog's. It has a fin on each side near the gills, two near the genital area, one at the tail and, largest of all, the dorsal fin behind the gills. It has another, medium sized, near the tail, in front of a smaller fin and pointing away from that one. The tail is big, thick, and scything, three or four times longer and wider in its upper part, and with small cavities near its base. Its small eyes are set wide apart, with a large pupil and a small, yellowish iris; its skin is like cartilage, which, when not relaxed, repels any weapon. Its back and sides are dark blue, its belly white.

Amazingly, the male has two genital members, bony, hollow, and white, one span long, equipped with three slightly long "points" instead of a glans, like blades that tear through anything that get in their way. This animal is destructive, ferocious, and man-eating; it is so lively that even when it is cut up into tiny pieces and placed on the grill, it still palpitates and seems to cling obstinately to life.

Like others of its kind, it is fair to eat when young, but the adults are tough, unpleasant, unhealthful, and liable to cause fluxes of the belly. It has just one very large intestine, which explains its terrible voracity. The heart is small, whitish, relaxed, made up of ventricles, and so lively that even when it is taken out and cut in pieces, it will go on beating a long time. The stomach is vast; the liver is white and divided into two lengths, each measuring four spans by ten inches. The spleen is the same length as the liver but only two inches wide.[1]

Atatapálcatl, or Pot Placed in Water

(14.29)

The Mexicans call this plant atatapálcatl, because it looks like the pots or jars that are placed on the waters of the lakes.

It is native to lakes, slow-flowing and stagnant water, the same as other species of water lily, to whose varieties this appears to belong, although the leaves are much smaller and lack stem and flower. The leaves have stalks like those of the navel of Venus, thick, round, smooth, reddish, twisted near the base. The roots sprout from the lower part like hairs, and become established in the mud, and almost in the water itself. The leaves are thick, round, medium-sized, deep green on top and paler on the underside; they float on the water like potamogeton [pondweed] or water lilies. It has no taste or aroma, and its temperament is moist and cold, so it is used commonly as a substitute for the common water lily. Applied, it gets rid of inflammations and erysipelas; taken in a dose of one dram, it reduces fever in children, and it is said to ease thus the head problem that causes eruptions; it helps to protect chastity, and finally, it combats all ills arising from heat and dryness. It lives all the year round and is picked and used throughout the year. Its native climate is moderate or slightly cold, like Mexico's, and it grows, as we have said, in lakes.

Ayotli, or the Nature and Different Kinds of Indian Squash

(14.33)

Among the different types of squash, which the Indians call ayotli, and omitting those that have already come to be familiar in our world, there are numerous varieties. The leaves of all of them are for the most part much the same, and would be like a grapevine if they were not so much larger. The flowers are yellow, in the shape of large oblong calyxes; but the fruits come in a great variety of names and shapes, and in what follows we are going to describe them as concisely and clearly as possible.

The first variety of squash is the tzilacayotli, or squash that makes a sound, also called cuicuilticayotli, that is, painted squash; it is hollow, as the sound reveals when it is tapped, and it is so huge that its circumference measures three spans. The seed is black and medium-sized; the pulp is white, filled with fibers, and almost adheres to the inside

1. Nieremberg added further description of the tiburon, taken from Acosta.

of the rind; the surface is smooth, with spots of bright and pale green.

The second variety, which some call cozticayotli, meaning yellow squash, and others call hacayotli and hoeyacayotli, because it is good to eat and has an oblong shape, has yellow pulp, as its name indicates, is four inches thick, has a white seed that is grooved or furrowed in places, like some melons, with deeper lines and deeper longitudinal channels. Its rind, though also at first intense and pale green, almost always turns yellow eventually, which is why it is called cozticayotli.

The third variety, known as tamalayotli, is much larger and round, which explains its name. Its skin is hard, the pulp is one span thick, yellow, and very pleasant to eat, and the seeds are white.

The fourth variety, also called tamalayotli, has a yellow rind, very bulky and wide, with light yellow pulp and a broad white seed. This squash is said to cure hemorrhoids and bloodshot eyes. There is yet another one with this same name, oblong, brownish, with edible red pulp and a white seed, which grows in warm places.

The fifth is the quauhayotli, which is melon-shaped, with red pulp two inches thick, a small, white seed, and reddish brown skin; I do not wish to speak here of the other variety that goes by this name, which, as it is a tree, will be reserved for another place. There is the tzonayotli, or hairy squash, so called for its very fibrous, inedible pulp, but the seeds are delicious; it is white, green, or yellow, although some say tzonayotli for the yellow tamalayotli, and use the name iztacayotli for the white tzonayotli. There is, besides, the iztactzilacayotli, with a broad white seed, white fibrous pulp two inches thick, which is edible and healthful. The tlilticayotli, with an elongated white seed, pulp three inches thick, brighter yellow and of medium size. The iztacayotli, one of the largest, has white skin and seeds, an oblong shape, and white, edible pulp three inches thick. To these can be added those that are not edible, but that belong to the species of squash, such as the atecómatl, like Spanish squash, which grows cultivated or wild, has no pulp, which is no good for eating, and which is used by the Indians only for carrying water, from which purpose it takes its name. Then there is the axicalli or water squash,

the size and shape of a shield, which has a thick skin and no pulp, which can be cut in half and made into two large vases, for use as containers or serving dishes. These same gourds, left whole and joined together in lines of seven, make rafts that are very good for transporting people, horses, or anything else. All of these have no pulp and cannot be eaten, the same as the allácatl, so called because it is used as a siphon or pump.

All of these varieties, like ours, have no taste or smell, supply cold and moist nutrition, good for the table and used to nourish those suffering from fevers or excessive heat in the kidneys, although, prepared with sugar they are less healthful and pleasant than ours. They grow in gardens, and in moist, cultivated places. The flowers and new growth on these plants are used by the Indians as vegetables, mainly with meat drippings. They grow at the onset of the rainy season, though during the rest of the year they do sprout and are used for food by the Mexicans. There are other types of squash whose nature is different, and therefore we shall speak of them separately in their appropriate places.

Atóchietl 3

(14.53)

The third atóchietl, also known as dictamum, we came across at the same time as others from the pueblos of Gutmano, near Michoacán. It is a herb with long purple flowers, a thick fibrous root, and small serrate leaves with the shape and smell of pulegium, of which it is undoubtedly a species. It was found that deer, shot by arrows and seriously wounded, run to this plant and eat it to recover their strength, and then run away at great speed; it is assumed from this and from experience that it is good for fresh wounds, especially poisoned ones.

Amohuitli of Yyauhtépec

(14.57)

This is an herb like the preceding one, but with cavities in the bigger axillae, and purple flowers, from which it takes its name. We are not aware of a single use for it, but we wish to record it among these descriptions because its smell is exactly the same as that Spanish supper dish that consists of lamb, eggs, pimento, and butter.

Mexixquílitl, Nasturtium or Iberis of the Indies

(14.58)

A certain species of nasturtium, very much like the one in our country, called mexixquílitl by the people here, grows spontaneously in Mexico, among the rubbish and on walls. It is a wonderful cure for pain from a cold cause, it reduces swelling of the legs when its decoction is rubbed on, and mixed with lime it clears worms. It is also used to make a medicine that is very effective against asthma, when equal parts of mexixquílitl, epazotl, seeds of green melons, quince seeds, black figs, and the gum of tragacanth are mixed together: all of this is pounded together into a liquid made viscous by the tragacanth gum and the quince seeds. One spoonful of this is taken in the mornings as needed, and it clears the affliction by expelling waste matter and phlegmatic humors three or more times on each occasion that it is taken. This remedy can be made stronger, if necessary, by increasing the proportion of stones. It is amazing that an herb so sharp and hot, mixed with unsalted cow's butter and applied, mitigates heat in the kidneys by reducing heat in the urine, as I have tested on myself with excellent results when I suffered from this illness. Some call it tlachhoihoilan.

Memeya of Tepecuacuilco

(14.60)

Besides the memeya described above, there is another, from Tepecuacuilco, which, though similar in properties to the other types of memeya or peplis,[2] I do not wish to omit on account of its beautiful red leaves. This is an herb one cubit high, with a fibrous root from which grow red or purple stems, narrow and cylindrical, and from them oblong, obtuse leaves tinged with red, in shape and size like those of the pomegranate. It has delicate, round, yellow flowers grouped at the tips of the branches. It is said to be cold like the plants related to it, and admirable for reducing fevers

and healing wounds, an opinion with which I must say I cannot agree until I have proved it from much more experience, for it seems to go against the judgment of Dioscorides. Tasting the sap these herbs exude, I could detect almost no heat; I did not perceive in the sap any bitterness or heat—or so little that it would be easy to believe that it is cold that predominates in such herbs. It could happen, though, that the herbs that Dioscorides refers to, because they are native [to Europe] give off more sap and so could be more bitter and of more intense heat, which could easily occur in some parts of that continent. But I desire to describe, with absolute accuracy, things belonging to this land. It grows in the warm region of Tepecuacuilco.

Mazacaxócotl or Cervino Plum Tree

(14.61)

Those fruits that the Indians call xocotl for their acid taste, and my countrymen call plums on account of the similarity not just of the fruit but of the whole tree, can be divided, as I have noted, into five varieties; but as the trees of all these varieties attain the same size, the same as Spanish plum trees, have the same wood, identical stems, roots, and leaves, let us treat all of them together in this chapter. One thing that is common to all is that they produce fruit that sticks to the branches before they grow leaves, which follow in very few trees. The leaves are used to make salsas and acidic condiments that loosen the belly and provide a food that is neither very pleasant nor very healthful. The ashes of these trees are used to dye the hair of young girls red. The plums of the first species (permit me to call this fruit plum, because there is no other name for it but the one the Creoles give it), called zacacoxotl, are red and oblong, the size of an average walnut, with a large, hard stone that is soft inside, striated and in the shape of a date pit. There is not much pulp, which is soft, succulent and yellow, as is the stone. They are used as food and many prefer their fine flavor over ours, but they are an acquired taste. They comfort the belly and have a pleasant flavor, sweet and acidic, yet in some ways, in my view, they compare with the delicate flavor of ours. The fruits

2. A name given to two plants, *porcilaca* and *meconion*, mentioned by Pliny, 20.20.81 210 and 27.12.93 119.

of the second kind, called atoyaxocotl, are much smaller, yellow, round, with a much better aroma, a smaller and rounder stone, and a more pleasant flavor. The third kind is the Haitian, which the Mexicans call cozticxocotl, which some—not without justification—classify among myrobalans and which, as the name indicates, is yellow. It has bigger markings, and more pleasant pulp, and is otherwise very much like the first fruit. The fourth type, called atoyaxocotlchichiltic, is red, and is the smallest one of all, but it beats all the others for its aroma, which is similar to the matzatli or pine, as the Spanish who live here call it, and which we will discuss in its place. The last variety of these fruits is larger than a walnut, the color of a raisin, and is known as chichioalxocotl, that is, sweat exuder, for it immediately tinges the hands of those who gather it. This one has more plentiful pulp than the other kinds, a smaller stone, and is otherwise like the others. The decoction of the bark of all these trees cures scabies and swellings of the legs. Its powder, which is cold, dry, and astringent, cures sores. It grows in any warm, humid place, wild or cultivated. There are many species that differ by color, which I do not think it seasonable to describe in detail.

Texócotl, or Fruit of Stone

(14.62)

This is a medium-sized tree with leaves like our apples, but rougher and serrate. It grows spontaneously in hilly places, and is covered in hundreds of thorns. The apples, like ours but smaller, no larger than walnuts, are yellow and very hard until they ripen, but then they turn as soft as butter. I think they taste nasty, but a lot of people like them. Each fruit has three crescent-shaped seeds, pretty much the size of the fruit, with two angles and one back, and they are as hard as rock. These apples are prepared with sugar or honey in many ways, and thus they mollify, and are just as pleasant as ours. The Mexican Indians sell them in the markets, picking first the ones that are just starting to rot so that they will lose their wild taste, and when they want them to keep for a long time they spray them with nitrate water. The shoots, pounded and taken with water, are said to cure exanthemas, and reduce heat, especially if they are mixed with shoots of capolin.

Zaqanquáhuitl, or Flag Tree

(14.79)

The zaqanquáhuitl, also called póchotl, is a large tree, spiny, with leaves like the olive almost always in groups of five, and fruit like a small melon in size and shape, lanuginous, white, bright, hardly any different from threads of spun silk, which can be woven very easily, as we proved in a test, and can be made into a soft cloth like real silk, but at a much lower cost and requiring less labor than our silk. But it is human nature to have a burning desire for something expensive rather than for something sold more cheaply. Amid the fibers there are round seeds, in shape and size like hemp, sweet, pleasant to taste, which are tasty raw or toasted, and are so good for fattening that emaciated people can quickly return to work. The flower is white, medium-sized, and shaped like that of the izcaxóchitl. There are some, as I said above, who call this tree póchotl because of the similarity of the leaves to the true póchotl, though the leaves of this one are smaller and it is neither spiny nor fructiferous. It grows in warm or mild climates, but prefers warm ones, in rural areas and hills, and practically everybody knows it.

Quauhtlatlatzin or Crackling Tree

(15.10)

This is a large tree with leaves like the mulberry but much larger, serrate, and with numerous veins; a brownish trunk, round fruit flattened on two sides, striated like a melon, and surrounded by twelve or more ridges, round, in shape and size like a silver *real* or the little wheels that make spindles turn. Three of these with a weight of one and a half drams will relieve a certain central, interior membrane that produces discomfort; they purge all humors by the upper or lower passages, especially the bilious and phlegmatic; it is a safe and effective remedy, moderately hot and very appropriate for illnesses from a cold causes. Toasted lightly and dissolved in water, they are taken in the morning. An amazing thing about this fruit is that when it is ripe, some of its striations produce shoots, open, and break out with such force and noise that it can be heard far away like gunshot. It grows in warm places, where it is very common.

Tlatlanquaye, or Long Pepper

(15.13)

The Indians of New Spain give the name tlatlanquaye to what Dioscorides called long pepper, although the method of keeping its fruit has never been known before now. It is a voluble, climbing plant with oblong leaves like the round pepper and with the same straight veins, long cylindrical fruit, and no flower. The fruit is sharp, by nature hot in the fourth degree, extraordinarily dry, and of subtle parts. The temperament of the leaves is gentler. The stems grow higher than a man. It grows in various sites in warm areas. The leaves, applied, are said to cure sores, especially malignant ones, and when the juice is pressed from the root and new growth, and taken or introduced, it is said to expel the inter-cutaneous fluid that accumulates with hydrops. Its decoc-tion cures edemas of the legs and phlegmatic humors; it provokes the terms, expels wind and the pains it causes, as it does those from a cold cause or the Indian plague. It is also said to resolve swellings of the throat or other parts of the body, especially if it is mixed with *centlinan;* it restores movement, provokes sweat, cures relaxation and convul-sion of the nerves, alleviates epilepsy with its aromatic smoke, relieves colds and chills, and provides a thousand similar cures that it would be a bore to enumerate, but they could easily be inferred from those mentioned here. It grows, as I indicated, in cold places, near water, walls or rocks, and some also call it quauhyauhtli and temozotl.

Itzcuinpatli, or Dog's Poison

(15.32)

This is an herb four spans long, which has oblong leaves, narrower and very angular, fruit that looks like a pine cone, green and yellow, numerous narrow roots similar to helle-bore, and covered, like cotton. Any part of this plant is lethal to animals that eat it, especially dogs, if some of it is ground into powder and added to their food. I have heard it said that six oboli of this herb, taken over nine days, cure lep-rosy, provided that during this time the patient rests and remains indoors. It grows in warm or mild places, such as Tototépec.

Axixpatli Ocimoide, or Diuretic Medicine with Leaves like Basil

(15.36)

Axixpatli ocimoide has thin white roots, delicate, round, brown stems and leaves like basil, from which we get its familiar name, but they are smaller and a little sinuous; it has a small purple flower near the base of each leaf, and mid-sized seed, white at first and turning black, contained in oblong capsules. The root, which is what is used principally in medicine, has no notable taste, except for being slightly sweet and juicy, and its nature is cold and moist. Taken in a dose of one dram with an appetizing drink or plain water, it eliminates urine, cleanses the kidneys, and removes heat from them and from the bladder; mixed with cacáoatl, it gently lightens the stomach. It grows on hills or mountains.

Axixpatli Cóztic, or Yellow ⟨Axixpatli⟩

(15.37)

The axixpatli cóztic—which, because of the shape of its leaves, some people call amamaxtla, or, as it were, "water lath"—is a lacustrine species of sharp sorrel, even though there are people who distinguish the axixpatli cóztic from the amamaxtla. The root is branched, completely yellow— from which the name comes—and very like that of the rhubarb called friars' ⟨rhubarb⟩ in its shape, color, and purga-tive properties, although it is more slender and branchy. Ground up and taken in a dose of two drams, it provokes urine extraordinarily and evacuates bilious humors. It grows in temperate or cold regions, near slow flowing or standing water. I know that the powder of this root, mixed in equal parts with manure from a horse, a dog, and a mouse and with the shells of eggs from which the chicks and mem-branes have been removed, marvelously breaks up kidney stones or bladder stones and expels them from the body after they have been broken up.

Axixtlácotl, or Diuretic Branch

(15.38)

The axixtlácotl, which is also called quapopoltzin and iztacxíhuitl, has slender, round, purple stalks growing from a fibrous root similar to that of the white hellebore, leaves like an alkanet's, but smaller, serrate, soft, delicate, hirsute, and streaked through by longitudinal veins; and flowers on almost all the branches: tiny, white with yellow in them and crowded together, fragrant, and of an acrid flavor. The root, which is what is principally used, has an aromatic taste, subtle parts, and a temperament that is hot and dry in the second degree. When the roots have been crushed and applied, they extract anything has been driven into the flesh. Taken in a dose of three drams, they notably provoke urine and clean out its passage, relieve those who are suffering from colics, get rid of spots on the face, cure the head rash of children and that of the entire body, get rid of fever by provoking sweat, reduce spleen, and ease pain. Mixed with cótotl and chichicxíhuitl, they get rid of flatulence, cure indigestion, and dissolve swellings. Nevertheless, the name they have given this herb only indicates its power to provoke urine, perhaps because this is its principal and most excellent property; or indeed because some of the Indian doctors who only knew of one or the other property of each herb—knowledge that they had inherited from their ancestors or from their own parents, also doctors—believed it efficacious only for evacuating urine, and thus have expressed it in its name: all of which I desire should be understood as well concerning the rest of the plants ⟨that I write about⟩. We have seen another herb of the same name in Cuernavaca with square stalks, crenellated leaves like a sage plant's and of a bitter taste, purple flowers disposed like spines at the ends of the stalks, and of a hotter and drier temperament. They said that it also cured fevers by provoking sweat, and that it grew in mountainous places; but since it differs little in its properties from that which we have described above, we have not taken pains to paint it. The former ⟨plant⟩ grows in mountainous and rocky places in Mexico.

Apancholoa, or Herb That Sprouts in Water

(15.39)

The apancholoa has roots like fibers, white, narrow and somewhat hirsute; stems about four spans long, narrow, round, purple, and woody, with thin, oblong leaves like the willow, purple or white flowers, long and wide, almost the length of each stalk. Its nature is cold, dry and astringent, for which reason it cures burns or mouth ulcers. The water in which the pounded roots have been left to soften, strained and drunk, detains fluxes of the belly, especially in children, and prevents abortion; but it is more effective if it is mixed with a plant called cozticpotoncaxóchitl, crushed and blended with it; it serves other very useful purposes thanks to its nature. It grows wild in mild regions, such as Tetzcoco, where we took care to have it painted, in humid or watery terrain, from which it takes its name.

Acxoyátic 1, or Herb like the Fir Tree

(15.40)

The acxoyátic is a root very much like a small pear in shape and size, with narrow, cylindrical green stems, on which grow thin, narrow, long, nearly cylindrical leaves, up to a point quite like those of flax, and arranged at intervals in groups of six or seven; next to each group of leaves grow red flowers contained in small calyxes, and from them grow berries, the size of chickpeas and full of seeds. It has virtually no taste or aroma, and is cold and moist in temperament. The pulverized root, taken with a suitably cold drink, reduces fevers, and they say also that it is intoxicating and that it can be mixed advantageously with medicines that relax. It grows next to the mountains of Chihuatla in Tetzcoco, in moist places, mild or slightly cold.

Acxóyatl, or Fir Tree

(15.41)

This is a tall tree with dense foliage, the same as our own native fir tree, or related to it. Not only does it exude resin, the same as ours, it also gives off an oil from little blisters on its trunk, very effective in easing pain, extracting cold, cleansing and purifying the large conduits of the body, taken in a dose of half an ounce if there is no excessive heat. It grows in cold areas, particularly in Tototepec, where there is another kind of fir known locally as axiuhócotl, tall, wide, and with extensive foliage, which exudes a similar liquid but has much smaller leaves, and of which we shall speak in another place.

Ahoapatli 2, or Oak Remedy

(15.43)

The ahoapatli is an herb four spans long, with rambling roots, which produce round, thin, ashy stems, leaves like nettles or ilex, from which it gets its name, and white flowers that separate into threads. The root, whose principal use is medicinal, is sharp, fragrant, and warm and dry almost in the third degree. It contains fluxes of the stomach, provokes urine, revives anyone suffering from cold, removes wind, strengthens the stomach and the brain, and also provides relief for any case where cinnamon would usually be used.

Totonilizpatli, or Fever Remedy

(15.46)

This is a small herb with roots like hairs, sinuous, long leaves in some respects like bracken, of which this may be a variety. It has no stem, flower, or fruit. The crushed leaves, dissolved in water and taken, reduce fevers, especially if mixed with mihuapatli and with ixicahui icalizpatli. It grows in rocky places next to water.

Acaxilótic, or Ear of Corn or Corn Stick

(15.50)

The acaxilótic is also called cexóchitl, or one flower, also nextamalxóchitl, or flower of Indian corn, or cooked corn; or teuhxóchitl, or prince's flower, or finally oloxóchitl or flower of olote (the Mexicans say olote for the spike or base of this grain, which gets narrower there). It has a long, quite thick root, which gradually narrows, and is fibrous and ramified. It has many straight stems, cylindrical, narrow, and of a brownish color, which grow mainly near the base of the leaves, which are like those of the yyauhtli or the polygonal, but larger, disposed in line on each side of the stalk, with a smell like a radish. Flowers grow at the ends of the stems to form a triple crown; blue, oblong, and crenellated at the edge. It tastes slightly bitter, and has no aroma. It is hot and salty. Taken or applied, it cures intermittent fevers. In a dose of three drams it kills tapeworm, and is extraordinar-

ily effective in purging bilious humors. It is commonly mixed in equal quantities with tlapalezpatli, cicimátic, pitzáhoac, tlalcacáhoatl, and eloxóchitl, and if they are all crushed together, they are taken in a dose of two-sixths of an ounce with water to retard excessive menstrual flow or a belly flux. It is native to moderate climes, either flat or slightly warm and hilly, like the land in Xochimilco, where the people know that this can be very good for reducing swellings; in those suffering from fever who have pustules on the whole body, perhaps expelling the humors through the skin; it fattens consumptives and, applied to the head, it helps the insane.

Chicomácatl, or Seven Sticks

(15.51)

This is a voluble plant that, although normally scarcely any bigger than a man, and the thickness of a thigh, will, if it grows near any tree, grow to the same size, wrapping its tendrils all the way to the top. Its stems are gray, the stalks green, leaves like the citron but larger, a very small white flower and no fruit. It has no discernible taste or smell, and is in nature cold and phlegmatic. The water extracted from the flowers is used to alleviate inflammations of the nose, mouth, and eyes. The leaves are taken in the quantity of half an ounce for dysentery, fatigue, fainting and coughing up blood. They prevent and contain inflammations when applied to the affected areas; they ease wounds and reduce fevers. It grows in mild or cold areas, in mountainous or flat terrain, such as Quauhchinanco, Quauhtépec, and Totolapa.

Ayacuicuéramo, or Painted Tree

(15.54)

The ayacuicuéramo, which the Mexicans, in whose land it grows, call tlacuilolquáhuitl, meaning painted tree, and others ocelolquáhuitl, meaning ocelot tree, grows commonly in the warm regions of the province of Michoacán. It is a large tree with dense foliage, whose leaves are like the elm but thinner, with wood of various colors, except that when it is in water, it sinks at once and goes all the way to the bottom. The wood is very good for fine carving and turning on a lathe. Its aroma and appearance are quite lovely. It exudes an oil that smells of styrax and gives off a pleasing vapor, very appropriate for all the remedies for which it is used.

Tletlematzin or Fire Tree of the Hand

(15.57)

This has a round root with many red fibers, long, brown stems with large, sinuous leaves, and a large red flower, dark outside, light inside. The root is hot and dry in the fourth degree, caustic, bitter, and endowed with subtle parts. Crushed and ground, it is an excellent remedy for sores caused by the French disease; taken in a dose of two drams it eases lameness; it cures itch, expelling the humors that cause it through the skin, and restoring the skin completely. They say it provokes more heat when applied than when taken. It grows in warm areas of Cuernavaca, in watery or moist places.

Atzóyatl, or Sweet-Smelling Herb

(15.58)

The atzóyatl has a large, gray, fibrous root, stems like the strawberry tree in size and height, long, soft, thin and purple, with leaves like the willow, but serrate, or rather, like the yyauhtli but longer, resembling it in having umbels of small, pale yellow flowers that separate into threads. Its nature is hot and dry in the second degree; it tastes strong at first, then turns sharp and sweet. Applied, the leaves reduce swellings, ease pains in the joints with amazing speed, and gout in the hands and feet; they remove stomach pains, clear swellings in the legs, provoke urine and sweat, induce abundant milk when applied to the breasts, are a noted cure for the French disease, and, finally, they provide all the cures associated with heat and dryness; and yet Mexican women, including those known as ticiti, use this herb to treat hot eruptions of the head in children, either because it has cold parts, or because, by removing and dissipating warm humors, it seems to refresh. It is native to a moderate climate, such as Mexico, and grows in flat and watery places.

Azpan, or Flag or Banner

(15.59)

The azpan is an herb two cubits high, with roots like fibers, leaves like the almond, serrated and a little smaller, and thin stems, at whose tips white flowers grow, which, before they open, are like a coriander seed, and when they bud, separate into threads; the indigenous people give the plant its name because of these slightly bending stalks full of flowers. Its taste is sharp, its smell strong, and its nature hot and dry almost in the fourth degree; it is thus said that the leaves, rubbed on the face, clean it very effectively, that it cures leprosy, rashes, and acne, and other such skin problems, and that, mixed with lime and fresh tlilzápotl, it cures impetigo. In addition, it is good for everything expected of such a temperament. The juice, either on its own or mixed with other purifying medicines, has the same applications. Its native climate is temperate, like the Mexican or Ichcateupan, and it grows wild. There is another herb called azpantli for the same reason as this one, similar to it except that the leaves are wider and not serrated, and it has the same nature and virtues, so some people call it azpan, like its relative that I have described here.

Ayecocímatl or Herb like Címatl

(15.60)

The ayecocímatl seems to belong to the types of beans that are innumerable throughout New Spain. It has a thick root, fibrous and short, thin stems, cylindrical, green, and voluble; medium-sized leaves like those of the pear tree, round, no different from those of the ololiuhqui, shaped something like a heart. Red flowers grow at the ends of the branches, like stars, which produce pods and seeds like broad beans. The root of this plant is used as a food by the Indians—these simple people will eat anything, for although its taste is not altogether unpleasant, it is difficult to cook and results in a hard and fibrous dish. This plant is in nature cold and moist with virtually no fragrance. Its juice benefits those suffering from inflamed eyes, and the raw root or its decoction evacuates the stomach and intestines by the upper and lower passages. It grows in the fields of Mexico almost all the time, in wild, moist places, and it flowers with the first rains.

Amohuitli, or Purple Herb Growing Next to Water

(15.63)

The amohuitli is a shrub with many stalks four cubits or more in length, nodular, and with leaves like the peach, red flowers, round, grouped in umbels, which produce a tiny seed. It is a bitter plant with whose decoction those with a cold wash themselves. It grows in flat, warm places in Hoaxtépec.

Axoquenietl or Heron Tobacco

(15.64)

This is a shrub with thin roots like fibers and stems with leaves like the peach, but larger. These have an almost bitter taste, pleasant aroma, and a temperament that is hot and dry roughly in the second degree. A decoction of the leaves is said to reduce fevers, but I do not see how it could do this effectively unless it does so by moderating more intense heat and reducing it to a lower degree, or calming the cold humors, or expelling the cause in some other way.

Tlályetl, or Small Yetl

(15.66)

The tlályetl, also called cioapatli of Tonalla, has a ramified white root, stems covered with whitish leaves, oblong, soft, serrate, and hirsute. The flower at the tip of the stem looks like that of manzanilla, but somewhat purple around the lip, the same as bellis, of which it is a type. The root is sharp, and hot and dry in the third degree; its juice, when drunk in a dose of two ounces, is extraordinary for soothing coughs and is especially good for new mothers. It grows in Xalatlauhco.

Tlályetl 2

(15.67)

The second tlályetl, which some call quaquauhtzóntic and others tonalxíhuitl, and still others micatlácotl and micaxíhuitl, has roots like fibers, thin, cylindrical, green stems, leaves like willow but smaller, tight, and compressed not far from the base, with three or four others, very small

and narrow, which sprout almost from the same place. Golden flowers grow at the tips of the stems, on small stalks, like chrysanthemums, and contained in round, green calyxes.

Amaquáhuitl or Paper Tree

(15.69)

This is a large tree with leaves like the citron, with white flowers and fruit arranged in corymbs, nearly tasteless and odorless, and of cold and dry nature. It grows in the mountains of Tepoztlan, where hordes of workers can often be seen making paper from this tree. The paper is not very suitable for writing and drawing, although dyes do not run on it, but it is ideal for wrapping, and more than adequate and useful among these western Indians for worshiping their gods, adding to their sacred vestments, and for funeral wear. Only the thickest branches are cut from the tree; new growth is left alone; they are macerated with water and left to soften overnight in streams and rivers. The next day the bark is stripped off and, once the exterior part has been cleaned, it is stretched out and thinned by being pounded with a flat stone, but it is slashed with a few striations, and then beaten with a willow branch doubled over into a circle, like a handle. This wood is soft and flexible. It is then cut in logs, which, beaten again with another, flatter stone, and polished, are finally split into leaves two spans long and about a span and a half wide, which is very similar to our thicker, smoother paper, but it is more compact and whiter, though not as good as our smooth paper. I know that other nations make paper from wood pulp, each in their own way; that the Chinese produce the thinnest and finest; which we have in our own country; that, like the reeds of an earlier time, paper in Europe is made today from pounded flax; but here we are referring only to Mexican paper.

Amázquitl or Papery Shrub

(15.71)

The leaves of the amázquitl are like the lemon tree's but with sharper points. This is a leafy tree appreciated only for its shade. It seems to belong, like the previous one [amacoztic] to the genre of itzámatl, since although its fruit is smaller, no bigger than hazelnuts, the fruit has the same white markings and contains seeds the same shape and nature as the fig; the wood is also light and little different from that of the fig. It grows in warm places, like Chietla, where we gather that the decoction of the outer covering of the root is very beneficial for fevers.

Itzámatl, or Papyrus of Knives

(15.72)

This is a tree of great size called thus for its similarity to the amaquáhuitl, from which paper is made, and because the leaves are shaped like the blade of a knife. The Haitians call this ceiba. There are two kinds, one with leaves like the citron, pale green on the underside and intense on top, round fruit marked with white spots and full of seeds like the fig, edible and with a flavor much like our figs, which is why the Creoles call this the Indian fig tree, and call the fruit Indian fig. One tree grows new leaves twice each year. When they are fresh and tender, the leaves exude a great quantity of juice. The other kind has much broader leaves, but they are more obtuse and darker, which is why some people call it tlilámatl, and with much smaller fruit. Both kinds have bland and sparse wood. As far as medical uses are concerned, I have ascertained only that the leaves are cold and dry and cure sores. Also, I collected from this tree, mainly in Hoaxtepec, manna, as the Arabs call it, very similar to ours in shape and properties, but slightly harder and more glutinous. In other places in New Spain, such as Cuernavaca, they sprinkle an excellent manna on sauces, just as good as what is imported from Campania.

Abaca

(15.83)

The abaca is a plantain like the others, but with narrower leaves and triangular fruit ten inches long, with white pulp and numerous black seeds, slightly smaller than chickpeas, blander and rounder. They make mats from this type of plan-

tain. It grows in the Philippine islands, where another kind grows too, with reddish blotches and small narrow fruit, of which there are three main varieties, called tolocdato, goyot, and bolongon, besides others that, although they have no names, would take too long to enumerate, and which have fragrant fruit, used to sweeten the breath, and a pleasant taste that, when the fruit is perfectly ripe, is not inferior to our apianas apples, just as green, various sizes, of a moderate temperament, or a little cold and moist. It produces flatulence and phlegm, calms the stomach and sweetens the breath. It is customary among the native population, after eating it, to abstain from all kinds of drink because with too much liquid it is indigestible.

The Indian Leaf, Which Is Also Called Malabathrum

(15.86)

The malabathrum is a tall tree, which the Indians call tamalapatra, not unlike the betre.[3] The leaves are narrow and compressed at the tip, green and soft, running the length of the branches; they are sweet smelling, somewhat redolent of caryophyllus. It provokes urine, expels cold, strengthens the inner parts; the juice strengthens the head, though more gently, pleasantly, and with minimal harm. It grows in many places in India, though mostly in Cambaya, close to water. This tree grows in New Spain, where they call it Tabasco pepper, and also caryophyllus, which we shall describe in the proper place, whose leaves are so fragrant that it compares favorably with malabathrum, or can be used as a substitute.

Purgative Tlatlanquaye

(15.88)

This tlatlanquaye or nodular herb has a round, fibrous root. The thin, voluble, spiny stems have tendrils that, when they touch the ground, take root. The tendrils are striated and have nodes at intervals of nine inches more or less, from which it gets its name, and at every node are leaves like the

---

3. Unidentified.

vine or squash. It is said to lack either flower or seed. The root, which is white and yellow, is bitter and hot; crushed and taken with water in a quantity of four drams, it purges both bilious and phlegmatic ⟨humors⟩ without any harm; but if the patient has difficulty taking it, it will produce the same result if introduced in a slightly larger quantity, and taken with some liquid. It is native to mild climes, such as those of Mexico.

Camotli, or Sweet Potato

(15.90)

The herb that the Haitians call the sweet potato, the Mexicans call camotli, for the shape of the root, which is the principal and most useful part; and even though it has been some time since its varieties began to be known to our countrymen, I do not wish to omit in this chapter what is told of its nutritious properties and of the manner of propagating and cultivating it. There are some varieties of this plant distinguished only by the color of the roots (since they all have voluble stalks, angular and round leaves, and flowers in the shape of white calyxes with purple in them). The root is sometimes red on the outside and white inside, and is called acamotli. If the outer skin is purple and the inner part white, it is called ihaicamotli. If the outside is white and the inside yellow with a reddish tinge, it is called xochicamotli. There are times when both the inside and the outside are red, or completely white, and then it is called camocpalcamotli or poxcauhcamotli: names bestowed many centuries ago according to the variety of the colors. All types have an oblong root, sometimes a voluminous one, according to the nature of the soil and of the various colors that I mentioned above. The said root is good to eat raw, roasted or boiled, and in various foods that are prepared with it; it has a flavor very like that of chestnuts, and it provides a similar food: good, albeit greasy and apt to produce flatulence. The stalk, as we have said, is voluble, cylindrical, and slender; it creeps along the ground; it has leaves similar to an eggplant's or to the insane fruit's, of a color that tends toward purple, and purple, small, oblong flowers. It is propagated in August by putting its vines in dug-up soil, and it is pulled up and the root used during the autumn, winter, and spring. It grows, if culti-

vated, in a temperate climate, or in a slightly cold or slightly hot one, but best of all in cultivated and moist soil.

Chichiccamótic, or Bitter Sweet Potato

(15.92)

The chichiccamótic has roots very like small sweet potatoes, white with purple in it and with soft pulp; and from them grow cylindrical, tawny-colored stalks nearly three spans in length, with leaves in the shape of a shield, or like an ivy's. The root is cold and moist, almost devoid of taste and scent, and rather glutinous; crushed and taken with water or some astringent drink, it stops dysenteries. It grows in the hot hills of Cocolan.

Charapu, or Crackling Tree

(15.94)

The charapu is a type of brasil or cotinus. It is the size of a peach, with leaves like laurel, and very small flowers at the tips of the branches, which bear berries very appropriate for making black beads, attractive to look at, the size and shape of spondilium or hazelnuts. The leaves have a certain sharpness with some astringency and bitterness, properties I have observed, but which will have to be investigated by those who come after me, for until now the natives have told me nothing about this tree or how it is used in medicine. It grows in warm areas in the province of Michoacán, where they say that a powder ground from it stuns river fish so that they are easy to catch, and that its fruit is used in place of soap to wash clothes.

Teuhtlacozauhqui, or Queen of the Serpents

(12.1)

Reptiles have their uses in nature: the Creator expressed his majesty no less in humble creatures. The teuhtlacozauhqui is a terrifying serpent, which the Creoles call the viper on account of the ferocity and venomousness of its lethal bite; it is four feet or more in length, and its body is one foot in circumference; it has a raised ridge on its back, a viper's head, a white belly with yellow markings, and its sides covered with white scales, but with blackish bands here and there; the back is gray with yellow crisscross stripes. There are many varieties of this snake, although the differences between them are small, and the bite of all of them is fatal if treatment is not available very quickly. If one of these snakes is disturbed or touched, it winds itself into a ball, twists and rattles violently, and jerks its neck to intimidate onlookers, but it does not bite unless it is attacked or irritated. It is considered effective to put into the ground any limb that has been bitten by this snake, cover it with earth, and keep it there until the pain stops entirely, and the sickness is then cured permanently and effectively, so they say. This snake slides across rocks very rapidly, but, strangely enough, much less rapidly across flat land and open spaces, so that some Mexicans have given it a name derived from their word for wind, calling it ecacóatl.[4] For each year of its age it has a noisy rattle on its tail, joined together in the same way as vertebrae. The eyes are black and medium sized. In the upper jaw it has two curved fangs from which it emits its venom, and five small teeth on each side of the same jaw, which are easy to see when it opens its mouth. Its movement is undulating.

Those who are bitten get cracks all over the body, and die, it is said, within twenty-four hours. The Indians who hunt these snakes catch them boldly by the tail and hold them upside down, but the snakes twist their necks and shake their rattles, and the whole body thrashes about in all directions as they try to retaliate against their captors. I have heard from people who feed these snakes and keep them in their houses that one snake can go a whole year without food or drink. In Pánuco they swear that ten days after the head has been cut off it becomes as thick as a thigh. Many have tried to domesticate this snake and keep it as a pet. It emits the poison through channels in the fangs, which are bone. Some affirm that it is viviparous, but they are in error, as I know from more reliable evidence.

With the fangs, which they keep as a medicine, Mexican doctors pierce the neck and nape of patients suffering from headache; and with the fat of this animal, almost the most harmful of them all, they rub the back to relieve pains, or on any other part of the body, and also to resolve tumors. The Indians eat its meat, and say it is absolutely true that it is better, and tastes better, than chicken. This serpent, wrapped up in thin linen, as thin as it can be, loses its ferocity to such an extent that a child could carry it without fear of harm. They say that if you hang this animal's head around your neck, the same as a viper's, it will alleviate throat problems and fevers. They cure the bites of all rattlesnakes with two ounces of human excrement taken in a little water, or with tobacco crushed and applied to the wound, and also with leaves of the hoitzmamaxalli (very common in the New World), mashed and applied, as I have noted in writing about trees. Also very good for these bites is chipáhoac, which some call acuitzehuaríracua, which we discuss in the study of herbs. ⟨The teuhtlacozauhqui⟩ is found in warm parts of New Spain.

4. That is, wind the noun, not the verb. (The association is with speed, not coiling.)

GEORG MARCGRAF

A volume on the natural history and medicines of Brazil, edited by Johannes de Laet, combined Georg Marc-graf's *Historia rerum naturalium Brasiliae* and Willem Piso's *De medicina Brasiliensi.* The book was published in 1648. A working draft of de Laet's complete edition of Marcgraf is preserved as British Library, MS Sloane 1554. In the printed text, Marcgraf included thirty-three of Hernández's descriptions of plants, taken from de Laet's Latin translation. In the 1648 edition Piso's text made no use of Hernández, but when Piso reissued the two works again in one volume, in 1658, he incorporated some material from Marcgraf, which he claimed as his own. Our translations are all taken from Marcgraf's 1648 text.

Mecapatli or Sarsaparilla

(1.7)

Mecapatli is the name given by the Mexicans to this famous medication, which the Spanish call sarsaparilla, and which is found in several varieties in New Spain. I would like to describe first that species that grows in Spain, and princi-pally in Andalucía, in valleys and hills, classified by expert botanists as *smilax aspera,* described by Dioscorides. It is found not far from Mexico City, in the pueblo[1] of Santa Fe, in cold and watery places close to the sweetest and most salubrious spring water, which is carried to the city by aque-

ducts. It grows very well in Tzonpanco and in the so-called Honduras, which the Mexicans call Hueimolan. I will not say anything about its form, since Dioscorides has described it magisterially. Its virtues are identical to those of the other species, though Dioscorides says nothing about its tem-perament or its properties. It provokes sweat, eases pains in the joints and other parts, and overcomes and destroys per-sistent and incurable illnesses. That alone is evidence of its property of combating poisons and it should be listed as an alexipharmic. That this is a species of sarsaparilla (although the Spanish who have never been to these lands can hardly

---

1. In Marcgraf's Latin, *pago* (from *pagus*), meaning in the village or town.

credit it) no one can doubt if they compare it with the other species that exist in these regions, even though the sarsaparilla of the Indies lacks a seed. But it is customary for men to marvel at such a foreign phenomenon, who cannot believe that something native to their own land is highly valued somewhere else. The nature of this plant is cold and dry, although it has mixed hot and subtle parts, from which it produces sweats, increases the heat of stomach, cleanses the kidneys and the flow of urine, and is diuretic.

Hoauhquílitl or Plant with Seeds Disposed in Tufts

(1.8)

In New Spain many species of wild orach,[2] which the Mexicans generally call hoauhtli or hoauhquílitl, can be found. They are sown and cultivated with great care in their gardens and nurseries, for example tlapalhoauhquílitl or tlapalhoauhtli, which the Spanish call by the corruption "quilites." It has a thick, short, fibrous root, from which grow red stems with red leaves, oblong and serrate, which are chewed cooked and taste good with oil and vinegar.

Xiuhquilitlpitzáhoac, or Narrow-Leaf Indigo, or Herbaceous Vegetable

(2.1)

The herb xiuhquílitl has only one ramified root with many straight stems, six spans high and the thickness of a little finger, ash-colored, round and smooth, sparse leaves like those of the chickpea, small white flowers tinged with red, and pods that hang in clusters from the stems, resembling fat little worms or maggots, and filled with black seeds. It is slightly bitter, with a sharp taste almost like a legume, and its nature is hot and dry in the second degree. Its powder cures old sores, first washed with urine, for which reason many call it palancapatli. It is said that the leaves, crushed and applied, or dissolved in water and smeared, relieve pain and reduce excessive heat in the heads of children. It grows wild in warm areas, in wild or hilly places, and although it is a herb, it still stays green and luxuriant for two years. The dye is known as cerulean, which the

Mexicans call mohuitli or tlacehuilli and the Spanish call azul. The way to prepare it is as follows: the leaves are torn into pieces in a pan or pot of water that has been brought to the boil and then allowed to cool to tepid, or better (as the experts say) cold without being heated at all; it is stirred vigorously with a wooden spatula, and the water gradually emptied as it is dyed, into a clay or earthenware pot, the liquid allowed to drain through holes at a certain height, and the extract from the leaves settles. This sediment is the dye. It is dried in the sun, put in a canvas bag, then formed into small wheels that are hardened by being placed on plates over the coals, and they can be kept for use throughout the year. It would be very convenient to sow this in Spain, in warmer areas such as Andalucía, or places on the Atlantic coast, in wooded or hilly places. The seed can be sown, like that of lettuces, in plowed fields, in January if the weather is mild or warm, and the soil moist and irrigated, otherwise in September or October. It can be transplanted at its due time, again like small lettuces, in more spacious fields, as long as the seedlings are kept free of harmful weeds, until finally it can be harvested and put to use.

Ichcaxíhuitl or Algodon

(2.2)

Ichcaxíhuitl, in Spanish algodon (that is, gossypium)[3] is very common in New Spain and many islands in the Ocean, and a good harvest is obtained from it year after year. It grows in warm and humid places, mainly cultivated. The shoots, ground and taken with water, are wonderfully effective, so they say, against scorpion stings, snake bites, and the venom of other poisonous creatures. The stalks seem to be cold, dry and astringent, and if they are reduced to a powder and applied externally, they cure ulcers; the leaves are naturally viscous.

Mecoztli

(2.16)

The yellow maguey, which the Mexicans call mecoztli, &c. is another species of maguey, whose leaves are yellow to the

---

2. *Atriplex mollis* (Chenopodiaceae).

3. Cotton.

edges, and have small, black spines; the leaves are likewise small in comparison to those of the preceding variety [i.e., the metl].[4] The stem of this one is two cubits high, one inch thick, and red; the flower is blue verging on red, and grows from the point of the stem; the root is woody. It grows on level ground in the woods in Mexico, at any time, although it flowers only in the summer. It propagates from suckers that grow on the stem. Three or four leaves in a decoction with just as many chili pods, gently expel, by sweat and urine, all kinds of gross and cold humors. The Indian doctors prescribe it for several days after childbirth, to comfort and reinvigorate. Wine squeezed from the half-roasted leaves is said to be good against asthma. This plant is cold and glutinous.

Xahualli

(3.1)

Xahualli is a very pretty tree, from whose wood people make long, handsome, robust spears. The leaves are similar to those of fraxinea, and the wood is heavy, its color gray tending to sandy; it bears fruit like the little head of the papaver, though without the corymb, and some people chew on the fruit when it is ripe. The Americans also squeeze a liquid from it, with which they wash their legs and, occasionally, the whole body, particularly when it is becoming weak from tiredness; it corroborates and invigorates, for the special quality of this is to be astringent and binding, and furthermore it tinges with a black color, for skin that has been washed with this liquid is perceptibly stained black, but in most cases the stain disappears of its own accord after fifteen days. Once stained, the fingernails never change color until they change by themselves. When the Indians are holding meetings, and when they set out from home to wage war, they paint themselves with this liquid to look more frightening to their enemies. What sometimes happens is that women harm themselves by washing their faces with this liquor mixed with rose water or some other water, and they apply remedies in vain, then they have to put up with a delay of two weeks.

Ixtlehuayopatli

(3.4)

Ixtlehuayopatli is a tree with leaves like the lemon tree, the underside white and villous, the top surface inclining to black. It bears tiny white flowers, and small fruit that is round, fragrant, and bitter to taste, much the same as the caryophyllus, with which it is interchangeable if need be, not only as a food but also as a medication. The bark is less hot though slightly bitter, the leaves not at all, though in aroma they scarcely differ from the bark. The pith, bruised, and in the quantity of two drams is diuretic as well as being a remarkable remedy for bloody diarrhea. It grows in the hills of Huitlango.

Papaya

(3.5)

Papaya is a mid-sized tree with large leaves like the fig and with many points, large oblong fruit, and a flavor that some people find pleasant, but it is generally not much valued as food. Before ripening, it exudes a sap that is good for treating rashes and swellings (from bites), worms, and skin diseases. After ripening, it exudes a juice that eases stomach pains. This tree grows on the island of Haiti, and warm parts of New Spain, such as Cuernavaca, Tlaquiltenanco and Yyauhtépec. From the unripe fruit they make a conserve that is wonderful for moderating excessive body heat, and it invigorates the heart. I experimented with it in the hospital at Hoaxtépec.[5]

Curaqua

(3.6)

The plant that is called curaqua by the people of Michoacán, quamóchitl and hoitzquáhuitl by the Mexicans, and brasil by the Spanish, is a thorny shrub with many branches and white roots, from which grow stems that are yellow on the outside and red on the inside, twisted and covered with almost heart-shaped leaves, but heavy at the tip, and with many veins that go obliquely from the back to the sides. It grows in the cool

---

4. LMS 6.12.

5. The last sentence is from Ximénez.

regions of Michoacán in wild or mountainous places, where other varieties grow, one of which is called pingüica and another uxaqua. Its taste is astringent and its temperament cold and dry. Its wood is used to dye thread red, since it is very much like the tree they call red sandal. The decoction is at first yellow and red afterward, and if it is boiled more the color intensifies to purple or, if alum is mixed in with it, a nicer red than cinnabar. This tree is refreshing, reduces fevers, binds, and is a tonic.

Nochtli or Species of Tunas

(3.15)

This plant, which the Haitians call tunas,[6] the Mexicans nochtli, and the ancients (some think erroneously) opuntia, indicating a fig tree, has been known for a long time and has begun to spread across the Old World many years ago, causing great amazement because of its monstrous shape and its weird assemblage of thick, spiny leaves; nonetheless, only among the Indians does it yield ripe fruit and wood, and it cannot be judged properly except where it bears fruit plentifully and regularly for the tables of the healthy and sick alike. Despite all of this I desire, without occupying myself with its form, already well known virtually everywhere, to enumerate its distinct varieties, to discuss its properties, and to give an idea of where it grows, the most suitable climate for it, when its seed should be sown, when it flowers and when it fruits. At times the varieties of tunas are distinguished by their flowers, which are first saffron-colored with white at the edges, then yellow on the outside, and inside the same color as the fruit, as can be seen in the tlatocnochtli, or deep yellow on the outside and white with red or also yellow on the inside. They differ also by the size and shape of the leaves as well as of the entire plant, though certainly all of them attain only the size of a shrub, with the exception of zacanochtli and the xoconochtli, which sometimes reach the height of a tree; as for the leaves, some of them are thick, others thin, some covered with spines, others having few, tiny ones; some are round, others square, some enormous, others minute. But it is the fruit primarily that distinguishes them, and that gives them their names, as we shall see in detail. In the province of Mexico, to my knowledge, there are seven species of tunas: the first, called iztacnochtli because its fruit is white, has round leaves, small and smooth, or with sparse spines, a yellow flower, thorny white fruit, and it is the size of a shrub. The second, which is known as coznochtli because of its yellow fruit, has broad, round leaves with many long spines, scarlet flowers with yellowish extremities, and scant yellow fruit. The tlatonochtli, or white tuna tending to red, has narrow, square leaves, extremely spiny and almost purple, which is peculiar to this one type, since all the rest have green leaves; the fruit is also spiny; the flower is yellow on the outside but inside it is the same color as the tuna. The fourth kind, known as tlapalnochtli, which is scarlet, has thin, narrow, square leaves, much smaller than those described above and less spiny, a small white flower with red, and fruit that is not very spiny and is scarlet and flame red. The fifth, called tzaponochtli because of its resemblance to a fruit that the Mexicans call tzápotl, has pale oval leaves, with some spines, and yellow flowers with white and some touches of scarlet. The zacanochtli or herbaceous tuna or wild tuna, reaches the height of a tree, and has round leaves, small and spiny, extremely spiny fruit scarcely bigger than a nut, and pale yellow flowers. There is also the xoconochtli, similar in form to zacanochtli, but with acidic leaves and fruit, from which it gets its name. The nature of all of them is cold in the second degree and moist, except for the seeds, which are dry and astringent. In addition, the leaves are cold and moist, and mucilaginous, for which reason juice squeezed from them and from the fruit is remarkable for cooling a burning fever; it assuages thirst and moistens dry bowels. If the fruit is eaten, seeds and all, as a normal food, it is said to prevent belly fluxes, especially if they are caused by heat. The fruit provides a foodstuff that is pleasant and refreshing, although it causes flatulence and is liable, like all fruit, to rot over time, and it is very appropriate for those suffering from a hot cause, which is why they are eaten with great relish and avidity in summer, mainly by those suffering from an excess

---

6. See LMS 2.6 and note, above.

of bile or hot distemper. They have a gum that moderates the color of the kidneys and the urine. The juice, or liquid extracted from them is wonderful against bilious and malignant fevers, especially when mixed with the juice of pitahaya. Its roots mixed with a certain species of geranium, a picture of which we also give in these books, alleviate hernias, cure erysipelas, mitigate the heat of fever or of any other cause, and they are a remedy for an excessively irritated liver. The Mexicans rub the juice of the leaves on the wheels of their carts to stop them overheating. They say also that the root, which is somewhat sharp, is wonderfully good for sores.

AFTERNOTE: ABRAHAM MUNTING

In *Naauwkeurige Beschrijving der Aardgewassen* (Utrecht and Leiden, 1696), Abraham Munting described one or two of the most famous and widely applied American medicinal plants, using Monardes and Hernández as his sources. Munting had access to both the Rome edition of Hernández and the *Quatro libros*. His descriptions blend quotation with paraphrase.

Guaiacum

The wood of this noble tree, the small guaiacum, is whiter, softer, more fragrant, more bitter, and has a smaller pith than the large one. It is extremely effective against all sorts of ailments of the human body, as noted here, but is a very powerful medicine for the Spanish Pox, hence it is known among the Spanish as *lignum sanctum,* or holy wood.[1]

Indigo

This shrub, dry and hot in the second degree, also quite bitter and sharp to taste, bruised and laid on the head, dissipates headache and heat: it also cures all wounds. The sap, boiled in wine, and applied to the hair, will dye it black.

Purgative Root of Michoacán

Named in Dutch as in Latin, Mechoacanna, after the American [i.e., Mexican] province of Michoacán, where it is native, and it was from this part of the world that it was brought to our country.[2] The Italians call it Indian Rhubarb. In the year 1652 I was fortunate to raise this plant from seed, and with diligent care enabled it to flourish.

---

1. The marginal reference is to "Francisc. Hernand. lib. rer. Med. Nov. Hispan. 3. cap. 29," which this passage does not actually quote but tersely summarizes. Guaiacum, or guaiac, was the standard cure for syphilis. The word itself is derived from the Taino word *guayacan.* See *QL* 1.2.29 above.

2. Cf. the fuller text for this entry in *QL* 2.1.38.

Virtues: The root of Michoacán is hot and dry to the third degree; such that it is a little too intense in nature.

Two drams of this root, dried and powdered, for an old person, but only one for a young one, and for a child just a half dram, taken in wine; or also the root may be steeped in wine.[3]

Tlalayótic

The root of nummularia americana, or American pennywort, or the sap of the same, is good against hot bloodedness of fevers, and only a little of it is taken, because it is dry and cold in nature. It stops all sorts of unnatural diarrhea; expels water; cures wounds, swellings in the mouth, and it relaxes tense nerves.[4]

Sarsaparilla

Boiled in water or wine, taken twice a day, in the morning and evening, six ounces at a time, hot, for forty consecutive days, the patient to be well covered up, and sweated. Otherwise, two drams of the powder of the dried root, taken with wine, is a very good remedy for the Spanish pox, chronic sickness, fevers, and nervous disorders. Moreover, very useful for all kinds of tumors and foul swellings; gross and viscous humors: an upset stomach, flatulence, cold humors of the mother, *harssenen,*[5] and many, many other complaints. It also dissolves hardness of the spleen, and causes sweating.[6]

---

3. The reference for the first paragraph is to "Rech. l. 5. rer. Med. Nov. hisp. c. 38," where the root is described as hot and dry in the third degree, but in the *Quatro libros* (2.1.38) it is said to be hot and dry in the *fourth.* The second paragraph appears to come from Dodoens (necessarily a late and posthumous edition), but the *Quatro libros* has advice on dosages similar to this, even though Hernández makes no distinction between dosages for old and young patients.

4. *Penningskruyd,* as it is called in Dutch, is cited in *QL* 2.2.58 as "Tlalayotic. . . ó numularia yndiana," also known as veronica.

Munting's reference is to "Recch. l. 6. c. 58," not the *Quatro libros,* and of the two sentences that constitute the last paragraph describing the virtues, possibly only the second comes from Recchi.

5. *Harssenen* is a variant of *hersenen,* brains, but Munting includes the word here in a list of maladies.

6. The virtues conflate "Recch. l. 8. Rer. Mexio.[sic] c. 42" and "Monard. hist. Nov. Orb. c. 22."

ITALY, c. 1580–1651

RERUM MEDICARUM NOVAE HISPANIAE THESAURUS: THE ROME EDITION

The text of the Rome edition of Hernández's writings on the natural history of New Spain is based on one of the manuscript copies of Nardo Antonio Recchi's selection and is organized the way Recchi had arranged it in 1580. Our selections are translated from John Carter Brown Library, Codex Latin 5, and from the 1651 edition. The Rome edition is not a particularly rare book, but complete copies are relatively scarce. Many copies have two title pages. Only one that we have seen has three indexes; many have two indexes, and some have only one. We have collated copies at the Biomedical Library, UCLA; the Henry E. Huntington Library; Madrid, Biblioteca Nacional (three copies) and Museo de las Ciencias Naturales (two); the British Library (two); the Facultad de Medicina, Valencia; the facsimile reprint of a copy originally in the library of the Accademia dei Lincei (Rome: Istituto Poligrafico, 1992); and Bethesda, National Library of Medicine (two). As explained in our introduction, the text block in all these copies is identical, even though some have title pages with different dates. We have not included any of the learned commentaries supplied in the Rome edition by the Lincei scholars.

Recchi divided his selection of plants into eight books. The first is a general treatise on plants, not represented here; books 2–8 correspond to the seven books and sections of the *Quatro libros,* with enough variations of selection and text to demonstrate that neither published text was drawn from the Brown Library manuscript itself.

All Hernández's descriptions of animals appeared in Johann Faber's *Animalia mexicana,* printed by Vitalis Mascardi in Rome. Only three separate copies of this work survive, with a title page dated 1628 (British Library, National Library of Medicine, private collection). Many copies of the Rome edition include, as they were meant to, Faber's text, bound in after more than 950 pages of plants, commentaries, and indexes. Faber's source text was the Lincei's manuscript copy of Recchi's selection. The animals occupy books 9 and 10 of the *Thesaurus,* with an extra section appended that includes some new material and some cross-references to these two books.

In an entirely separate, earlier publication, Fabio Colonna included one chapter in his *Minus cognitarum stirpium* on the *cempoalxóchitl,* more a paraphrase than a citation but interesting for the recognition he grants to Recchi, though not Hernández.

Texaxapotla

(2.3)

Texaxapotla, or perforated stone, which is also called tzimpalihuizpatli, or sneeze mover, is an herb bearing leaves like fine flax with delicate purple stems that extend into the ground. It has many small yellow flowers and thin roots. The whole plant smells like the citron and has a similarly bitter taste. It grows in warm places in Cuernavaca and Tlaquitenango and on rocks in the countryside of Huaxtepec. It is hot and dry almost in the fourth degree.

Chichicpatli 7

(2.18)

Chichicpatli is an herb also called techichic with rough leaves like a wall germander's, yellow flowers clustered at the ends of the stalks and contained in oblong calyxes, stems almost four spans ⟨long⟩, and a ramified root. The root is devoid of bitterness; it is fragrant, sharp, of a hot and dry nature and subtle parts. It grows in Itztoluca, in the sown fields. It is an extraordinary medicine, used a great deal by the natives, for the crushed roots stimulate the appetite, ease bellyache, combat cold, get rid of flatulence, cure an itchy scalp, and kill lice. A handful of crushed leaves dissolved in water resolves swellings.

Iztactlatlacótic, or White Herb with Long Leaves

(2.21)

This herb is thirty-six inches long; it has oblong, rough leaves, small white flowers contained in calyxes, and a ramified root whose cortex is gray. It is highly esteemed by the people of Tlacotepec, in whose lands it grows. The root is hot, dry, fragrant, resinous, of subtle parts and the same temperament as the amamaxtlácotl, which exudes blood; crushed and taken in a dose of three drams it admirably eases pains.

Iztacquauhxíotl, or White Quauhxíotl

(3.19)

The iztacquauhxíotl, also called quauhxíotl, is a medium-sized tree with round leaves and reddish stems and stalks. It exudes a white gum with an acrid taste. It grows in the warm areas of Itzocan. The gum is clearly hot in the third degree. It binds loose bowels when taken with water in a dose of one scruple, and is a good cure for dysentery. It also eases, when smeared, pains and swellings; the water it is mixed with becomes milky. There is another type with the same properties and appearance, called tlatlahuicquauhxíotl, but its resin is reddish as its name indicates.

Ezquáhuitl 2

(3.23)

I found too, in the fields around Cuernavaca that belong to Tepequacuilco, a tree very much like the ezquáhuitl of Cuernavaca, but with rounder leaves, hirsute and rough, with a thick bark and ramified root, which grows near water and is also astringent, aromatic, bitter, hot, and useful for the same things. If cut, this gives off copious amounts of sap, which is especially notable for reducing inflammations of the eyes. It is cold, dry and astringent, which is not surprising since, whatever hot parts it has, with cold in it like this, it will have these effects. It grows in warm places in Cuernavaca and Yacapichtla.

Ezquáhuitl [or Dragon's Blood]

(3.32)

The ezquáhuitl is a large tree with large, angular leaves like the mullein. It exudes a sap known as dragon's blood, from which its name comes, for ezquáhuitl means "tree of blood." It grows in Quauhchinanco. The nature of this sap is cold and astringent; it makes the teeth fast, prevents fluxes, and possesses, in sum, the same virtues, same appearance, and same applications as the dragon's blood of the Canaries. There is another tree of the same name that exudes a similar sap, which we shall describe elsewhere, and we may add something separately about the trees of the Canaries.

Izquixóchitl

(3.37)

The izquixóchitl, or plant that has flowerlike corn kernels that burst into stars when heated, is a tall tree with leaves like the citron. The flower seems like the wild rose in shape, and has the savor of a Spanish rose. It is lovely in appearance and highly valued for its extremely fragrant flowers, and would make a fine adornment to the royal gardens, if it were not native to hotter places. It grows wild in Cuernavaca and Hoaxtepec, but it is better cultivated. Its temperament is somewhat cold and astringent. It grows in hot areas, although it is also found in cool ones, thanks to the care of the kings and human labor, and it flowers year-round. Applied, the flower eases toothache; taken, it cures surfeits and chest problems, aids digestion, and it is mixed with cacáhoatl drinks to sweeten the breath.

Achíotl or Good Medicine for Dye

(3.41)

The achíotl, which some people call chacanguarica and others pamacua, is a tree whose size, trunk and shape are about the same as the citron, with leaves resembling those of the elm in shape, asperity, and greenness; the color of the bark of the trunk and branches is deep yellow; inside it is greener; the wood is white and prickly; it has large star-shaped flowers, with five petals, white with some red, and prickly fruit in the shape and size of small green almonds, with four spines running lengthwise. When the fruit ripens, it dehisces to reveal in its cavity several egg-shaped grains, completely red. It grows in warm regions, and thrives better in dry places than in humid ones. It is cold in the third degree with some dryness and astringency. The Indians value this tree highly and customarily plant it near their houses. It has leaves all year round, and bears fruit in the spring, when it is usually harvested. The wood is good for kindling fire, like flint, when two pieces are rubbed together; the bark is used to make rope that is stronger than any made from hemp; painters use the seed to get the color scarlet by mixing it with moderately cold water; and it is just as useful to doctors for, taken or applied, it brings down high fevers, alleviates dysentery, and clears tumors, for all of which reasons it can be conveniently mixed with cataplasms, with those refreshing drinks known as juleps, and with any cold nourishment or medication. It is added to cacao as a refresher and to enhance its color and flavor. It takes away toothache if the cause of the pain is hot, and strengthens the teeth; it is diuretic, thirst quenching, and for some people it takes the place of saffron. To prepare the dye, take ripe grains, put them in hot water, and stir them constantly and in one direction until all the dye has leeched into the water. When the liquid has cooled, drain the grains out and form them into rolls, like indigo or mohuitli, which is produced from the xiuhquílitl, and save them for later use. This dye is so tenacious that a mere dab will not wash out, and mixed with urine it is indelible. It is a little astringent, so that mixed with resin it cures scabies and ulcers; it strengthens the stomach, retards fluxes of the bowel, and increases milk if mixed with the bark of cacao, which it neutralizes however much is taken, for milk is commonly digested with the help of achíotl without the slightest harm.

Tamarind

(3.50)

The Eastern and Western Indians, just as many other nations ⟨do⟩, contrary to the usage of the Greeks and Latins, give names only to fruits and flowers, leaving the plants themselves without a denomination. Such is the case with the tamarind tree, which has no indigenous name given it by the Mexicans (since it was brought to these lands only a little while ago); whereas its fruit has received not just one, but many denominations. Thus, the Malabarese call it puli, the Guzaratos ambili, and the Arabs tamarinds, or Indian dates: not because this tree resembles the palm or its fruit bears any likeness to dates, but because they want to call it that or perhaps because it has a certain shape like fingers, although it is thicker and generally longer ⟨than a finger⟩. It is a tree the size of a walnut or an ash, with small branches like a palm's, filled with tiny leaves similar to those of the rue, but larger, or to those of the so-called mesquite, to those of the hoaxin, or to those of the quauhnacaztli. It has hard wood and has pods in the shape of a bent finger or a bow, whose skin is green at the beginning and ash-gray at maturity and can be peeled off easily. The fruit encloses smooth, tawny-colored seeds a little larger than those of the lupine; when these have been removed, doctors use the pulp ⟨of the fruit⟩, which has a sweet, acidic, and agreeable flavor. The said pods have the particular quality that at night they protect themselves from the cold's rigors by hiding themselves among the leaves, whereas during the day they stretch themselves out and come forth from amid the foliage. The leaves are acidic and have an agreeable flavor; and thus, where these trees are abundant, they are used for sauces, without the need for vinegar.

From the drawing and true image taken from nature that we give of this tree, as from our description, it should be clear and beyond doubt to everyone that the oxyphoenica of the Greeks is not the tamarind tree; for these ⟨fruits⟩ are not dates, but rather, as we have said, pods resembling bent fingers. The Arabs are so mistaken and modern people are so confused in their description, that because of it the tamarind tree can thus be judged the same ⟨as the oxyphoenica⟩ by those who have not seen it with their own eyes, as we have. It grows at the port of Acapulco and in Cuernavaca, not far from Mexico City, where we took care to paint its image; and we have caused it to be sowed from seed in various places and to be brought to Spain, hoping that very soon great benefit will be derived from this excellent medicine.

It is of a cold and dry temperament; it digests bile, it stops mucus, it mitigates heat and it purges the said humors, but especially bile. Some people give the green pods to sick persons to eat, with only the skin taken off and with sugar, to digest the humors and to prepare them for their evacuation, with better results than if they had used vinegar syrup. Others, with the water or the liquid in which they have been squeezed after having been soaked for a time, purge the bilious humor and thin out gross humors; and, in short, others take this water mixed with the so-called Indies nut-oil, in

order to evacuate [these humors] more gently and safely. Also they make drafts with vinegar, above all from those ⟨pods that are⟩ already mature, and they apply the crushed leaves to erysipelas with great benefit. Those ⟨pods⟩ that are carried from the East to Spain and the other regions of the world are not pure, but rather have been prepared with salt so that they may not spoil or rot because of the sea and the long voyage. A preparation is made from the fresh ones, sticking them together with sugar, with which the said humors are digested and evacuated without discomfort and very effectively.

Ahoapatli of Tlilanco

(3.65)

This is a large tree with spiny leaves like the holm oak, but a bit longer, with smaller, yellow and round flowers, and fruit that eventually turns black. The stems are yellow inside. It grow in the hills and flat places of Upper Mixteca. They say that a decoction of its scrapings greatly benefits the jaundiced and those suffering from heart trouble because of excessive bile.

Ahoéhoetl, or Water-Drum

(3.66)

This tree was called ahoéhoetl by the Mexicans because it usually grows on riverbanks or near streams, and because the Indians customarily make their drums out of it, which they call hoéhoetl or teponaxtli. Some people, nevertheless, are of the opinion that its name does not come from this—considering that drums are better made out of tlacuilolquáhuitl or capolinquáhuitl wood—but from the fact that it is near the water and that, when it is stirred by the breeze, it makes a sound. The Spaniards who have emigrated to these lands call it a savin, and also a cedar, for the red color of the wood; but it should be classified among the types of fir, for in addition to the fruit and general aspect that entirely justify our opinion, the wood is soft and flexible and very prone to deteriorating and rotting, above all if it is driven into the ground (contrary to that of the cedar, which is said to be highly durable and almost immortal), although in water it remains whole for a longer time: for which reason Mexican chieftains and kings have been in the habit of putting it down as the base and foundation of the buildings they make in this lagoon. In Michoacán this tree is called pénsamo. There are, as I understand, four varieties that are distinguished by size, color, and fruit. For some exceed the tallest pines in height and girth, have white wood, and at times reach a thickness of twenty-four feet or more. Others, whose wood is also white, with a red pith or heart, are smaller in size and produce cones filled with resin, no larger than ordinary olives; which I wanted to paint because in their shape the shapes of all the others are pretty well represented. There are others, even smaller, with red wood and a rounder top. The last ones, which are the smallest of all, scarcely exceed even common cedars in size and have red wood with a white pith. All have red bark and leaves like a fir's, albeit smaller and more slender; resin flows from them all, if not spontaneously, certainly when it has been melted by fire. Its shape would be the same as our fir's, if it were not that the leaves, as we have said, are more slender, the branches more drooping, and the tops sharper. Chips of the wood, when put into the fire in clay pots with the lids on, produce resin; but this does not flow spontaneously, nor does anything well out of these trees similar to the so-called oil that distills from the blisters on the branches of Indian firs—which, nevertheless, according to some people's opinion, differ not at all from our own firs. The taste of this tree with which we are dealing presently is acrid and astringent, with a certain bitterness and agreeable scent. Its temperament is hot and dry in the third degree, although its resin is much more acrid and much hotter than the fir's and has much stronger properties, as we have said. When burned, the bark is astringent and heals burns and chafed and eroded skin. Together with litharge and powdered incense, it cures sores; and mixed with myrtle ointment, it helps the formation of scar tissue. Ground up with cobblers' ink, it keeps sores from spreading; it makes the entrails costive, provokes urine, and its smoke draws out fetuses and afterbirths ⟨from the womb⟩. The leaves, ground up and rubbed on, cure scabies and swellings of the legs, ease inflammations and get rid of the wounds that caused them. They prevent toothache when one washes one's teeth with them dissolved in vinegar; they keep away fears that are vain and without foundation; and in a dose of six oboli with honey water, they help people who have liver complaints. The resin is highly acrid, with an extremely strong odor, hot in the fourth degree; it cures pains from a cold cause and rapidly alleviates disorders of the joints that proceed from the same. It expels flatulence, dissipates swellings of phlegmatic origin, eases sinews that have been strained by thick humors and purifies and strengthens them. In short, it usually helps all those upon whom other, gentler medicines have been tried, with little or no relief. They grow in all areas, so they could be easily transplanted to Spain, being propagated from seed, cuttings, or roots near streams and stagnant or standing water; even though the smallest variety usually grows and thrives far from water as well. They grow in every season, and resin is gathered from them all year long; but at no time and in no place are they seen to blossom.

Enguamba

(3.75)

The enguamba is a mid-sized tree covered with bark like the cork tree, but yellow and reddish, of gray wood with yellowish pith, oblong sinuous leaves, whitish underneath but whose veins are yellowish purple; its flowers are green and white, in corymbs; the fruit is sour and black, from which a yellow oil is extracted, wonderfully efficacious for resolving tumors and clearing ulcers. It grows in rocky places in Uruapa, in the province of Michoacán.

Intzimberaqua

(3.78)

This tree is slightly larger than the peach and is quite shady, with leaves like the lemon, thicker, smaller, and more fragrant, more pleasant to taste than bay leaves, with a seed resembling coriander but a little larger, green to begin with and then black. It should be classified among the laurels. It grows in cold places in Tancítaro, in the province of Michoacán, and in the convent garden there. The leaves, taken with water in a dose of two drams, control diarrhea, and applied they relieve pains. They say that the leaves cure coughing, whether they are taken by themselves or cooked with meat and the broth is taken. They are hot in the third degree and very astringent.

Atlepatli, or Igneous Medicine

(4.1)

The atlepatli is a species of our ranunculus, with small heart-shaped leaves, crenellated, with long stems that grow from hairlike roots; it has slender, green, and delicate stalks, and abundant yellow flowers no different from the heads of wood asparagus. It is caustic by nature. In the form of an ointment it cures leprosy, ringworm, worm, and rashes. It eats away superfluous flesh and ulcerates healthy flesh. It is native to mild regions, like Mexico, and grows near running water throughout the year.

Xonequilpatli

(4.7)

This is a shrub with ramified roots, gray stems with willow-like leaves, but smaller and narrower, and tiny yellow flowers in the form of small calyxes. Its nature is hot and dry in the third degree, astringent, and it burns the throat even though at first it seems sweet, with the flavor of licorice, and gives virtually no sensation of heat. The crushed leaves, dissolved in water and taken in a dose of half an ounce, ease pains in the joints, or any others from a cold cause, and pains caused by tension; they induce sweat, strengthen weakened nerves, and cure, so they say, almost all illnesses from a cold cause. It might be the same as macuilpatli.

Iztacpatli of Tepéxic

(4.9)

The iztacpatli of Tepéxic, which is also known as tlanoquilonipatli, is a shrub with very small leaves that resemble a bird's feathers, or rather like tlalmizquitl, and yellow flowers. It grows in the mild regions of Tepéxic. It is sharp, and in temperament hot and dry in the third degree. The skin of

the root, ground and taken in a dose of one dram, is said to purge all humors, especially the phlegmatic, and to clear buboes, from which it gets its second name.[1]

Axixpatli of Texaxa

(4.15)

The axixpatli of Texaxa is a voluble shrub with a ramified root, with five-sided voluble stems and leaves like those of the vine. They have a bitter taste and a warm temperament. Its juice, taken, provokes urine and is wonderful for curing the jaundiced. It grows near water in warm places.

Ecapatli, or Small Elder

(4.16)

The ecapatli, which some call tlalhoaxin, others totoncaxihoitl or hot medicine, others xometontli or small elder, and others xiopatli, is a hispid shrub with leaves like the almond, flexible stems, narrow, purple and round, and medium-sized yellow flowers on the outermost branches, from which grow narrow pods, cylindrical and long, and full of purple seeds like lentils, but much smaller. It has a strong aroma and bitter taste. It grows wild in warm or cool areas, though it is also cultivated as a medicinal remedy in houses and gardens. Its nature is hot, dry, and somewhat astringent. It cures tumors and ulcers; its leaves, crushed and placed on the stomach, help children who are vomiting milk. Applied or rubbed, they remove headache, and applied to the whole body or taken in the quantity of one handful they stop hot and cold shivers in fevers. Some say that in this way they also cure surfeits, and that, applied, they alleviate ringworm and leprosy, which the Indians call xiotl, rubbing it first with lichen.

Huitsiqua

(4.17)

This plant, known in Michoacán as huitsiqua, is called xoxouhcapatli by the Mexicans. It is a large herb or shrub with oblong serrated leaves the size of the citron, but with

---

1. The people of Michoacán call it *hoximo*.

small ones as well. Seeds and flowers grow around the bases of the leaves. It grows in warm, damp places, such as those to be found in Mexico. The leaves are hot, dry, and somewhat astringent, and they smell like French lavender. The ground leaves cure putrid sores and facial swelling; applied to the head, it cures discharge from the eyes, and instilled in the nostrils it stops nosebleeds; it cures alopecia, alleviates dysentery, and either resolves tumors or ripens and opens them. Its juice helps the eyes, and steam from its decoction with iztáuhyatl is a very effective remedy for pains in the joints and any cold conditions.

Izticpatli

(4.21)

The izticpatli, also known as tezonquílitl, has a thick, long root, white inside, soft and succulent; purple stems, seven-pointed sinuous leaves, a small, oblong white flower, and round fruit almost like a hazelnut. It grows in the hills of Huitzoco. The root, which is extremely refreshing, stripped of its bark and powdered, is commonly taken for fevers. Its decoction, taken with plain water, is optimal and also corrects any hot distempers. No plant of this type is more esteemed for reducing heat, indeed in this respect it is incomparable.

Coatli, or Water Snake

(4.25)

The coatli, or water snake, which others call tlapalezpatli, or red medicine of the blood, is a large shrub with leaves like the chickpea, but smaller, or like rue but larger. It has a small, pale yellow flower, elongated and disposed in spikes. Its nature is cold and moist, and it lacks any notable aroma. It grows in mild regions, like Mexico, and sometimes hot ones, such as Quauhchinango. The water in which pieces of the stems have been soaked for a while takes on a blue hue, and when drunk, cools and cleanses the kidneys and bladder; it reduces acidity in the urine, reduces fevers, and cures colic. All this can be proven effectively if it is mixed with the roots of the maguey, though they loosen the bowels, as I confirmed several times by testing myself, and it is

confirmed by the testimony of many others. They say also that its resin reduces inflammation of the eyes and clears away growths there. Some time ago I began to prescribe this wood to the Spanish, who expressed wonder that the water turns blue. There is another type of this plant with the same properties, but it does not dye water at all.

Tzontecpatli, or Medicine for Wounds

(4.35)

The tzontecpatli is a shrub with voluble stems of bright green, cylindrical, narrow and long, with leaves like basil, but entire, and fibrous roots. It grows in Tenanpulco, in high or flat places. The shoots, when cut off, exude abundant, milky sap, which, applied to recent wounds, closes them and produces a scar in no time. The sap is hot and dry in the third degree, bitter and sharp to taste.

Ezpatli of Cuernavaca

(4.38)

The ezpatli of Cuernavaca, also known as quauheztli, or blood medicine, is a shrub with leaves like rounder mullein leaves, but hairy, fleshy, soft, and almost heart-shaped. If it is cut it exudes a red sap, from which its name is derived, and gives off a strong smell of French lavender. The bark is hot, aromatic, resinous, dry, astringent and bitter; it is hot in the second degree or greater. A decoction of the roots, which are red and ramified, introduced or taken, cures dysentery, and the liquid exuded from the branches cures chronic wounds. It grows in warm areas such as Cuernavaca, Temimiltzinco, and Teucaltzinco, where I saw it in rocky places.

Yamancapatli, or Mild Medicine

(4.42)

The yamancapatli is a shrub with stems that are soft, thick, gray, and succulent; they are smooth where there are no shoots, but rough and nodular where twigs grow. The leaves, which are like portulaca, split into two sections when they are older; the root is fibrous, thick, and long. Wherever it is broken or cut, it gives off a viscid liquid that tastes and smells much like tecopalli or incense in our own country. It grows in Mexico, where they swear that the powdered root cures ulcers that are putrid, malignant, and cancerous. It also grows in Pánuco. Its nature is hot, dry, aromatic and astringent. They say that the liquid from this shrub is good for making the teeth firm and easing pain in the gums; it also cures burns, and the root, taken in any quantity, alleviates disorders of the joints and looseness of the vertebrae.

Xiopatli, or Cure for Leprosy

(4.43)

This is a shrub with woody, ramified, abundant roots, white inside, brown outside, from which numerous nodular stems grow, soft, green, cylindrical, an inch thick and four cubits long; the leaves are like the mulberry, but much bigger, rougher, and serrate. Crushed and applied, the leaves cure leprosy and make it disappear, also ringworm, especially if, after this treatment, the patient is taken to the bath the Indians call temazcalli. It grows in Hoeitlalpa, in humid places and mountain passes, near water. Its nature is cold, dry, glutinous and somewhat astringent.

Ahoapatli of Yacapichtla or Oak Remedy

(5.1)

The ahoapatli is a shrubby herb, with a thick, fibrous root from which spring abundant purple stems, leaves like those of the ilex, and small, yellow flowers at the tips of the stalks that do not wither. It has a sharp flavor, a pleasant aroma, and is hot and dry almost in the fourth degree. A decoction of the juice kills lice; the smoke drives away bugs. When drunk, it eases stomach pains from a cold cause, removes flatulence, helps prevent diarrhea, and taken as an infusion it relieves colic and intestinal disorders. The root is the part that is mainly used. It grows in temperate or slightly hot regions, such as Yacapichtla.

Acxoyátic 2

(5.2)

The acxoyátic, also called tlachpahuáztic or scopas or tlalcócol or "undulating" because of its misshapen root,

called by yet others pipitzáhoac or iztacpatli pipitzáhoac because of its small size, is a tiny herb with narrow shoots one span high, in groups of three or four with leaves like the fir tree, hence its principal name. Flowers at the tips of the stems grow in spikes, small, delicate, and seeds at first white, turning to gray. The narrow root is three times as thick as the stems. The root is twisted or knotted, and white. It grows in a moderate or cool climate, such as Mexico, so I hope that, if the seeds are taken to Spain, and sown, it will be grown there. The root, which is the part principally used for medicine, has a slightly bitter taste and no smell; it is hot and dry in the third degree. Coarsely mashed and taken in the morning in a dose of six oboli on an empty stomach, and mixed with some suitable draft for curing an indisposition, it will purge all humors, especially phlegmatic and bilious ones, by both upper and lower passages, without causing any harm. Thus it is said to be great for hydrops, asthma, impediments to movement, bodily pains, and mange. Whether the patient has a fever or not, the root can be prescribed fresh or dried, though it is wiser, if using dried root, to reduce the dose a little. If the humors that have to be purged are too numerous, it is necessary when taking this medicine to fast for half a day. This root, ground and mixed with human urine and applied in drops, cures eye trouble and clears up cloudy vision.

Chilpatli, or Chili Medicine

(5.5)

Chilpatli is an herb with a fibrous root, green nodular stems six to eight cubits long, and on them leaves like basil but larger, whole and whitish on the underside; mid-sized flowers, yellow shading into red and disposed in corymbs, from which at the end berries form, looking much like black pepper or hawthorn berries. It grows in the warm regions of Pahuatlan, Papalotícpac, and Hoeitlalpa, in flat places and on mountain slopes, and it is sown and cultivated in gardens for medicine. It is bitter, hot and dry in the fourth degree. At first it tastes of resin, then it reveals its astringent nature. The leaves in a dose of two scruples, ground into powder and mixed with ten ounces of atolli, purge the body of all humors with admirable speed and efficacy, and cure quartan fevers principally; any larger quantity is dangerous. Applied, they cure toothache and ringworm, chapped skin, and itch; made for some time with a potion of corn, they alleviate putrid and cancerous sores. Its juice destroys warts and opens tumors. They say that five leaves, taken, will cure dysentery, perhaps cleansing the blood or because it is not entirely devoid of astringency; the leaves are also said to cure pains in the joints. Some smear their arrows with its juice instead of poison, and fell deer and wild animals that way.

Cococtemécatl, or Bitter Twisted Cord

(5.8)

The cococtemécatl, which some call cococtemecaxíhuitl, has a fibrous root, red voluble stems, and on them leaves like those of basil, only much bigger, more angular and crenellated; flowers on the topmost branches, small, pilose, white with purple, and they break out into threads. It grows in Yacapichtla and Quauhquechulla, in warm and rocky places. The leaves are glutinous, so that, crushed by the fistful and taken, they cure dysentery. The root and stems are dry and hot in the fourth degree and of subtle parts; they cure loss of alopecia and ringworm. Two drams of the root, taken, ease stomach pains and cramp, are diuretic, are good for women at childbirth, alleviating illnesses from a cold cause, and they ease wind pains.

Cococxíhuitl of Teocalzingo

(5.10)

The cococxíhuitl of Teocalzingo has a ramified root, gray stems, on which are sharp, mintlike leaves, oblong, whitish and serrate, and green and yellow fruit at the extremities of the stems in the form of rosebuds. It grows on hilltops in warm areas. It is hot and dry in the fourth degree, and burns the tongue when it is tasted. It gives off a smell of cumin; it combats cold and dissipates flatulence from a cold cause, eases sharp stomach pains and stimulates the appetite, whether the herb itself is eaten or its decoction is taken; it provokes the terms and urine, opens obstructions, cures

paralysis, aids digestion, cuts gross humors, restores feeling to parts of the body that are numb from cold, and is useful for things like that.

Ololiuhqui, or Plant with Round Leaves

(5.14)

The ololiuhqui, which others call coaxíhuitl, that is, the serpent herb, is a voluble plant with thin green stems and green leaves, which are heart-shaped. The flowers are white and elongate. Its seeds are similar to coriander, from which its name is derived, and the roots are like fibers. It is hot in the fourth degree. It cures the French disease and also calms pains that come from exposure to cold. It dispels flatulence and resolves tumors. The powder of this plant is mixed with resin and is very good for broken bones. It strengthens women's "relaxed" waist. Its medicinal uses are limited to the seed, which is ground and rubbed into the head and on the forehead with milk and chili. It is said to cure eye diseases. If it is eaten, it excites the sexual appetite. The seed tastes bitter and, like the rest of the plant, is very hot. When the Indian priests wanted to simulate conversations with the gods, and when they wished to receive answers from them, they would eat this plant in order to induce delirium, and thus see a thousand phantasms and figures of death. Its properties can be similar to the solanum manicum that Dioscorides described.

Tzahuéngueni or Filipendula of Michoacán

(5.20)

Tzahuéngueni is an herb whose roots resemble those of the oenanthe in our country, but are a little larger, full of fibers, five or six joined together, and from each one grows only one stem covered with long, narrow leaves, and flowers that are yellow in the center and purple at the edges. It grows in cold places in Michoacán, such as Pátzcuaro. The root tastes like the copal, is hot and dry in the fourth degree and somewhat bitter. Applied, it is said to get rid of scabies and cure the pustules that come from the French disease; it is said also to expel flatulence, expel cold, provoke sweat, bring warmth to cold parts of the body, and relieve chest problems. It has subtle parts, for which reason it is easy to infer its many other uses.

Zacatlepatli 2

(5.27)

The zacatlepatli, also known as tletlatía or burning medicine, is an herb with abundant roots like the asphodel, from which come leaves like barley or grass, yellow flowers in calyxes, and a small round seed. It grows in cold places like Huexotzinco and Xalatlanco. The roots mixed with lime are said to cure chronic ulcers, especially those that open like a honeycomb; these are dilated and cleaned, and eventually disappear; applied the roots are also said to cure mumps, to break and open tumors, to cure tetters and when necessary to corrode and penetrate healthy flesh. It is hot in the fourth degree and is by nature caustic, hence its name.

Axixcozahuilizpatli, or Yellow Diuretic Medicine

(5.28)

This is an herb bearing almost yellow leaves, from which its name is derived, in the form of shields or like ivy, and lined with numerous veins. The root is very short, quite thick, fibrous, and from it come round, woody stems. The root has a pleasant taste, is slightly bitter, and is hot and dry in the third degree, and of subtle parts. The decoction of the leaves taken daily in the morning provokes urine and gets rid of kidney trouble. It grows in valleys in cold regions and in wild places in Yancuitlan, in Upper Mixteca.

Epázotl or Aromatic Herb

(5.32)

This is an aromatic herb with roots that branch out, stems that grow out in the shape of a large elbow; oblong and reddish leaves. The seed is spiny. This plant grows in temperate and warm regions. It grows in gardens in those areas and in many others. It is cultivated because of it usefulness. This herb is bitter, aromatic and hot in the third degree. It is edible raw and cooked and, when added to foods, it fortifies the body. It helps asthmatics and those

who suffer from problems of the chest. It also offers an agreeable nourishment. A decoction of the roots controls dysentery; removes inflammations and expels worms from the bowels.

Phehuame, or Good Medicine for Childbirth

(5.36)

This plant, which the people of Michoacán, where it grows plentifully, call phehuame, is called by our Dioscorides aristolochia clematis; but as it has never been seen by Europeans whether painted or with their own eyes, while it is familiar in the New World, I took care to have it painted and to mention here the uses to which these people put it, and which I have proved myself now, from my personal experience. It is a voluble plant with heart-shaped leaves and purple flowers like other varieties of aristolochia, a thick root, long and covered with a skin like a cork tree. It is the root that is used mostly for medicine, since it is very fragrant, sharp, hot and dry in the third degree and of subtle parts. Its decoction, prepared in exactly the same way as the china root, or sarsaparilla, or mixed with them, and prescribed with a regimen of like alimentation and other things called the non-naturals, is a wonderful cure for any illness from a cold cause, or for the Spanish plague, alleviates chronic coughing and asthma, expels kidney stones, cures bladder infections from a cold cause, corrects loss of color, provokes the terms, induces childbirth, clears obstructions, and expels cold. The root in a dose of two drams, purges gross and viscous humors, especially phlegmatic ones, just like the roots of all its family, which, I think, was not known to the ancients. This plant is held in high regard by the Indians, and counted among the most healthful. It grows in mild or cool areas in Michoacán.

Teocuilin or Rock Worms

(5.39)

This small herb has a remarkable form, for it has stalks like nodes or scales, surrounded by circles like palms, and when they touch the ground, the little hairs that grow all over it take root. The heart-shaped leaves are sparse; and there are some shoots or fruit, if it can be called that, much like long pepper. The taste of this herb is aromatic, sharp, and hot and dry in the third, or perhaps the fourth, degree. It can be ground, and its powder is an effective cure for wounds; it also expels wind. When introduced it eases stomach pains, drives out cold in the bowels, cures hydrops, provokes urine, and is good for other similar purposes. It has subtle parts, and grows on rocks in humid, warm places.

Iztactexcaltlácotl, or White Stick of the Rocks

(5.42)

This is an herb with purple stems, cylindrical, four cubits long; serrate leaves like the nettle, and at the tip dense clusters of pilose white flowers tinged with purple, and which do not fade. It grows in rocky places in Xalatlauhco. Its savor is exactly like anise; its temperament is hot and dry in the third degree, and it has subtle parts. One handful of the crushed root, taken with water or wine, provokes sweat in those suffering any pain and in this way eases it admirably.

Atzóyatl 2

(5.47)

The herb atzóyatl has roots like fibers, from which grow numerous stems divided by red knots and hirsute leaves, pale and heart-shaped, but elongated. The flowers are red outside, white inside, four inches long, with elongated calyxes. It has the taste and aroma of anise with a touch of bitterness. It is native to hilly places and it flowers in September. It is hot and dry with some gross parts and some astringency, for all which reasons it stops diarrhea, strengthens the stomach, dissipates flatulence and eases pains from a cold cause.

Tlacocoltzin, or Small, Twisted Herb

(5.52)

Among the people of Tetzcoco I found a species of tithymalus, which seemed to me to be the *helioscope;* but as its form was not identical, I had it depicted. Tlacocoltzin, also known as cucultzin, is a small herb with leaves like portu-

laca, narrower, longer, and more pointed, of a diffuse green color, alternating on the stems. Between these can be seen three or four large leaves like anagallidis, where the branches start, pale yellow at the base, purple at the tip. It has four or five stems, red near the root, full of copious sap, a long root contorted at its extremity, and fibrous, covered by a gray-black skin. It grows anywhere, but mainly in warm places. Its roots and leaves are prized by the Indians for purging phlegmatic humors and both biles, taken in a dose of one dram, as well as for curing the French disease, to such an extent that they keep this like a secret, not readily revealed to anyone.

Ixtenéxtic or Ashen Eyes

(5.59)

This has a thick root full of branches, purple stems that are thin, round hispid and one cubit long, full of leaves the size and shape of the lemon but serrate, hirsute, rough and whitish, with flowers like chrysanthemums. It grows in the cold region of Xalatlauhco, in the hills and valleys. The root is somewhat bitter, sharp, diuretic, and the throat is immediately sensitive to its nature. It is aromatic, dry and hot in the fourth degree, and of subtle parts. Crushed and applied, it resolves scrofula, clears leprosy and ringworm, and to cure the illness that the Mexican Indians call tzatzayanaliztli, in which the whole body gets chapped, the resin is applied first, then the powder from the root, and chicken feathers are placed on top. This medicament is much prized by the Mexicans.

Axixcozahuilizpatli of Yancuitlan, 2

(6.3)

This has a ramified root, narrow, cylindrical, nodular stems with tiny leguminous leaves, small yellow flowers that somewhat resemble those of chickpea, but a little smaller. It is bitter, hot and dry in the third degree, though in the end it seems to have a certain sweetness like licorice. It is said that the decoction cures hoarseness, eases pains of the stomach from a cold cause, provokes urine, and cleans the urinary tract, from which it gets its name.

Coaquíltic, or Serpentine Vegetable

(6.9)

The coaquíltic, also called tzatzayanaquíltic, or herb like laurel, has a large ramified root, white and covered with a thick skin, hollow white stems tending to purple, long, crenellated, sinuous leaves a bit like the second sysimbrius, and a seed like fennel in the shape of a fly. The root is very succulent; it is bitter with some sharpness, in nature hot and dry in the third degree. It grows in the gentle and temperate climate of the hills of Culhuacan. It is hot, as said above, and of subtle parts. It provokes urine, dissipates flatulence, warms the stomach, loosens the bowels, cures afflictions of the womb, and, taken in a solution with water, it is a cure for intermittent fevers. It is commonly given to children with fevers, and also to adults, in whom it can help to burn off or destroy the cause of the illness. The decoction of the root frees the milk of wet nurses in cases of obstruction.

Nahuitéputz, or Four-Sides

(6.12)

This is a multiplex. First, it has a single thick and fibrous root, many stalks nearly three cubits long, a little thicker than the little finger, deep yellow and pennate, with certain foliaceous appendages that extend lengthwise to four sides, from which the name comes. There are upon them rough leaves similar to arrowheads but much larger, and yellow and stellate flowers larger than a chrysanthemum. It grows in temperate regions, such as the Mexican one, but it does not refuse ⟨to grow in⟩ hot ones, high places, or the countryside. The root's fibers are hot and dry in the third degree, fragrant, acrid, bitter, resinous, and of subtle parts. Crushed and taken in a dose of a half dram with wine or some other liquid, they cure indigestion, evacuating the disordered foods by means of the lower passage. Ground to a powder, they alleviate the pustules that arise from the French disease, if these are washed beforehand with a decoction of ahuácatl and xalxócotl; and they open and clean out boils. They say also that the same root, taken in a dose of an ounce, softens the bowels and provokes urine. According to some people, it should be taken in a larger amount; and there are

those who swear that it provokes sweat, heals colds, and—by evacuating the cause—cures fevers' highest pitches and the fevers themselves; that it gets rid of headache and dissipates eye inflammations; that it heats and strengthens a stomach weakened on account of cold; that it opens obstructions in the viscera, hurries up slow menstruation, alleviates cachexia, and helps a cold indisposition of any abdominal organ whatsoever. A decoction of it is introduced into women giving birth; and the leaves, applied, bring swellings to a head or dissolve them. An herb similar to the preceding one seems to be of the same species: with a large yellow flower with purple ⟨in it⟩ but almost without taste or odor, of a cold and humid nature, which improves those who have a fever and cures eye inflammations; for which reason some people call it ixpatli, even though in Chiauhtla, where it grows, they sometimes call it pitzahoaccacaxpatli and more frequently cacaxtlácotl. I have seen also another variety of nahuitéputz among the Itzocanese, with roots like the hellebore's: acrid, hot and dry in the third degree, and very efficacious in containing digestive fluxes—which I have not bothered to paint, since it did not have leaves when we saw it. There is yet another variety, of a cold temperament and very efficacious in mitigating the excessive heat of the liver.

Tzonpotónic or Fetid Hair

(6.16)

There are two kinds of tzonpotónic, which some call tlacochíchic, that is, bitter stick, and others call bitter flower. The first kind has serrate leaves, quite long like the willow, straight reddish stems as thick as a goosefeather, and at the tips white, downy, fragrant flowers, something like those of the elder. The roots are fibrous, and look like fibers. It grows in moist places, near running water. The root is fragrant and resinous, somewhat hot and dry in the third degree, somewhat astringent and with a bitter taste. It cures surfeits, stimulates the appetite and provokes the terms. Some say that the decoction of the juice cures chest problems and itch. There is another species called iztactlacochíchic among the people of Hoexotzinco, with narrower leaves, and it is useful for all the same things.

Xararo

(6.24)

This herb has black, fibrous roots, cylindrical brown stems, with leaves like the willow except that they are rough, serrated, and whitish underneath; at the tips, pilose yellow flowers contained in scarious calyxes. It grows in mild, hilly, and rocky places in the province of Michoacán. It looks like the chichianton and the malacaxóchitl. The root is bitter and fragrant, and therefore hot and dry in the third degree; they say that, taken in a dose of one dram and a half, together with half an ounce of curitzeti, it purges all cold humors gently and safely, and that on its own it cures fatigue and does everything one would expect of its temperament.

Yolmimiquilizpatli

(6.25)

Yolmimiquilizpatli is an herb with long, narrow leaves and long stems adorned with small, pale yellow flowers; the roots are thin. It grows in Oaxaca. The root is bitter, sharp, and hot in the third degree; taken in a dose of three drams it is said to cure syncope caused by gross humors, and to purge phlegmatic and bilious humors if it is taken twice a day.

Ixpatli, or Medicine for the Eyes

(6.26)

Ixpatli is a small herb with long, narrow leaves, stems about four inches long, a medium-sized purplish flower, and a round root, slightly larger than a hazelnut. It is the parsley described by Dioscorides or something closely related to it. It grows in cold, moist, rural places in Upper Mixteca, also in the fields around Oaxaca. The root is mucilaginous, somewhat bitter, hot in the third degree, and it burns the throat. It cures the eyes and consumes their growths; it also cures hydrops and syncope, and, taken in a dose of two drams, it purges bilious and phlegmatic humors by the upper and lower passages, and so alleviates disorders of the heart, and removes the French plague.

Zacahuitzpatli, or Spiny Grass Medicine

(6.29)

This star-shaped herb has short stems that trail on the ground, with numerous small leaves, delicate and grouped in clusters along the length of the stem; in the center of the herb are long white strands. The root is small and fibrous. It grows in cold parts of Yalhualiuhcan, in arid valleys. Its roots are kept for year-round use; mashed and taken with wine made from maguey, or with water in a dose of three drams, they are said to purge bilious and phlegmatic humors by the upper and lower passages. It tastes bitter, burns the throat, and is hot and dry almost in the fourth degree.

Zayolpatli, or Mosquito Medicine

(6.30)

This herb has deep yellow stems and a thick, long root, leaves like mint, whole, in groups of three or five, flowers like fennel or the acocotli, and around the umbel are seeds the shape and size of black peppercorns. It grows in warm, hilly places in Hoitzoco and Texaxáhuac. The seed is aromatic and slightly bitter. The root is at first sweet, then sharp, burns the throat, gives off juice and is warm and dry in the third degree. The bark is good for the skin and resolves tumors. Smeared on, the root cures itch and other things; the seed cures other infections, though less effectively. It cleans swollen parts of the body, especially the stomach, taking one ounce of the root with wine, and is the remedy for chronic sores.

Apitzalpatli Tzontololotli

(6.31)

The apitzalpatli tzontololotli—or astringent remedy with round threads—is an herb known in Michoacán, where it grows, as zazaltzin because it is viscous. It has numerous, serrate, almost round leaves (from which the name comes) similar to those of the oak but bigger, rough, hirsute, and ash-colored. At the ends of its slender, hirsute, round stalks are pale yellow flowers similar to a chrysanthemum, medium-sized and crowded together in large numbers. It grows in the hills in hot areas. The ramified root is fragrant and slightly bitter to the taste, hot and dry almost in the third degree, viscous, and of a rather bitter and resinous flavor. When it has been ground to powder, mixed with turpentine, and applied to the knees, it rids them of cold, eases their pain, and strengthens and invigorates them if they have been weakened by an excess of labor. Its decoction firms the teeth and tightens the gums, helps those who have dysentery ⟨and⟩ looseness of the uterus and the kidneys, ⟨and⟩ in ⟨cases of⟩ fractures and fatigue. The Mexican kings and high noblemen used to take the ground bark with water, in a dose of half an ounce, after the national game of batey—which we call the ball game—in order to prevent the illnesses that generally follow extreme fatigue.

Tlalayotli or Small Squash

(6.35)

The tlalayotli has heart-shaped, medium-sized, and sharply pointed leaves, and voluble nodular stems that trail along the ground. Its little gourds are the length and thickness of a fist, with marks of ash and green intermixed, full of lanuginous seeds, and the root is long, fibrous and round. It grows in the warm region of Yacapichtla, where the Indians cure bloodshot eyes by rubbing the eyelids with its leaves until the blood is all gone. The taste is bitter and its temperament a little hot. The root, taken with water in a dose of two drams, is said to purge thick and viscous humors by the upper and lower passages, and, applied, it ripens and opens swellings and cures sores.

Zayolpatli of Oaxaca

(6.36)

The zayolpatli or mosquito herb is a tiny plant, so fragile that the earth drags it down. It is covered with white star-shaped flowers, with small, narrow leaves and roots, and nodular stems. It grows in warm, shady places in Oaxaca. It is somewhat hot and bitter; the decoction of one ounce to twelve ounces of water, reduced to one third, purges, when drunk, phlegmatic and bilious humors by the upper and lower passages, stimulates the appetite and is antiemetic; it should be taken in the morning for four days, or more if necessary.

Cozolmécatl, or Cradle Cord

(6.57)

The cozolmécatl, also called olcacatzan, seems to belong to the species of Mexican china, for it has a thick, round, red, fibrous root, heavy when fresh but lighter as time goes by. The red stems round the root are knotted, narrow, spiny, reedy and flexible, full of tendrils, and twining; they climb to the tops of nearby trees. The leaves are round and medium-sized with three longitudinal veins; the fruit is like the myrtle, with a lot of seeds. The plant grows in the towns of Juan de Cuenca, a warm area, at high or low altitudes in Mecatlan, and also in Totonacapa, where they say there are two types of this voluble plant: the one, which we have described, fruit-bearing, very healthful, and from whose arundinaceous stems they make very attractive walking sticks with alternating red and black stripes, and another that bears no fruit and should be classified more accurately as poisonous. Marvels are attributed to this plant by those who have experienced its effects: it cleans bloodshot eyes very quickly; just one leaf applied to the eyes will restore their luster; it cures mouth ulcers; the powdered root consumes excrescences and restores healthy flesh where the genital area has been infected by the French disease; although its temperament is moderate, by certain unknown virtues it combats hot illnesses as well as cold, and not just by topical application, but also by being taken. Both the leaves and the root are used, being innocuous whatever quantity is taken. It is said, further, that it augments and reestablishes weakened strength by mere contact, similarly restores semiextinct heat, and revives the moribund; that the leaves, applied, miraculously relieve toothache, headache, pains in the joints and other parts of the body, and if they adhere to any place that is painful, one can expect a certain return to health, for they will stick only when the pain is relieved: otherwise they fall straight off. It is said also to excite sexual activity extraordinarily, to comfort the head, and to help induce sleep; when drunk with wine it cures colic, expels wind, combats poisons, is a tonic, and aids digestion; it returns strength in a remarkable way to those weakened by too much sex: they lie down on it. And, finally, it is said that among the great multitude of illnesses there is scarcely a single one that this plant is not good for, and so they say that just by having discovered this one plant and by having passed on knowledge of it to the Old World, the royal efforts have been a success, the expense has not been wasted, nor has so much labor been in vain. Time and an exact knowledge of things will confirm all of this and make it manifest.

Caquiztli

(6.62)

The first caquiztli has red roots like fibers, square stems and at intervals opposed leaves like basil, but fewer, resembling oregano but not serrate; blue, slightly elongate flowers in groups of three, and accompanied here and there by two smaller leaves. It grows in the mountains of Mexico. It is bitter, sharp, and hot and dry almost in the third degree. They say that the leaves, mashed and dissolved in water, then smeared on the skin, cure the itch. A decoction of the leaves, taken, provokes sweat; and I am assured too that those who pass blood in the urine have their health restored if they are given the vapor of wine from maguey (called white pulque) in which this herb has been cooked, and as soon as they have inhaled the smoke, they go to bed, wrap up warm, and sweat.

Ixtomio, or Lanuginous Herb

(6.64)

The ixtomioxíhuitl, also called tomioxíhuitl, memeya, quapopolton, and quapopoltzin, has hirsute, uneven, spiny leaves, resembling those of ox-tongue, a yellow stem two cubits long; small white flowers in small calyxes, which break up into threads, and numerous roots like fibers. Taken in a dose of two drams, the roots are said to purge all humors by provoking vomit. They are in nature hot and dry with some bitterness. Eaten, they calm coughing and help chest infections, cleanse the kidneys and bladder, clear putres-

cent sores in the genital areas of women and men, cure hemorrhoids and, purging the cause of the flux by the upper channel, they also cure diarrhea. It grows in valleys and flat places in cool areas, and its root is pulled up and kept for use throughout the year.

Tlalixtomio or Small Ixtomio

(6.65)

The tlalixtomio has quite thick roots, ramified, purple cylindrical stems, covered with leaves like portulaca but a little larger, and flowers, also purple, at the tips of the stems. The roots, ground and taken in a dose of two drams with water, purge phlegm by the upper passage, cleanse the intestines and, when introduced, cure colic. They are very bitter, and hot and dry in the third degree.

Herb of Paradise

(6.66)

This herb takes its name from its leaves, which look like the plumage of a bird of paradise. The leaves are hispid and tawny. The stems and roots are fibrous. It grows between Chocándiran and Atapan, in the province of Michoacán. It is very bitter, and hot and dry in the third degree. It cures skin diseases, kills worms, expels wind, cures indigestion, and clears obstructions.

Pacxantzin, or Sedimentary Plant

(7.3)

The pacxantzin is also known as tenextlácotl, meaning "lime stick," or tlacocacalaca. It is a branchy herb with stems two cubits long, cylindrical, woody, striated with an ash color tending to purple, from which it takes its name. The sparse, rough leaves look like sage, whitish underneath and green on top, fiberlike roots, large yellow flowers that grow from tiny scarious calyxes. Its nature is hot and dry in the second degree, with an assertive taste and smell. It is native to a mild climate, such as Tepoztlan, and it flowers in September. The decoction of the roots cures surfeits, strengthens a weak stomach, and brings heat to the chest. It is also prescribed for those recovering from any grave illness who are taken to the baths. The crushed leaves, mixed with equal parts of chichiantic and tlatlaolton, and applied to bruises, dry up and expel all the humors that accumulate there; but the Indian doctors customarily instill at the same time, in the nose, powder of tlacoxiloxóchitl.

Tlalcoatli or Small Coatli

(7.5)

The herb tlalcoatli has thin nodular stems covered with small, delicate leaves like heather; the flowers are white, elongate and like a flock of wool; it has many long, narrow, fiberlike roots. It grows in the hills and plains in cold areas, such as Huexotzinco. Its nature is hot in the second degree and phlegmatic. A decoction of the juice of the roots is prescribed for those experiencing pain or difficulty urinating, for it calms the pain, cleanses the tract, and expels both the urine and anything else that is retained.

Tlalzacamecaxóchitl, or String Flower of Land Pasture

(7.6)

This herb has a transverse, fibrous root, from which grow many stalks with leaves like a willow's or an olive's, and at their ends white flowers with red in them, densely clustered, delicate, and medium-sized. The root is hot and dry in the second degree, and fragrant; when taken in half-ounce doses, it cures intermittent fevers and returns consciousness to those persons who have lost it in some fainting spell.

Ixiayáhoal of Chapultépec

(7.7)

Ixiayáhoal seems to be a species of nepeta or calamint unknown in Europe. It has small, serrate, slightly serrate leaves, almost heart-shaped, and woody stems three spans long, numerous white and mid-sized flowers, and a long fibrous root. It is native to hilly and mild places, such as Tetzcoco and Chapultépec, for which we have given it its sub-

title, for ease of distinction. It is fragrant, hot and dry in the second degree. The root taken with water controls diarrhea, ripens and opens tumors, combats colds and intermittent fevers, induces sweat and urine, and expels from the stomach all viscous humors.

The Peruvian or Large Chimalácatl Which Some Call the Sunflower

(7.15)

This Peruvian chimalácatl might also be called anthilion or sunflower. It has roots like fibers and only a single straight stem, which reaches a height of fifteen feet and is as thick as an arm, round, hollow, and green. The large leaves are serrate, white underneath and in the shape of the nettle, and the round flowers at the tips measure more than one span; they are golden with some reddish color in the center. The seeds are concealed like those of the melon but are cylindrical in shape and are similar to the melon seeds in their white color, in their temperament and almost in all of its nature even though, when they are eaten in large quantities, they can cause headaches. However, they can help pains in the chest and even take away these pains and heartburn. Some people grind the seeds and roast them and make them into bread. It is said to excite sexual appetite. It grows in Peru and everywhere in the American provinces in plains and the woods. Its grows best in wooded areas and in the places where it is cultivated.

Tlalcapolin, Small Cherry, or Chamaecerasus of Atlapulco

(7.19)

This is a small herb, measuring one span, with serrate, oblong leaves spaced out in groups of four or five, and purple stems. At the ends of the stems are small red flowers, and fruit very similar to our cherries, though smaller, hence the name. The ramified white roots are hardly thicker than a goose feather. It grows in hilly and cool places in Atlapulco, in groves. It is hot, dry, and astringent. The dried root can be kept for use throughout the year. When it is powdered, it cures dysentery.

Tlalcoxóchitl of Anenecuilco

(7.20)

The tlalcoxóchitl of Anenecuilco, which some call tlacoxi-huitl, and which in Hoaxtepec they call tlacopatli, has leaves like the willow and, growing from some of the roots as if they were fibers, tawny stems at whose tips there are small white flowers tinged with red, elongate and disposed in groups. It grows in warm, flat places. I have been told that this plant was brought from the South Sea to Anenencuilco, because it is such an excellent remedy. Its nature is hot, dry, and astringent, and it is thus prescribed for those suffering fatigue, since it is said to strengthen and revive them. They also affirm that the powdered root is an effective cure for old wounds.

Chiantzotzolli, or Plant That Swells in Humid Conditions

(7.26)

The herb known as chiantzotzolli has leaves like ivy, only larger, square stems of one and a half spans, small white flowers in oblong calyxes that at the end produce and contain the seed, which is white and flattened like a lentil, and ramified roots. It smells like our thyme, but it loses its aroma at once; the leaves and roots seem completely devoid of heat or a certain astringency and sharpness. The seed is cold or moderately warm with a certain viscosity and slimy nature, and is commonly taken with water in a dose of one ounce each morning and evening against fevers, dysentery, and other fluxes, with wonderful results, whenever a poultice made with cobwebs, red wine, and fresh eggs is applied two or three times to the stomach. With this seed they make a condiment with sugar and honey, with shelled almonds or melon seeds or other plants, very pleasant relishes and refreshing drinks like the so-called chiantzotzollatolli, which is very effective in reducing feverish heat and constitutes a good and pleasant food. It was highly esteemed in time of war, when anyone equipped with a bagful of it believed that no other nutrition was necessary. They mixed the seed with roasted corn to make flour, and ground it so that it would keep longer, and when occasion demanded they would prepare a drink to which they usually added the boiled juice of the maguey, which is perhaps not as good as our honey, and a little pimento. This plant grows wherever it is sown, mainly in cultivated, irrigated places.

Tzopelicxíhuitl

(7.35)

This herb has leaves opposed at intervals, the shape and size of basil, but with other, smaller ones that sprout from the same base. The stems are thin and round. White flowers grow on elongate peduncles, which look like small oblong vertebrae, and the thin roots are like hairs. It grows in warm, humid places, hilly or flat, and in the mountain passes in Pánuco. The leaves of this herb are so sweet that even honey, sugar, and other sweet substances seem inferior, as if it was nature's desire with this plant to see how much sweetness could be packed into natural things. It is useful, too, for the leaves taken with water reduce fevers, and its juice relieves coughing and hoarseness and stimulates the appetite.

Cececpatli of Acatlan

(7.38)

The herb cececpatli of Acatlan has many leaves, like rue but smaller, and long narrow roots, from which the stems sprout. It grows wild in hot places, mainly in lower Mixteca, where it is sometimes called charapehuari, or xoxocpatli, and also querámbeni. The root is sweet, astringent, and moderately hot, but they say it kills worms in the stomach, cures dysentery, itch, pustules and wounds, cleans the jaundiced, purges bilious and phlegmatic humors, and eases stomach pains if taken in a dose of one ounce.

Cozticmecapatli of Tilanco

(7.39)

This herb has small, round leaves like a pulse or pennywort, stalks an inch and a half long, at the tips, purple flowers in spikes, and a pale, fibrous root. It seems to be moist and moderately hot in nature. It grows anywhere cold in Tilanco. Applied, it is said to cure snake bites and other poisonous animal bites.

Acuitzehuaríracua or
Herb That Counters Poisons

(7.53)

This herb, which the people of Michoacán, in whose lands it grows, normally call acuitzehuaríracua, or huichoquachaqua, the Mexicans call chipaoacíztic for its cool nature and the whiteness of its root, and others, for the same reasons, call enemy of poisons or antidote. This miracle plant's leaves are like those of sorrel; from the rounded root that looks like a small quince (only it is white on the inside and yellow on the outside), soft stems grow, about an inch and a half in length, and at the ends are small flowers, white with red, and grouped in little circles. It grows in temperate or slightly warm regions, in humid and flat places. This root, which is the principal part used in medicine, is moderate in nature, or a little cold and moist, and has a pleasant, sweet taste. Its sap, or the liquor distilled from it, drunk in the desired quantity, reduces feverish heat, and strengthens the heart, and is a very fast and safe remedy for poisonous potions and stings, especially those of scorpions; it serves as an excellent preventive and antidote, above all if the crushed root is also applied in the form of a poultice or a plaster. It reduces heat in the kidneys, soothes sore throats and chest pains, diminishes acidity in the urine, stimulates the appetite, and by a wondrous and mysterious virtue, it is a remedy for all these illnesses however it is used. I have heard it said that in the lands of the Michoacán another variety of this herb grows, with leaves like the baccaris, called ocuro by the natives and, erroneously, scorsonera by others, but I have still never seen an example of this one.

Tlalchipillin of Hoexotzinco

(7.54)

Tlalchipillin is an herb with somewhat serrate leaves like oregano, stems one span and a half tall, round and narrow, white flowers from which capsules are produced, which, when they open, reveal a small, round, white seed, and a fibrous root. It grows in the rainy season in humid parts of Hoexotzinco. The root is somewhat hot and moist; taken in

a dose of two drams, it is said to purge all humors very effectively by the lower passage, and it is a remedy much prized by the natives.

Iztaololtzin of Cholula

(7.56)

Iztaololtzin is an herb with a milky root like scammony, to which it perhaps belongs, and voluble stems with leaves resembling those of this same herb, but more curved at the base, and oblong flowers, white with red and contained in calyxes. It grows in dry places in cold areas, as in Cholula. The root has a slightly sweet flavor, yet they say that taken in a dose of half an ounce, it purges the body.

Zocobut of Pánuco 2

(7.57)

Zocobut of Pánuco has leaves like the peach, but wider and thicker, voluble stems, and a round root the shape and size of a small ball, soft, with a sweet and pleasant aroma. They say that this herb bears neither flower nor fruit. The root is applied to ripen and open buboes and swellings. Taken, it provokes urine, expels gravel and retards excessive menstrual flow; applied to the forehead it cures migraine, and taken or applied it combats poisons and poisonous stings and bites. For all these reasons it is highly esteemed by the natives, and it is not easy to get them to tell you its properties.

First Acacóyotl or Fox Stick

(8.2)

Acacóyotl or fox stick is an herb that produces a long stem, reedy, thicker than a man's thumb and an intense green; leaves wide, thick, and long and with many delicate veins that extend obliquely from the central dorsal vein to the edges of the leaf; flowers are disposed in corymbs on the tips of the stems, somewhat elongate, gold in color and pretty to look at, each one of which produces dun-colored seeds that are hard, round, a little smaller than hazelnuts, and which some of our compatriots, whose time to leave is fast approaching,[2] are accustomed to call the tears of Moses. But there is nothing special about it apart from the extraordinary width of the leaves and the golden flowers. The seeds are extremely tough and of a remarkable roundness. It grows in moderate or slightly warm climates.

Coaxíhuitl, or Viper's Herb

(8.8)

The herb coaxíhuitl, or viper's herb, also called chalcuítlatl, has leaves like St. John's wort, but smaller and not pierced. The thin, red, round stems are two cubits long and the root is thick and fibrous. Purple, oblong flowers grow in calyxes near the base of each leaf and along each stem. It is native to a moderate climate and mountainous places, and it flowers in September. It is almost devoid of taste and smell, and its nature is cold and glutinous. A decoction of the root cures dysentery, alleviates asthma, eases pains, reduces fevers, and, instilled in the nostrils, stops nosebleeds.

Teómetl or Maguey of the Gods

(8.19)

This is a species of maguey that should be included with the rest of the descriptions, almost the same in shape and virtues, with a long fibrous root and delicate spines; the leaves are at least two spans long. Its juice, taken or applied, reduces fevers. It grows in cold or hot places, high or rural.

Quilamolli, or Amolli Herb

(8.26)

Quilamolli is an herb with a narrow, long root, voluble stems, white flowers, very long, and in the form of calyxes, and medium-sized, heart-shaped leaves. It grows in the warm hills of Iztlan. It lacks any notable taste or smell, and its nature is cold and moist. The leaves, dissolved in water and applied, cure inflammations, relieve headaches, reduce excessive heat, and alleviate inflammations in children's eyes, dye the hair darker, cure ringworm, and relieve itching. The juice, taken, purges bilious and phlegmatic humors by the upper passage, and new growth, introduced in the penis, provokes urine. There is another herb with the same name and equivalent properties, and as can be imagined, it is related to this one, but its leaves are not distributed around the stems. The Indians call our briony chichicamolli, and say that its decoction, introduced, purges phlegmatic humors very well and cures the French disease and other illnesses that impede movement, as well as old and persistent ones.

Tlaquilin

(8.29)

This herb has a large, fibrous root, stems three or four cubits long with a great number of branches, leaves like solanum but larger, and long flowers of several colors. The nature of the root is cold, moist, and phlegmatic, so it is taken and applied for cooling. It grows in various parts of Mexico, and is cultivated in gardens as an ornamental and for its flowers. Some call it teotlaquilin.

Tlallantlacuacuitlapilli 3

(8.31)

The leaves of the tlallantlacuacuitlapilli are like basil in groups of three or four; the stems are three spans long, woody, smooth, and red in places; the fruit is shaped like acorns, ripe and red in parts, full of medium-sized seeds, and the flowers are red and star-shaped. It has a distinctive taste, is mucilaginous, piquant, and of a cold and moist nature, like the plants known as quequéxquic. The root is fibrous, ramified and thick. It grows in warm areas of Tepoztlan. It cures cough and other chest illnesses and seems, to the taste, to be chewable like the gum of tragacanth. Some say that it restores strength to women after childbirth and to those suffering from fatigue, and that it eases pains.

---

2. It is not clear if Hernández means people returning to Spain or about to die.

Apitzalpatli 2

(8.36)

The second apitzalpatli, which some call tlaelpatli, or remedy for dysentery, is an herb with a round and fibrous root, stems a little bigger than a palm, cylindrical, narrow and whitish, with opposed leaves, small, serrate, almost round, and spaced out; there are tiny purple flowers at the tips of the branches. It grows in the lands of Xalatlauhco and is native to cold areas and wild places. The roots have no noticeable aroma, nor do they taste very astringent, yet a dozen leaves mashed and taken with water are said to contain diarrhea and dysentery, reduce fever and restore strength to weak limbs.

Coatli Xochitlanense or Coanenepilli

(8.58)

The coanenepilli[3] is also known as iztaccoanenepilli, or coapatli, or coatli xochitlanense. Its leaves are the shape of half moons or horseshoes, studded with yellow splotches. The stems are voluble and round, adorned with multicolored tendrils and flowers like betony but much smaller. The long, twisted, fibrous root, which is the thickness of one's little finger, is the part used in medicine. It grows in many places in the Mexican fields, but mainly in Xochitlan, where its properties were first investigated and understood. The root is somewhat sweet, fragrant, hot and dry almost in the second degree; they say that, crushed and taken in a dose of three drams, it cures spleen, restores movement that was impeded, relieves pains, stimulates the appetite, provokes urine, reduces heat, eases stomach pains, and releases unejaculated semen, and semen already almost ejaculated from its proper place by dreams; it is said to combat snakebites and is a powerful antidote to poisons of all kinds, expelling them at once by the lower passage. It is said to protect, the day it is taken, against sorcery, traps,

and the snares of prostitutes. Some believe that the flowers are similarly effective.

Peruvian Coca

(8.59)

This is an herb, so they tell me, about four spans long, with pale green leaves like the myrtle, only a little larger and softer, and shaped (as shown) like another small leaf; it has a seed and racemes that, like the myrtle, turn red as they begin to mature and eventually turn blackish, that being when the leaves are cut, put out to dry on racks and kept for future use.[4] As far as cultivation is concerned, the seed is sown in seedbeds and then transplanted to well-worked soil, laid out in rows like beans or chickpeas. The leaves are crushed and mixed with a powder of burned shells; this mixture is formed into pills, which are left to dry, to be used later. When these pills are taken orally, it is said that they quench the thirst, nourish the body amazingly, reduce hunger when there is not much food or drink to be had, and eliminate fatigue on long journeys. These pills are also commonly mixed with yetl for pleasure when people stay at home, to help get to sleep or to induce total relaxation, tranquility, and oblivion of all cares and troubles. Coca serves likewise as money, in such a way that in the markets there is a brisk trade in this plant.

Cozticxíhuitl

(8.60)

This herb has long narrow leaves like flax, thin stems of an inch and a half, a yellow flower, and a round seed at the end of the stalks, and a long, narrow fibrous roots. It grows in the hills and cold parts of Chalco. The crushed root, taken with water in a dose of half an ounce, purges bilious and phlegmatic humors. The root is very sharp, hot and dry in the third degree, and tends to burn the throat.

---

3. The geographical report for the Mines of Tasco (Relaciones geográficas del siglo XVI, 7:129) records this and other local plants: "There is a root, which the natives call cohuanenepilli, that is used as an antidote to poison; *cardosanto,* myrtle, laurel [and] *estafiate* [and] artemisia; and many others are described and pictured by Dr. Francisco Hernández, His Majesty's protomédico, who came

to ⟨New Spain⟩ for this purpose [i.e., to describe such things]." The report was probably written in 1577.

4. A French translation of this text appears in Claude Duret, *Histoire admirable des plantes et herbes esmerveillables & miraculeuses en nature* (Paris, 1605), 195. Duret named Benzoni, da Orta, Monardes, Oviedo, Cieza, Rouille, and Acosta as his sources.

Qualancapatli, or Medicine for the Angry Man

(8.64)

Qualancapatli is an herb with leaves like the willow, twisted stems, cylindrical and narrow. It grows in Hueitlalpa. It is cold, moist, and virtually tasteless and odorless. The crushed leaves, dissolved in water, are prescribed for anyone suffering from an insult or injury, hence its name.

Tlalcuitlaxolli, or Guts of the Earth

(8.67)

Tlalcuitlaxolli, also called yahuacapatli, has leaves like oregano, but longer, narrower, and entire, and round fruit all the way along the stem, on both sides of the base of the leaves, and thin, long, white roots. It grows in Atlapulco, where they instill the juice in the nostrils to purge phlegm in the head and rid headache, and also to cure facial swellings. They hold it in great esteem. The roots taken in a quantity of two drams purge all humors by inducing vomit and loosening the bowels. It is a safe and harmless remedy, although it does sometimes cause anxiety. Dry, and taken with warm water, it is gentler than if taken fresh.

Cozamaloxíhuitl or Rainbow Herb

(8.75)

The cozamaloxíhuitl is a little herb with a thin, quite long root, stems with leaves like rue that cover the stem like threads, all over it, and flowers of an iridescent whiteness, shaped like those of the hoaxin. It grows in warm or mild hills in lower Mixteca. It is cold, dry, and astringent. It cleans the teeth, restores flesh to damaged gums, and gets rid of all pus, for all which reasons it is a remarkable medicine when it is crushed or chewed, or just its juice taken. It also cures sores in the genital area, and is especially helpful in many other ways.

Tepari, or Fat Plant

(8.79)

Tepari is an herb with wide, serrate, oblong leaves, looking like the point of a spear, spiny and with a sharp down like the nettle. The stems are long, round and hollow with nodes at intervals of four inches, a fibrous, tapering root. It grows in Pátzcuaro. Dried and ground, the leaves cure sores, the same as the decoction of the root, which when taken also eases pains and reduces fevers, and applied with an unguent it cures arthritis. It is a tasteless herb, without smell, and by nature cold.

Ayotochtli, or Rabbit with a Hard Shell, Called by Others Tatou or Armadillo

(9.1)

The ayotochtli or rabbit with a hard shell, is a monstrous animal naturally covered with hard plates, the size of a Maltese terrier, but with a much longer tail. The paws are like a hedgehog's, and so is the snout, though it is narrower and longer. This animal is protected all over by its hard shield of individual, movable plates, with which it can cover itself in a ball, if necessary, which is why the Spanish call it armadillo, meaning armor-plated or armed, or as the Portuguese say, covered. The ears are like a mouse's, but longer and much thinner; the long, nodular rounded tail, is also covered with plates; the white belly is covered with soft skin like a human's, with quite long, thin, sparse hairs. It hunts ants by drawing in its shoulders and putting its tail in its mouth, and so the insects that come crawling there fall into its trap, becoming food for the wily beast. There is surely no other animal with its resources and skill in defending and feeding itself. When it needs to go downhill, it tucks its head and tail into its belly, withdraws into its shell, forms itself into a ball, and rolls down. And if anybody should persist in pursuing it, the armadillo will turn against him, even killing him by striking fiercely against his chest with its back. It is found in marshlands. It feeds on grubs, fish, and worms, as well as on some berries and fruits, in addition to ants, as we have mentioned. Its meat is extremely greasy and sweet; it is a phlegmatic, laxative food. They used to use the tail to strengthen and protect blowpipes (which used to be very widespread) and the shell had many uses, relative both to warlike noises and to the serenity of peace. It is said that the shell, ground and taken in a dose of one dram with a decoction of sage, is of great help in treating the French disease, by inducing sweat. It lives in warm places, like Yyauhtépec and, as we have said already, marshland, and beside lakes.

Axolotl, or Water Game

(9.4)

This is a type of lake fish covered with white skin; it has four paws like a lizard, and it is one span long and an inch wide, but it can be found up to one cubit in length. The vulva is like a woman's, the belly has gray splotches from halfway down the body all the way to the tail, which is very long and narrow at its tip, tapering; it has a short, wide, cartilaginous tongue. It swims with all four legs, which have fingers very similar to a frog's. The head is flattened, and large in proportion to the body. The mouth is half open and black. It has been observed many times to menstruate like a woman, and eating stimulates sexual activity, not unlike skinks, which some call crocodiles, and which perhaps belong to the same species. It makes a wholesome and tasty food, similar to eels. It is prepared in many ways: fried, roasted, or boiled. The Spanish season them generally with cloves and chili, the Mexicans only with chili, chopped or whole, their favorite and most popular condiment. Its name comes from its strange and exotic shape.[5]

Axin, or Worm Grease

(9.5)

In the trees called quapatli or in others that the Spanish call plum trees (because that is what they look like—although they seem more properly to belong to the Arabic myrobalans) certain hispid worms grow, called axocuillin, meaning that which contains axin. They are yellow, barely two inches long, and the thickness of a goose feather. The natives shake them down from the trees, then cook them in water until they shrivel, and fat of the same color called axin floats on the water. They keep it for many uses, forming it into slabs rather like cow's butter. It has the smell and smoothness of oil, and is very effective for all the same things that oil is good for, but it has never been used as a food. It relieves pains in any part of the body, relaxes and eases tense

muscles, resolves swellings or, if it is more appropriate, brings them to a head. It alleviates erysipelas, ulcers, convulsions, and also hernias, when it is mixed with resin and tobacco, and promptly reduces or resolves all kinds of abscesses.

Manatee

(9.13)

There lives in either ocean and in the lakes a fish that the Haitians call the manatee, an animal almost the same in form as a calf, with a bulky head and front legs like a goat's. It is gray, covered with sparse fur, and although it is fierce it does not bite. It lives in the sea and on the shore, sometimes coming out of the water. It feeds on marine plants and some kinds of marine fruit. Its transverse tail is rounded; the head and snout are like a calf's; it has large nostrils, teats, and ears, and small eyes and teeth, coarse lips, and a thick hide even tougher than a bull's. It has two forearms, each with five nails like human ones in the shape of quills. The navel and anus are large, the vulva like a woman's, the penis like a man's. Its fat and meat are like a pig's, and the meat is pleasant to taste whether it is eaten fresh or salted, and especially harmful to those with the French disease. The ribs and viscera are like those of the bull and are similarly huge. It mates the same way humans do, the female lying supine on the sand, with the male quickly mounting her. They give birth to only one calf, but it is very large—so large that anything bigger would be a monster. One finds in the head of this animal a little rock that, when powdered and taken with water or some other liquid, is said to expel retained urine and any obstruction in the urinary tract. The stone found in the male is white and is used for men; the yellowish stone in the female is useful for women.

Bird of Paradise

(9.6)

Humanity has found the true nicknames that for so many centuries had been hidden from men. What did those sailors who went to the Moluccas discover but these birds, which

---

5. Its paronomasiac name means "sport of the water."

do not have the use of their feet, like the oldest species in the world, but these ones are absolutely devoid of feet: instead, in their place they have some feathers, which are orange, hispid, thin, two spans and four inches long, and which grow from the middle of the body like a very thick mane. They use these feathers to hang from trees (when they have stopped flying), since they cannot roost; they also use them to embrace one another when male and female are together, after laying the eggs in a hollow in the male's back, where they are incubated and protected, hugged in the frontal cavity. Some say that they fly continuously, that they always stay up high, and if by some accident they fall to earth, they are easily captured by children. It is not difficult, given its small body and large feathers, for them to stay airborne and rest on the wing, as if they were roosting in the branches of trees or on the ground. They are barely bigger than a gold-finch or a tarin,[6] while the length of their plumage is two spans, five inches, no smaller than an eagle's. This plumage is thin, white tending to reddish, and the feathers grow out of the back and the rest of the body, not from the shoulders or the arms, since they have none. The beak is black, almost two inches long, and somewhat curved. The head and neck are like those of the dove, but that is partly gold and partly royal blue. The neck is royal blue underneath and gold on top. The breast and back are golden with a deeper yellow pattern of semicircles. Toward the tail the feathers, which are short in comparison to the other plumage, is orange tending to gray. It lives on dew, vapor, and minute animals, or the smallest creatures at the highest altitudes, for nature has ordained that a creature that lives entirely in the air needs no food, or what little can be found there. Yet even though it is perpetually fasting, its little body has plenty of meat and fat on it. The Indians use the dried bird to make headdresses, which they use for the beauty of its plumage, the variety of its colors, and the unusual form and beauty of this bird.

Cercopithecus

(9.7)

The cercopitheci are found in the warmest parts of New Spain, where they are called ozumatli by the Mexicans. They come in different sizes and colors: black, yellow, and gray; large, medium, and surprisingly small, some with a head like a dog's. Almost all carry their young on their backs, where they cling. It is a thing worthy of poetry that they climb trees, and aim and throw branches at passersby; they cross rivers in a file, each holding the tail of the one in front, or swinging from tree to tree; but especially wonderful is the way they treat wounds from arrows or other weapons, by applying leaves or moss to the wound, to stanch the flow of blood and thus, if possible, save a life. They give birth to just one baby, which holds on tightly as they carry it everywhere and tend it with lavish attention and love, in mountain passes, all the way up to the highest peaks. There, hunters construct a pyre around which they scatter corn, and in which they place a stone called cacalotetl or crow, which has the property of detonating and jumping when it gets hot. The cercopitheci gather the corn and then fall to eating it but, alarmed by the noise of the stone, they then behave as if they were blind, forgetting their young, abandoning their offspring and leaving them to be captured by the hunters. Everything else about their nature is so well known that it would be superfluous to repeat it here. But I do not wish to neglect to say that the bones of the cercopithecus, ground and taken, ease and expel, by provoking sweat, the pains that come from the French disease.

The Mazame, or Deer

(9.14)

Among the kinds of deer that can be found in New Spain (apart from those that are completely white, which the Indians consider kings of the deer, and which they call iztac-mazame because of its color), the first are the acuillame, much like Spanish deer in shape, size and disposition. Smaller than the Spanish are the quauhtlamazame, but unaware of fear to such a degree that, when men attack them, they wound and even kill them quite frequently. Next to these in size are the tlalhuicamazame, which would be identical in shape and behavior if they were not more timid. The smallest of all are the temamazame; but those, and the other

6. A small finch.

kinds, among them the teuhtlalmazame, are more accurately classified among sheep. It seems to me opportune to say here that some deer or bucks have growing inside them the stone known as bezoar, or lord of poison. We have heard seasoned hunters say that they have found these stones many times when they opened up these animals, the same stones that are found in Peruvian sheep without horns called vicuñas (there are other, horned, sheep called tarucas and guacanas) and also in the teuhtlamazame, which are the size of an average goat or a little larger, and are covered with whitish gray and brown fur that comes off easily, but have white belly and sides, so the Creoles call them berrendos; the horns are wide at the base and branch out slightly, they are small, round and sharply pointed; the ears are under them; we give an image of it here. Some of the bucks, called mazatl chichiltic or temamazame, have very short, pointed horns, brown and gray but white underneath, and this too is pictured. Bezoar are also found in the chamois, which are numerous here, the same as Spanish deer, common in these lands. Equally in hornless goats, common in Peru, and, in sum, there is hardly a species of deer or goat in whose stomach or other intestinal cavity this stone does not form and grow slowly, from food residue. This is the same stone that is found in bulls and cows, consisting of onionlike membranes that grow in layers one on top of another. However, these stones are found only in very old animals, those about to die of old age; they are not found in animals just anywhere, either, but only in certain well-defined areas where there is plenty of the right food; all of which explains why in Spain and other countries they are not particularly easy to find. But not all the stones are beneficial, good for protecting health and eradicating illnesses: only those that are formed from very healthful herbs eaten by the animals; it is thus not only difficult to judge if the admirable virtues, which in our time are attributed to these stones and propagated everywhere, but also to know how they should be selected, which ones are useful and which are not; about all which nothing can be affirmed with any certainty. It is said, however, that they make a very effective remedy for all kinds of poisoning, that they cure syncope and epileptic fits, that, applied to the fingers they induce sleep, increase energy, excite sexual activity, toughen all the faculties, and relieve pains; that if some part of them is consumed or even held in the hands, they break up and expel stones in the kidneys and bladder; that it alleviates the flow of urine, helps with childbirth, favors conception, and that, in short, there are few illnesses that these stones do not cure, to the point where some people, relying on this stone alone, come to be—in their own opinion—perfect doctors, and shamelessly pass themselves off as such. These stones come in a variety of shapes and colors, some in brilliant white, others gray, others yellow, some ash-colored or black, or polished like glass or obsidian. Some are ovoid, some round, some triangular. Some of them have near the bottom or in the middle a kind of ball, which seems to shift because of the nucleus which accumulates and grows within the crust, like the stones known as aetites[7] (or perhaps these are aetites, which eagles steal and take back to their nests), and others have powder or gravel. There are so many in New Spain that they are sold very cheaply, one or sometimes two for a single escudo, while a few years ago one average stone fetched two hundred escudos or more. I was told all this and warned about it, to avoid becoming a victim of fraudulent people who live by theft and break all laws, provided that by doing so they will increase their fortune, and who, by having such an abundance and enormous quantity of these stones, do not need to fake them or adulterate them—yet plenty of counterfeits are to be found. As for fossilized stones to which some Arab peoples give the same name, for their ability to counteract poisons, they are here too, mainly on the banks of the river Tetzhuatlan, of various shapes and colors, since its waters abound with stones; but one does not find the ones that these people say form in the corners of the eyes of these animals, when, by way of treatment, after devouring serpents that have come out of their caves, with the force of their breath or some other mysterious power, they are submerged in the rivers. I was also shown some small stones said to have been eaten by the deer to facilitate the birth of their young, and which were found later in the stomach. Of all this, if God permits me, we shall speak in due course.

7. Also known as eaglestones, after Pliny 10.3.4 12 and 30.14.44 130.

Tlacuatzin (Possum)

(9.18)

The tlacuatzin is an animal the shape and size of a small dog, two spans long, with a narrow, elongated, hairless snout, a small head, and very thin and soft ears, almost transparent. It has long white hair, but gray or black at the tips, a cylindrical tail, two spans long and very similar to that of snakes, gray but with a white tip; the tail holds on tightly to everything it catches. The body and paws are like a badger's. When it gives birth, its litter is four or five pups, born already formed, still small but protected by a pouch in the belly that has been provided for by nature as a pocket or extra flap of skin, made so precise and symmetrical that it seems to be stuck on to the belly by the wonderful artifice of nature, such as is not found in any other animal. The eyes are black, small, alert, and open. It climbs trees with incredible agility, and hides in caves for long periods. It feeds on small fowl, like the fox and wild weasels, whose heads it chews off to drink the blood. With respect to everything else, it is an innocuous, inoffensive animal, although because of its instinctive cunning it plays dead when it cannot otherwise escape human pursuit, or to fool its predators and then bite them. The tail of this animal is an excellent medicament: it is ground in a dose of one dram and drunk with water, after fasting. It cleans the urinary tract admirably, provoking urine and bringing with it gravel and anything else obstructing this conduit. It excites sexual activity, produces milk, cures fractures and colic, brings on childbirth, provokes menstruation, comforts the belly, and, pounded and applied, it can extract thorns stuck in the flesh; perhaps no other medicine is more efficacious in these respects. The animal lives in warm places and eats meat, fruit, bread, vegetables, grains, and all kinds of food, which we were able to prove by experiment, feeding it everything we had in the house.

Citli, or Hare

(Animals 1.3)

New Spain also produces hares like ours in appearance and in value as food, but with exceptionally long ears in relation to body size, and wider, too. The Indians weave the skins of these animals in their clothing and in the linens they use to make capes, and so do the Creoles, the same way they use rabbit fur and the feathers of various birds. So great is the industry and minute care of these people in making good use of the most trivial things.

The Bulls and Cows of Quivira

(Animals 1.30)

When the Spanish penetrated as far inland as these regions, they found, among other wonders, herds of wild cattle of medium and short stature, arched back, luxuriant mane, and a long, curly, brown, shaggy coat all over the body.[8] The meat is just as tasty and healthful as beef in our country. The natives eat it raw, drink the blood, and wear the skins to keep warm. I have been told that one of these animals was sent to King Philip, and that farther from the river Aconquis[9] there is a race of hunchbacked people, but this I have not been able to prove beyond a doubt.

The Skull Found in Chalco and the Bones of Giants That Have Been Discovered

(Animals 1.32)

The above descriptions of these exotic animals seem to require that I give here some account of the human skull found in Chalco at the digging of a well. The skull had two faces, four eyes, two noses, two pairs of jaws, and sixty-four teeth, which were fully grown, but worn and decayed by long years of use. We are not amazed by such an adrogyne, which either antiquity produced or Plato imagined, to fit his philosophy. Also, in recent times, many enormous bones of giants have been discovered, in both Tetzcoco and Toluca, some of which have been shipped to Spain while others have been preserved by the viceroys as marvelous rarities. I know that among them were some maxillary teeth, five inches broad and ten inches long, from which one may deduce the size of the head they came from, which would have to be at

---

8. It is not certain where Quivira was, but present-day New Mexico seems likely (see *Antiquities* 1.1). Hernández appears to be describing and illustrating the North American bison.

9. Unidentified, unless Hernández means the Aconchi, in northern Mexico.

least the size of a man's outstretched arms. All this is too familiar for anyone to credit it, and yet I know for certain that there are people who deny the possibility of many things until they have seen them with their own eyes, to such an extent that what Pliny said is true, that "the power and majesty of nature are continually unbelievable." Perhaps they came from other lands in this region, these men of abnormal size (for around Cape Horn there are Patagonians of giant stature) and were killed by the natives, or perhaps by some freak of nature they were born here, and the natives, fearing that they would multiply, persecuted them and exterminated them completely.

Maquizcóatl

(Animals (Reptiles) chapter 22)

Maquizcóatl is also known as tetzauhcóatl or rare serpent, because it is indeed very seldom seen; in fact, it is almost a miracle when somebody does see it: the maquizcóatl is only moderately long, the thickness of a man's little finger, and silvery colored, translucent almost to the point of transparency. It moves, according to some people, either forward or backward, even though it does not have more than one head; perhaps it is the ancient amphisbaena.[10] There is another snake known by the same name that also moves in either of two directions without also having two heads: this apparently

has never been seen either, unless it is the same one we have reported, which we found in Itztoluca and took care to represent in a drawing.

Itlilayo Teoquetzaliztli, Also Called Kidney Stone, and Third Mexican Jasper

(10.7)

There is another species of green jasper that is exceedingly common here, but which has small white and gray spots, and is called itlilayo teoquetzaliztli, or dark emerald, classified among the emeralds. It is said that when it is tied on to the arm or applied to a painful kidney, it cures kidney pain and breaks up kidney stones. It is diuretic, and expels all waste matter; but it is used in the following manner: when pain strikes, it is applied to the affected area, and once the pain has gone, it is tied to the metacarpus on the same side as the affected kidney. They say that by cleansing the urinary tracts, it prevents stones from forming or it dissolves them and stops gravel from coming together in a lump, because of its viscous humor, and flushes it out with the urine. This stone is found in various shapes: fish, bird's head, parrot's beak, more commonly in the little perforated balls that the Indians like to string together as necklaces. The most highly prized is the brightest green, the most brilliant, spotted with white.

10. A two-headed snake. Snakes are sometimes found with two heads growing side by side, though they do not survive long in the wild. The amphisbaena, however, was supposed to have a head at each end of its body.

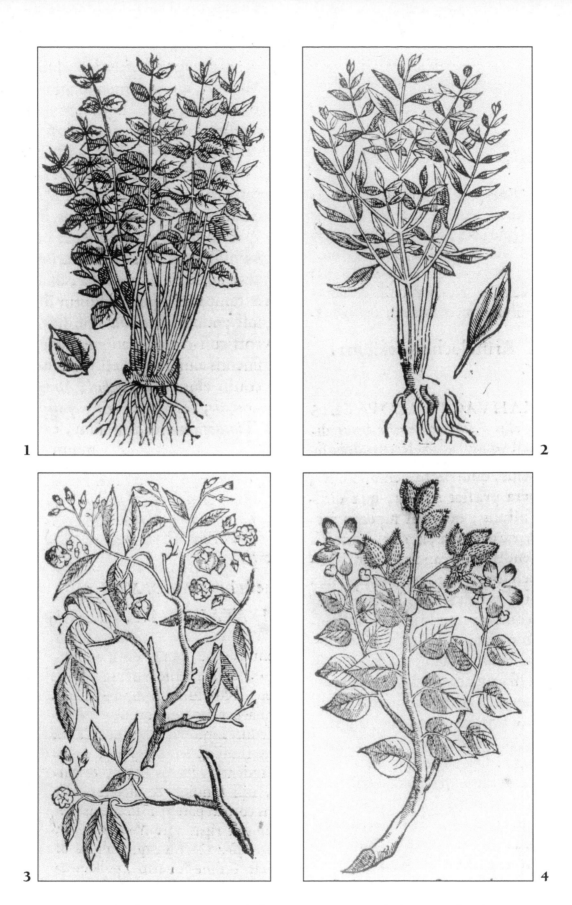

1 Chichicpatli • **2** Iztactlatlacótic • **3** Izquixóchitl • **4** Achíotl

Illustrations from *Rerum medicarum Novae Hispaniae thesaurus* (Rome, 1651)
History and Special Collections, Louise M. Darling Biomedical Library, UCLA

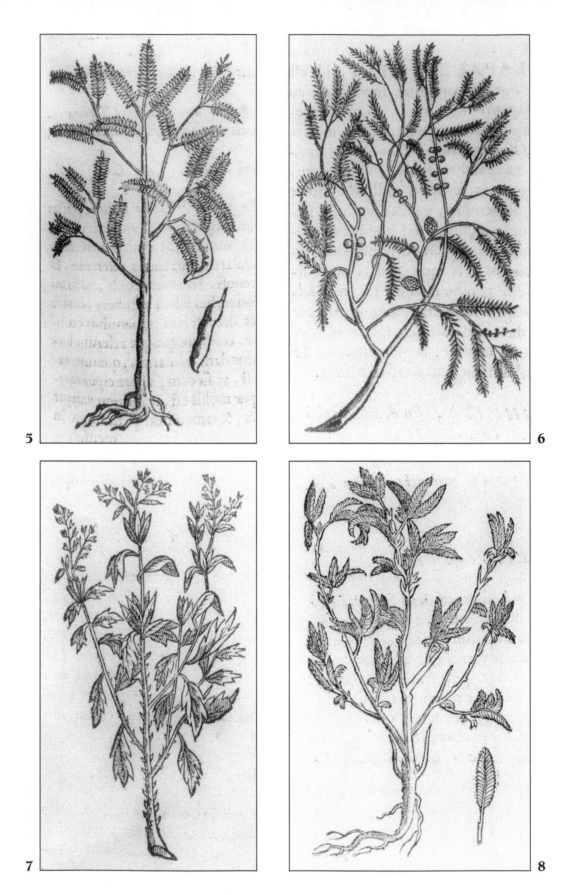

5 Tamarind • **6** Ahoéhoetl • **7** Enguamba • **8** Iztacpatli of Tepéxic

Illustrations from *Rerum medicarum Novae Hispaniae thesaurus* (Rome, 1651)
History and Special Collections, Louise M. Darling Biomedical Library, UCLA

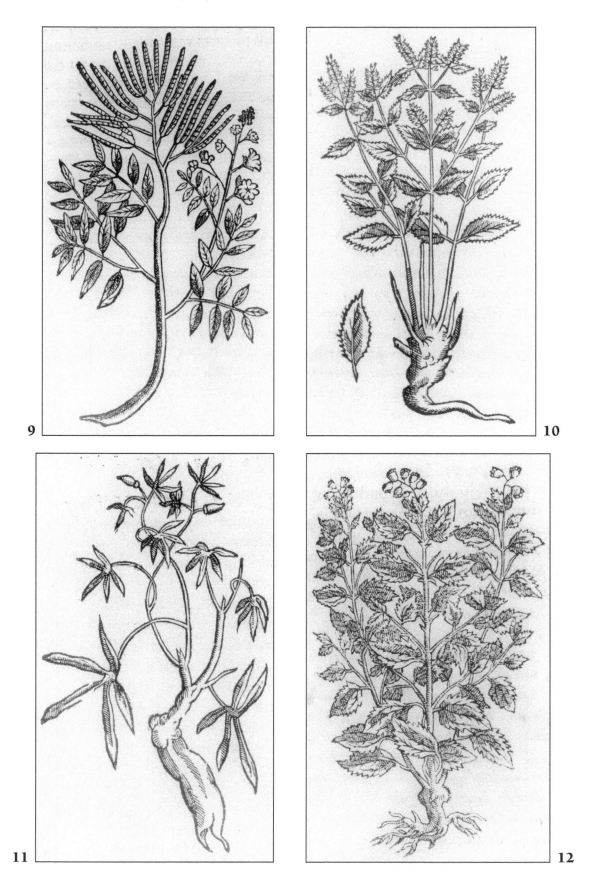

9 Ecapatli, or small elder • **10** Huitsiqua • **11** Izticpatli • **12** Ahoapatli of Yacapichtlan

Illustrations from *Rerum medicarum Novae Hispaniae thesaurus* (Rome, 1651)
History and Special Collections, Louise M. Darling Biomedical Library, UCLA

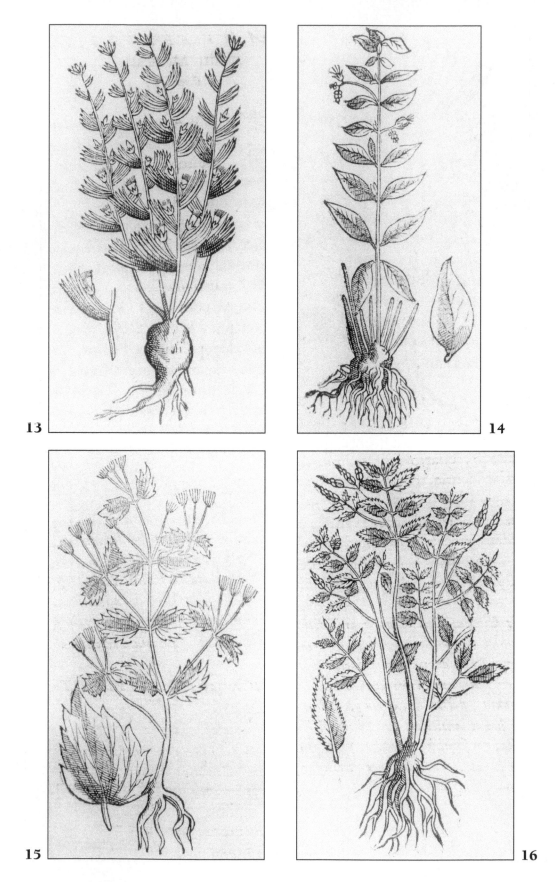

13 Acxoyátic • **14** Chilpatli • **15** Cococtemécatl, or bitter twisted cord • **16** Cococxíhuitl of Teocalzingo

Illustrations from *Rerum medicarum Novae Hispaniae thesaurus* (Rome, 1651)
History and Special Collections, Louise M. Darling Biomedical Library, UCLA

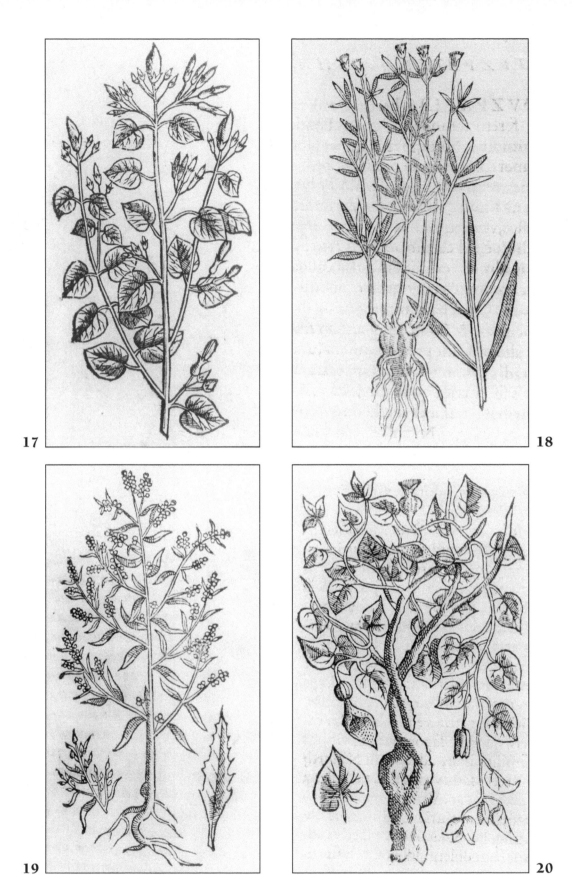

17 Ololiuhqui, or plant with round leaves • **18** Tzahuéngueni or filipendula of Michoacán
19 Epázotl or aromatic herb • **20** Phehuame

Illustrations from *Rerum medicarum Novae Hispaniae thesaurus* (Rome, 1651)
History and Special Collections, Louise M. Darling Biomedical Library, UCLA

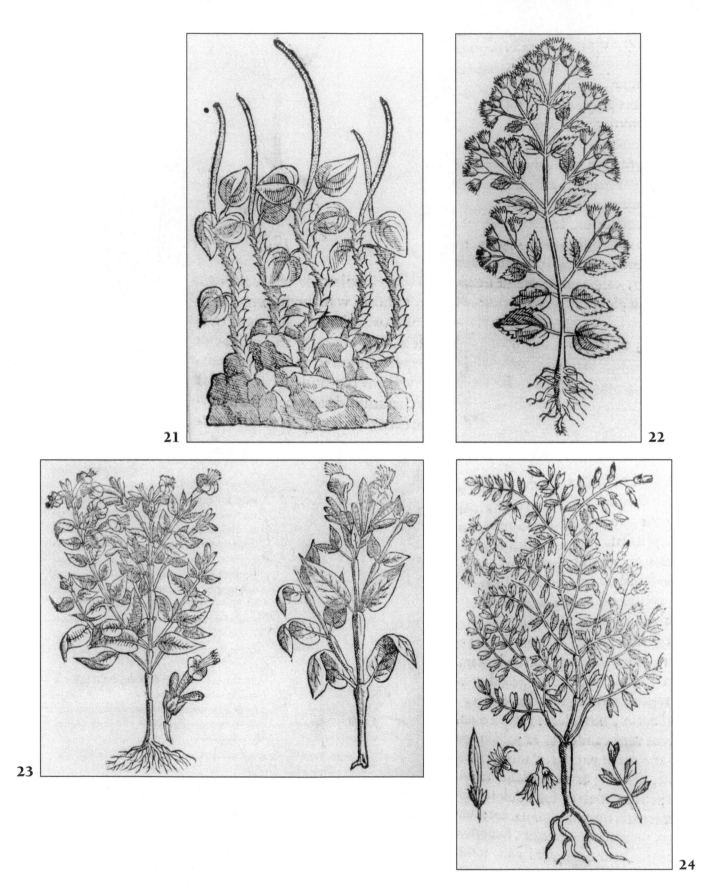

21 Teocuilin or rock worms • **22** Iztactexcaltlácotl, or white stick of the rocks
23 Atzóyatl • **24** Axixcozahuilizpatli of Yancuitlan

Illustrations from *Rerum medicarum Novae Hispaniae thesaurus* (Rome, 1651)
History and Special Collections, Louise M. Darling Biomedical Library, UCLA

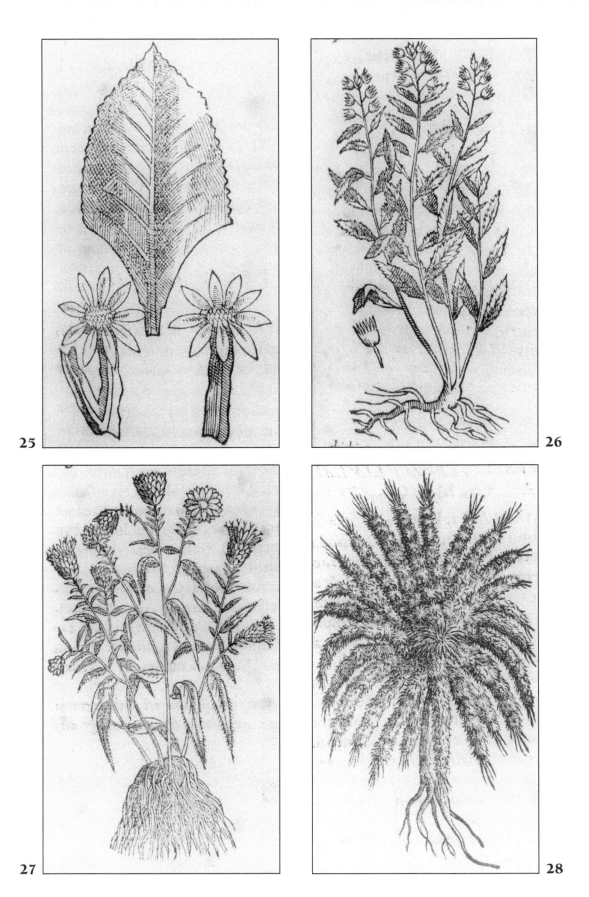

25 Nahuitéputz, or four-sides • **26** Tzonpotónic or fetid hair
27 Xararo • **28** Zacahuitzpatli, or spiny grass medicine

Illustrations from *Rerum medicarum Novae Hispaniae thesaurus* (Rome, 1651)
History and Special Collections, Louise M. Darling Biomedical Library, UCLA

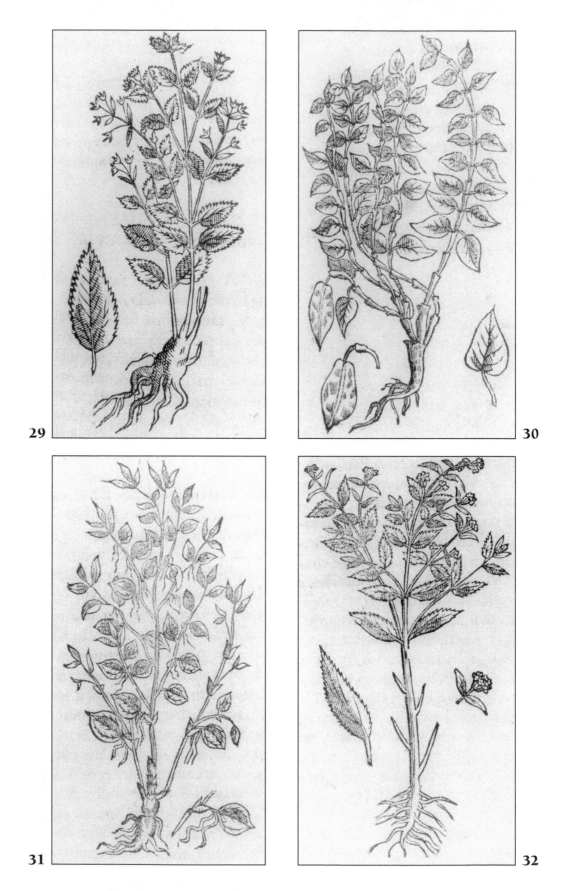

29 Apitzalpatli tzontololotli • **30** Tlalayotli or small squash
31 Cozolmécatl, or cradle cord • **32** Ixtomio, or lanuginous herb

Illustrations from *Rerum medicarum Novae Hispaniae thesaurus* (Rome, 1651)
History and Special Collections, Louise M. Darling Biomedical Library, UCLA

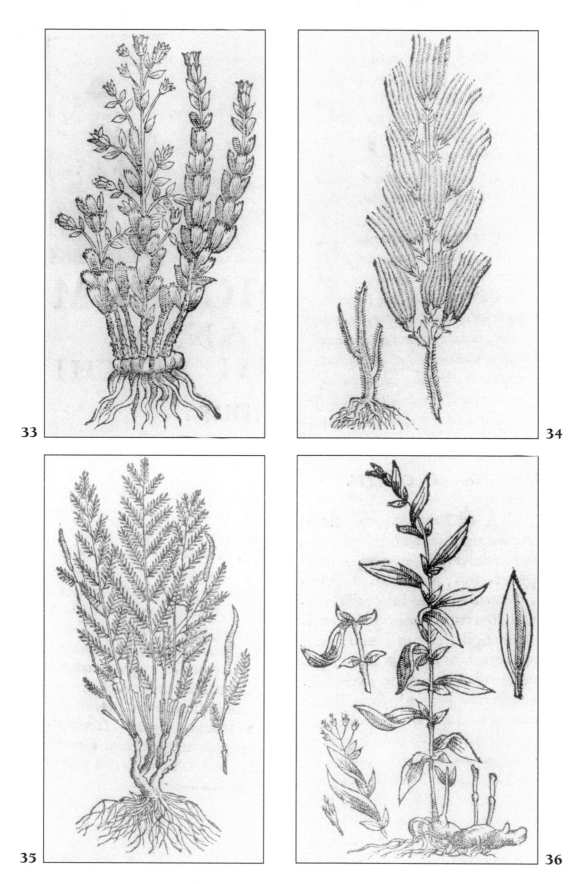

33 Tlalixtomio or small ixtomio • **34** Herb of Paradise • **35** Tlalcoatli or small coatli
36 Tlalzacamecaxóchitl, or string flower of land pasture

Illustrations from *Rerum medicarum Novae Hispaniae thesaurus* (Rome, 1651)
History and Special Collections, Louise M. Darling Biomedical Library, UCLA

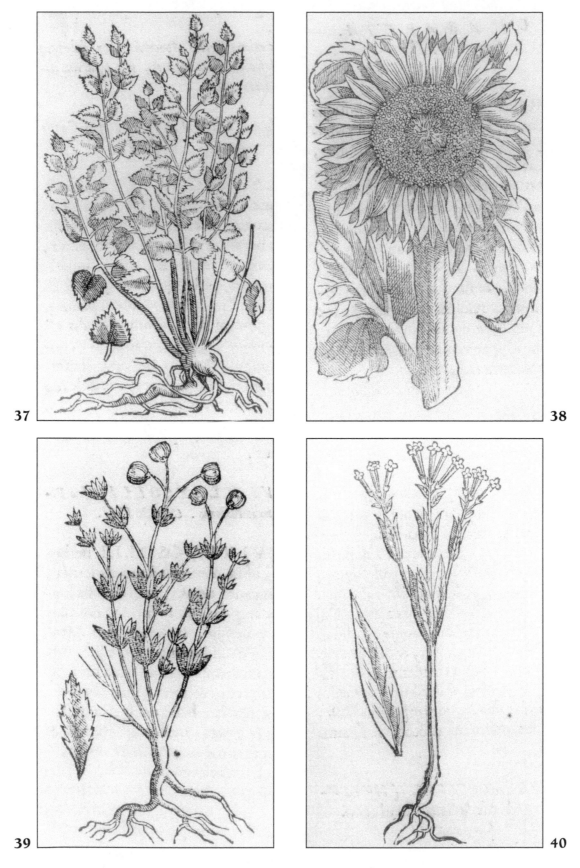

37 Ixiayáhoal of Chapultepec • 38 The Peruvian or large chimalácatl which some call the sunflower
39 Tlalcapolin, small cherry, or chamaecerasus of Atlapulco • 40 Tlalcoxóchitl of Anenecuilco

Illustrations from *Rerum medicarum Novae Hispaniae thesaurus* (Rome, 1651)
History and Special Collections, Louise M. Darling Biomedical Library, UCLA

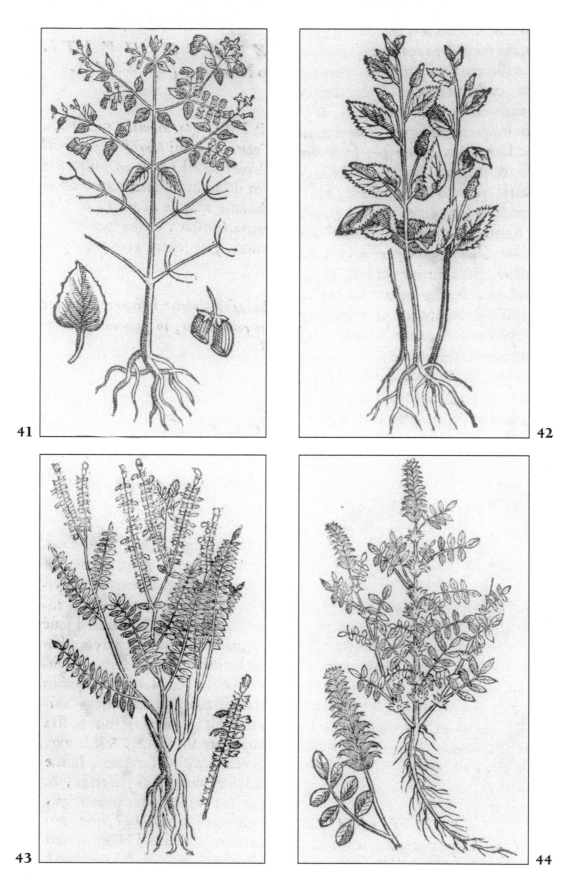

41 Chiantzotzolli, or plant that swells in humid conditions • **42** Tzopelicxíhuitl
43 Cececpatli of Acatlan • **44** Cozticmecapatli of Tilanco

Illustrations from *Rerum medicarum Novae Hispaniae thesaurus* (Rome, 1651)
History and Special Collections, Louise M. Darling Biomedical Library, UCLA

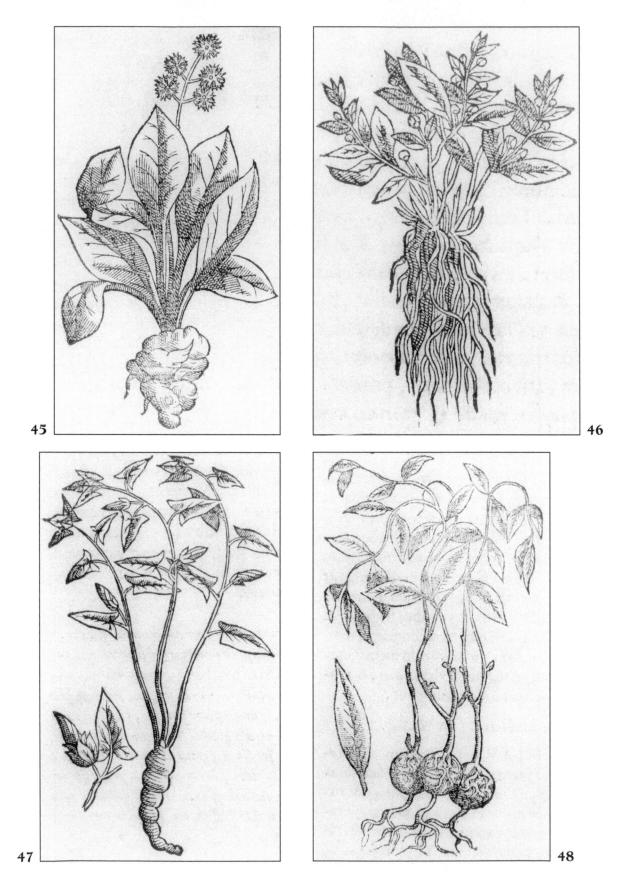

45 Acuitzehuaríracua or herb that counters poisons • **46** Tlalchipillin of Hoexotzinco
47 Iztaololtzin of Cholula • **48** Zocobut of Pánuco

Illustrations from *Rerum medicarum Novae Hispaniae thesaurus* (Rome, 1651)
History and Special Collections, Louise M. Darling Biomedical Library, UCLA

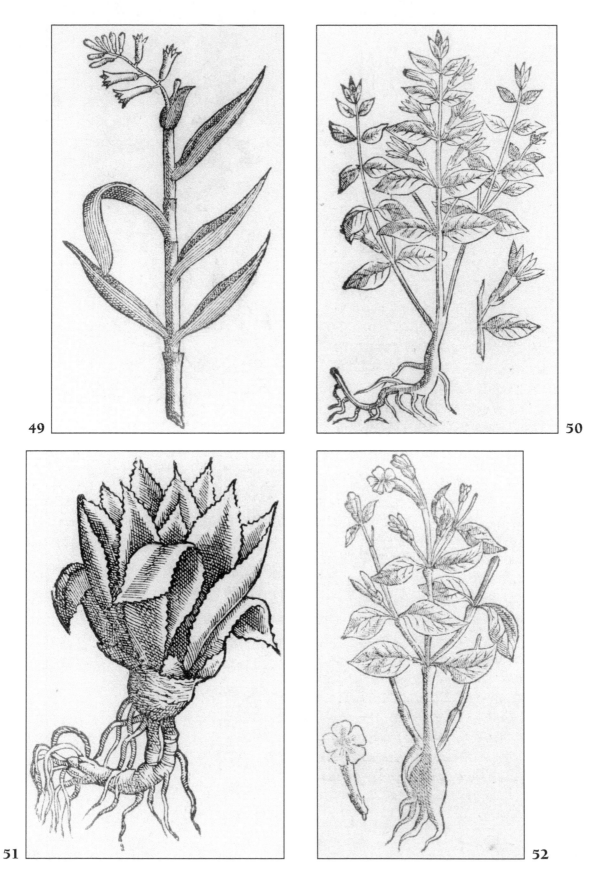

49 First Acacóyotl or fox stick • **50** Coaxíhuitl, or viper's herb • **51** Teómetl or maguey of the gods • **52** Tlaquilin

Illustrations from *Rerum medicarum Novae Hispaniae thesaurus* (Rome, 1651)
History and Special Collections, Louise M. Darling Biomedical Library, UCLA

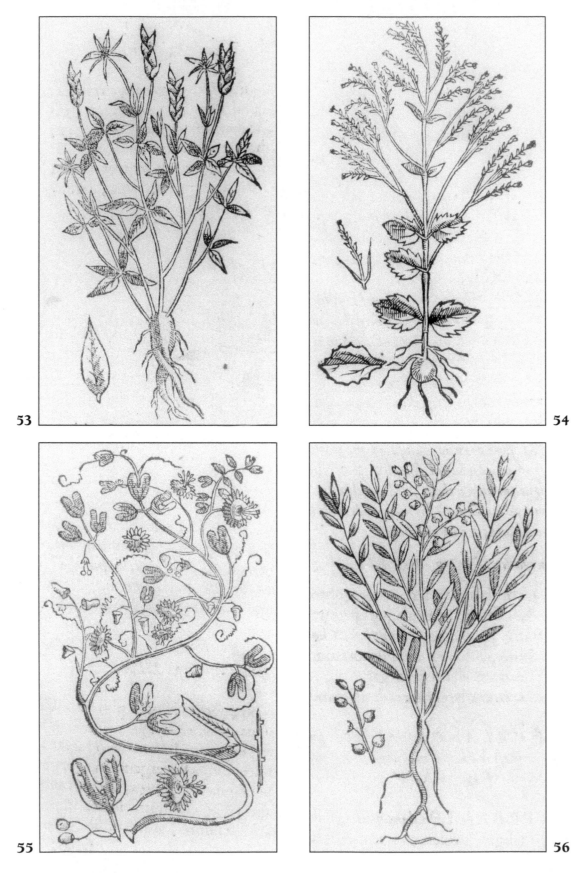

53 Tlallantlacuacuitlapilli • **54** Apitzalpatli • **55** Coatli xochitlanense or coanenepilli • **56** Cozticxíhuitl

Illustrations from *Rerum medicarum Novae Hispaniae thesaurus* (Rome, 1651)
History and Special Collections, Louise M. Darling Biomedical Library, UCLA

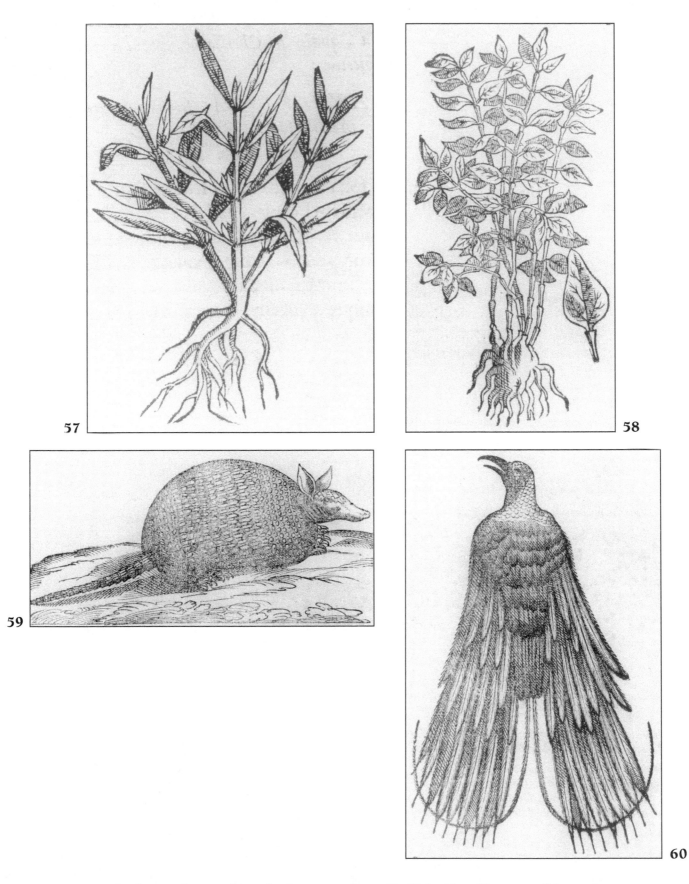

57 Qualancapatli, or medicine for the angry man • **58** Tlalcuitlaxolli, or guts of the earth
59 Armadillo • **60** Bird of Paradise

Illustrations from *Rerum medicarum Novae Hispaniae thesaurus* (Rome, 1651)
History and Special Collections, Louise M. Darling Biomedical Library, UCLA

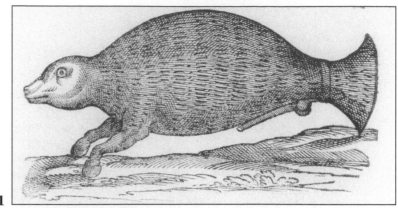

61

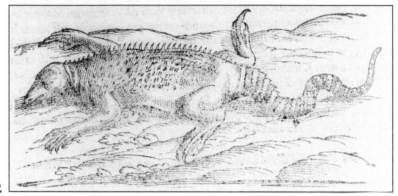

62

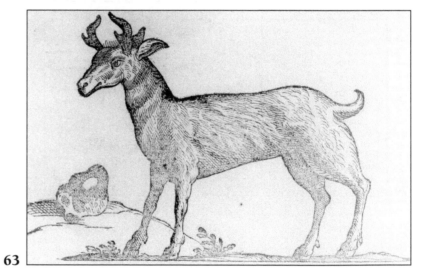

63

61 Manatee
62 Axolotl, or water game
63 Mazame, or deer
64 Bezoar stones

Illustrations from *Rerum medicarum
Novae Hispaniae thesaurus* (Rome, 1651)
History and Special Collections,
Louise M. Darling Biomedical Library, UCLA

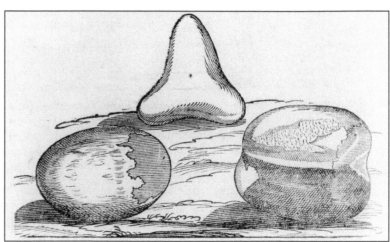

64

ENGLAND, 1659–1825

SEVEN ENGLISH AUTHORS

The sources for this section are (in chronological order):

Robert Lovell, *Pambotanologia. Sive, Enchiridion Botanicum* (Oxford, 1659)

Henry Stubbe, *The Indian Nectar* (London, 1662)

John Chamberlayne, *The Manner of Making Tea, Coffee, and Chocolate* (London, 1671)

Hans Sloane, *Natural History of Jamaica,* 2 vols. (London, 1707–25)

James Petiver, *Hortus Peruvianus Medicinalis: or, The South-Sea Herbal* [London, 1715]

James Newton, *The Complete Herbal* (London, 1752)

Erasmus Darwin, *The Botanick Garden* (London, 1825)

Robert Lovell's thick little volume, *Pambotanologia. Sive, Enchiridion Botanicum* (Oxford, 1659), contains an appendix "concerning such Trees, Shrubbs, Plants and Fruits, which grow in the East and West Indies &c. Shewing their Temperature, Vertues, Use and Danger." This appendix includes summary extracts, in English, of Hernández's descriptions of ninety-five plants, with the abbreviations T and V (for temperament and virtue). Although Lovell did revise other parts of his text for the second edition of his book (Oxford, 1665), this appendix remained textually identical. Hernández is mentioned nowhere, nor are his manuscripts or printed books that contain his texts. Lovell used the *Quatro libros* for the first three plants and either that text or the Rome edition of Hernández for the remainder. Richard Pulteney, in *Biographical Sketches* (1790), recognized the ninety-five Mexican plants in Lovell as drawn from the work of Hernández and wrote a short paragraph on Lovell, viewing him more as a curiosity than a botanist. Otherwise, Lovell himself remains obscure and his book little known.

Henry Stubbe's book is devoted to chocolate and thus includes descriptions of cacao and the ingredients commonly added to it—*achiotl, orejuelas,* cinnamon, and so on. On a smaller scale, the same applies to John Chamberlayne's account of chocolate, which was a translation of the famous treatise by Antonio Colmenero de Ledesma, with additional passages taken from Hernández and inserted by Chamberlayne.

Sir Hans Sloane published a paper on allspice and wintergreen, in which he made use of Hernández's descriptions (*Philosophical Transactions,* no. 191 [December 1687]). But Sloane's ambitious work the *Natural History of Jamaica* contains some forty-eight extracts and quotations from Hernández, together with a sprinkling of allusions. Sloane is rare among the scholars and writers represented in this volume, because he is forthright enough to condemn some of the images and identifications of Hernández as erroneous or inaccurate. For example, in his discussion of yucca (also known as cassava or manioc), Sloane declares, "The Plant figur'd by *Hernandez* and *Terrentius,* under the Name of *Hiuca sive Mizmaitl,* seems not this *Cassada,* but rather a *Serpentaria* by its Figure, but I am notwithstanding apt to believe, considering *Hernandez's* Errors, this may be it" (*Jamaica,* 1:131).

James Petiver's *Hortus* is an extremely rare, very brief, large-format pamphlet. His interest in Hernández is attested by his extensive marginal annotations to his copies of Nieremberg and Marcgraf. It is also possible that Petiver owned the Latin translation of Hernández by de Laet, the manuscript acquired by Sloane and represented elsewhere in this volume. Petiver's *Hortus* is the only evidence in print of his familiarity with Hernández.

James Newton's *Complete Herbal* contains an appendix entitled *Enchyridion Universale Plantarum: or, An Universal and Complete History of Plants, with Their Icons, in a Manual,* with six varieties of apple taken from Hernández or Nieremberg.

A distorted statement about *manzanilla,* probably adapted from Sloane's translation and paraphrase of Hernández, appears in a footnote to Erasmus Darwin's poem *The Botanick Garden,* pt. 2, *Loves of the Plants,* canto 3, line 188. We include it as a curio.

Robert Lovell

Axixtlácotl

Diureticall red, *Axixtlacotl, Virga diuretica.* T. the flowers are sharp: the root (which is chiefly used) is odoriferous, of thin parts, hot and dry [in the second degree]. V. Being stamped and applyed they draw forth things fixed in the flesh. [Three drams] thereof drunk expell the urine, and helpe the collick, spots in the face, and scabs in the heads of children, or in any part of the body. It helps feavers, lesseneth the spleene, easeth paine, and with other remedies discusseth flatulencies, helps the stomack and dropsie, and discusseth tumours.

Hoitzxóchitl

Launce-leaf'd tree, *Hoitzxochitl, Arbor lonchifolia.* T. the flower is hot and dry [in the second degree] and very astringent, first seeming sweet, and then bitter. V. Drunk it helps the diseases of the wombe, corroborateth the heart, and serveth in stead of saffron in meates, the fruit relented in water and taken into the nostrills helps the paines of the head, and paines of the teeth being applyed thereunto.

Zazalictlacopatli

Cinamon bindweed, *Cacalic tlacopatlis, Convolvulus cinnamomeus.* T. Is hot and dry. V. [one ounce of the seed] taken evacuates urine, and helps the cold fits of quartane agues. Also it helpeth the dropsie, and grief of the stomack. It reduceth the wombe, and cureth the convulsion taken in wine, and helps the inflammation of the eyes.

Caninga

Caninga-tree, *Arbor caninga.* T. the bark is hot and dry almost ⟨in the⟩ [fourth degree], sharpe, of the taste of cloves. It purgeth the bloud, and resists poyson, it helps paines of the belly, and discusseth flatulencies. The decoction helpeth the griefes of the joynts caused by cold.

Quauhxiloxóchitl

Hairy flower, *Xiloxachitl, Flos capillaceus*. T. Is cold *sc*. The bark, almost without sapor or odour. V. It helps the ulcers of the gums, taken in water it expells urine, and cleanseth the reines and bladder.

Tlalámatl

Vomiting tree, *Tlalamatl, Arbor vomitoria*. T. is cold, astringent, and glutinous. V. the leaves bruised and a pugill taken in water, evacuates all humours gently, and without trouble; the roots applied help ulcers.

Quauhxílotl

Muske cucumber-tree, *Quauhxilotl, Arbor cucumeris moschati*. T. Is hot and dry [in the first degree]. V. the decoction of the leaves helpes deafnesse caused by cold, being dropped into the eares.

Coacamachalli

Snakejaw-tree, *Coacamachillis, Maxilla colubri*. T. the leaves are astringent, sweet and a little glutinous, moderately hot. V. the leaves applyed helpe the paines of the French disease and tensions.

Cocoquáhuitl of Huaxaca

Cordiall tree, *Cocus quahuitl, Arbor cordiaca*. T. Is cold and dry. V. [One ounce] of the juice taken twice every day helps the syncope, and lassitude.

Tlacoxiloxóchitl

Bearded-flower, *Tlacoxiloxochitl, Flos barbarus*. T. The bark of the root is sharpe, hot [in the thrid degree], dry, astringent, and a little glutinous. V. the flowers stamped, mixt with water and instilled, help the griefes of the eyes. They restraine inflammations, consume superfluous flesh, and help the argemata. The decoction or infusion of the root stops the flux of bloud and dysenterie, and helpeth the decayed appetite. Some say also that it lenifieth the breast, looseth the belly, expelleth choller by vomit, and helpeth the cough.

Tlacoxóchitl

Red haired shrub, *tlacoxochitl, Capilli rubei*. T. the root is bitter, odoriferous, hot and dry [in the third degree]. V. the decoction therof [*sic*] helpeth the dysenterie, and griefe of the joynts.

Chichictlapalezquáhuitl

Bitter bloud sweating-tree, *Chichictlapal ezquahuitl, Arbor rubri sanguinis amara. Sanguiflua*. T. Is hot, glutinous, resinous, odoriferous and astringent. V. the barke of the stock being stamped drunk in the quantity of 6 [oboli] in water, helpeth the haemoptysis or spitting of bloud, and helpeth the inflammation of the eies.

Bitonco

Bitoncus. T. The root is hot and dry [in the third degree], a little bitter, odoriferous and sharpe. V. It corroborateth laxe members and the stomacke, it strengtheneth the head. It is a little astringent, yet it purgeth gently.

Zacapipillolxóchitl

Hanging flower, *Cacapilol xochitl, Herbosus & flos pendens*. T. is cold and moist. V. [Half an ounce] of the bark of the root taken helpeth feavers.

Xalquáhuitl

Spotted shrub, *Xalquahuitl, Stypes punctatus*. T. is hot [in the fourth degree], and dry. V. the decoction taken doth corroborate, discusse, provoke the menses, and help fulnesse.

Coacihuizpatli

Tooth-curing herb, *Coacihuizpatli, Dentium medicina*. T. The root is bitter, sharp, hot and dry [in the third degree]. V. the root helps paines, chiefly of the teeth, and contractions of the nerves, 2 [drams] being drunk once a day.

Tlalquequétzal

Earth-feather, *Tlalquequetzal. Penna terræ*. T. Its bitter with a certain acrimonie, odoriferous of thin parts, and hot and dry [in the third degree]. V. The juice drunk provoketh urine, evacuates the menses, strengtheneth a cold stomack, discusseth winde, and helps the diarrhoea, and ulcers, of the secrets. It helpeth tumors and obstructions, chiefly of the womb: so applied. As a pessarie applied it helpeth the scab, it stops the belly and helpeth the cough.

Zacachíchic

Bitter herbe, *Cacachichit, Herba amara*. T. it's very bitter, hot and dry [in the third degree]. V. [One ounce of] the juice [of the seed] thereof purgeth all humors, but chiefly flegme and choller by vomit: it cureth fullnesse and causeth appetite, it helpeth the itching of the eies and cough and discusseth flatulencies.

Tlaquauhtilizpatli

Venerious herb, *Tlaquauh tilizpatli, Medicina venerea*. T. it's of a sweet taste, like Licorice, hot and moist [in the second degree]. V. Applyed and drunk it couseth [*sic*] venery and helpeth the diearrhoea in children 2 [drams] of the powder being taken. It also purgeth the urinarie passages, and expells the stone of the reines.

Acuitzehuaríraqua

Alexipharmick herbe, *Acuitze huariacua, Herba adversa venenis*. T. the root (which is chiefly used in Physick) is somewhat cold, and moist, and of a sweet taste. V. the juice thereof drunk helpeth the heat of feavers, corroborateth the heart, and resisteth poyson. Drunk and applyed it helpeth the heat of the reines, and acrimonie of urine, and causeth appetite. It helpeth the tumors of the jawes, and paines of the breast, and is a panacea.

Atehuapatli

River herb, *Atehuapatli, Herba nascens juxta rives*. T. It's cold and moist, with a little astriction. V. the root drunk causeth fecundity, and preventeth abortion.

Oceloxóchitl

Tiger flower, *Ocoloxochitl, Flos tigris*. T. the root is cold. V. 1 [dram] of the root drunk in water helpeth the feaver, and causeth fecundity. It's of cold and pleasant nutriment, loosening and helpfull to the breast.

Omixóchitl

Bonie flower, *Omizochitl, Flos Osseus*. T. the root is cold and moist, salivous and lubricous. V. the root applyed repelleth tumors: drunk it helpeth the heate of feavers, and fluxes of a hot cause.

Hoehoetzontecómatl

Old mans head, *Hoehoetzonte comatl, Caput senis*. T. the root is cold and moist, and strengthening. V. Applyed it helpeth tumors. Drunk it helpeth feavers.

Coacihuizpatli

Anodyne herb, *Coaciuizpatli, Medicina doloris*. T. it's a little hot, and without much taste. V. the decoction thereof helps the French pox: three handfull of the leaves being boiled in 3 [pounds] of water, and drunk. Also it helpeth all paines, especially of the joints, 10 [ounces] thereof being drunk every morning.

Henry Stubbe

Mecaxóchitl

This sort of *Spicery* is hot in the first Degree, and dry in the second; it is Cordial, good against Wind, and Poyson; it brings away the dead child, it provokes Urine, and the Terms; it gives quick delivery in time of a hard labour; it opens Obstructions, and strengthens the body with a moderate adstriction; it repairs the decay of natural heat, and fills with nourishment passing to each part with new spirits, it strengthens the Liver, and is of an excellent temper, and Aromatique mixture.

Xochinacaztli

There is no Ingredient in *Chocolata* of greater esteem, by reason of its Aromatical and Cordial virtue, and excellent smell: it is *hot* in the third, and *dry* in the second Degree, it strengthens the Heart, and Vital parts, it begets many and strong Spirits, and especially the Vital Spirits of a strong mixture, not dissipable: and it hath an excellent taste.

John Chamberlayne

Achíotl

⟨This⟩ is [Hernández] says a Tree, in greatness, body, and shape very like the *Orange* Tree, its Leaves are like those of the *Elm* in Colour and roughness, its Bark, Body, and Branches are reddish drawing to a Green, its flowers are large, distinguished or divided into five Leaves in the shape of a Star, of a whitish Purple Colour, its fruit is like the outward Shell of a *Chesnut,* of the form and bigness of a little green *Almond, Quadrangular* or four Square, which being ripe opens it self, containing certain grains or Stones like those of the *Raisins,* but much, more round. The Savages and Natives of the Country have it in great Esteem; and Plant it near their houses, 'tis green all the year round, and bears its Fruit in spring time, at which time they have a custom to lop it, for out of its wood they Strike Fire as with a Flintstone, its bark is very proper to make Ropes, which shall be stronger than that which is made of Hemp it self, of its seed they make a Crimson red tincture, which the Painters imploy in their Colours, they make use of it also in Physick, for being of a cold quality, and being drunk with some Water of the same Nature, or applyed to the outward parts, allays the ardour and burning of the Feaver, hinders the Dysenterie or griping of the Guts, lastly they mix it with great profit and success in all the cooling potions, whence it happens that they mix it with the drink of *Chocolate* to cool, and to give it a taste and fine colour, *sed haec obiter.*

Hans Sloane

Tomahuactlacopatli

The Root is bitterish, hot in the third Degree, smelling sweet and rosiny. If put in form of a Poultess on Swellings it Cures them. It eases pain, and puts off the cold fit of an Ague. It strengthens the Heart, Stomach and Brain. Cleanses the Stomach and Breast, and stops Fluxes.

Piña de las Indias [pineapple]

It corrodes a Knife in a night, if it sticks in it. *Xim. Laet.* It is cold and dry, it is given to those in Fevers to cool, and excite Appetite, though apt to turn to Choler. A slice held on the Tongue quenches thirst, and moistens the Tongue. *Hernand.*

Cococxíhuitl

It is hot and dry in the fourth Degree, with some Adstriction. The Twigs bark'd take off spots and marks from the Eyes, The juice consumes Wind, cures Tetters as well as the Fruit, and eases pain from cold Causes. The Leaves cure old Sores, being applied to them. They take off Warts, especially

those of the *Præputium* and *Pudenda,* which has been found by most certain Experiment. It is likewise called *Quauhchilli,* from being as sharp as *Indian* Pepper, and was planted by the *Indian* Kings in their Gardens.

Chicállotl

The Seed powdered and taken to the quantity of two Drams, purges all Humours, especially Flegm from the Joints. The Milk, with a Womans Milk that bore a Female, dropt into the Eyes, Cures their Inflammations. It is good against intermitting Fevers. The Flower applied Cures the Scab. The Tast is bitter, and it is hot and dry. Its distill'd Water, with the tops of *Mizquitl* takes spots out of the Eyes, and eats Proud Flesh, takes away pains of the Head, and helps other such Diseases.

Olcacatzan pahuatlánico

It yields a Gum called *Tzitcli,* which the *Indians* chaw to strengthen the Teeth. The Decoction is good against Chronical Distempers, against the *French Pox.* Oriental *China* has a lighter, not so firm, tenderer, and less Adstringent Root, and yet this Kind does the same with it, *Sarsa* or *Guajacum,* if the same methods are followed. It is Cold, Dry, and Adstringent, but bitterish, and of subtle parts, strengthening the Stomach, expelling Wind, voiding by the Pores Melancholick Humours and Flegm, which eludes other Medicines, thereby giving ease.

Tozcuitlapilxóchitl

This Plant repels Tumours, for the Root which is used is glewy, of a sweet tast, and cold and moist.

Iztaccíhuatli

The Decoction is given to Women in Childbed. It dissipates Wind, provokes the *Catamenia,* is good against Convulsions, takes away Gripes, and is a remedy against all sorts of Cold, for it is hot and bitter.

Chichicahoazton

I question not this being the Plant mentioned by *Hernandez,* called *Cohayelli,* every thing agreeing to it. He tells us that,

It is hot in the fourth Degree, tasts like Skirrets, though a little sharp and smelling. The Root powdered, and taken to the quantity of three Drams in ten Ounces of water, strengthens the weak and cold Stomach, eases pains of the Belly and other parts from Colds, dissipates Wind, is good for Colick and Iliack Diseases, is Diuretick, and helps the *Catamenia*, cures Surfeits, incites to Venery, and is good against the Bites of Venemous Serpents. It has a better effect, if it be given out of a hot and strengthening Liquor, it dissipates preternatural Tumours, and humours in the Joints, and remedies all cold intemperatures.

It is called *Itubu* in *Surinam*, or *Fuga Serpentum*, because they come not where it grows. 'Tis *Alexipharmic* from its volatile Salt, and the smell of the Leaves cures Hysterick Fits.

Xiuhquilitlpitzáhuac

This seems to be the *Xihuiquilitlpitxuahuac, Hernandez* and *Xim,* tho' there be a very ill or improper Figure, as may appear by their saying that it is *Ciceris folijs*, these Leaves being not at all like them, 'tis hot and dry in the second Degree. The Powder heals old Sores if they be wash'd with Urine before; bruis'd and put to the Head, they cure its aching, as does their Decoction. They thinks [sic] it would grow well in *Spain*.

Ichcaxíhuitl

The Shoots being stamp'd and drunk with Water, cure the Stinging of Scorpions, Vipers, and other venemous Creatures. The Stalk is cold, dry, and adstringent, powder'd and strew'd on Ulcers, it heals them. The Leaves are also healing.

Xocoxóchitl

Every thing in this Tree agrees with the Description of the *Xocoxitla*, or *Piper Tavasci*, of *Hernan.* and *Ximenes* in the Spanish Translation of *Hernan.* printed at *Mexico, f.* 2. only the Flower, which he describes to be scarlet and like Pomgranates [sic] with the Smell of Orange-Flowers, no way agree to this.

It may supply the Place of Pepper and be used for *Carpobalsamum* or *Carpesium*, it strengthens the Heart and Stom-ach, helps the Mother, expels Wind, the cold Fit of Agues, opens Obstructions, is diuretick, is good for the Colic and Iliac Passions, excites Venery, and cuts gross and tough Humours.

Zayolizcan

This agrees to *Hernandez* and *Ximenes* their Descriptions who say, that the Decoction of the Bark of the Roots and Trunc drank, is good for Uterine Diseases, is diuretic, and cleanses the Body, and that the Roots, Bark or Leaves apply'd, open, cleanse and dissipate Swellings and Ulcers, and heal Burns.

Guayacan

The Flower when dryed turns pale, and does not keep its blue Colour, whence *Jo. Terentius, Lynceus ap. Hernandez* describes the Flower to be of that Colour; in other Things the Description is good, and the *Icon* of the Fruit exact; but there seems to be great Confusion and very few certain Marks between *Guayacan* and *Lignum-Sanctum*, as may appear to any perusing *Hernandez Ximenes* and *Terentius*.

James Petiver

Caranna

Flows from the Trunk of a *Tree* like a *Palm*, which grows plentifully in *New Spain*. Mr. *Lemery* says it's so call'd from *Carthagena* in the *Spanish* West *Indies* where it grows in plenty. It's so famed a *Cephalick, Arthritick* and *Vulnerary*, that it's usually said what *Tacamahac* cannot cure, *Caranna* can. *Hernandez* says it's a large *Tree* with longish L[eaves] growing *Star-wise*.

Tlapalezpatli

Nephritick *Wood.* By reason it's a Sovereign Remedy for the *Stone, Gravel,* and Difficulty of *Urine*, it's also good in *Obstructions* of the *Liver* and *Spleen.* Grows in *New Spain* and chiefly about *Mexico. Hernandez* says it's a large Shrub with little roundish Leaves, its *Flower* yellow, long and little, growing in *Spikes. The Mexicans* call this Tree *Coatli* and *Tlapalz patli.*

James Newton

Huitztomatzin

Huitz-Tomalzin, [or] Tomal spinosa, Recchi. The shrub with a thick root and spinous stems, 4 spans high; the leaf somewhat like Spinach—leaf on the under side hairy and whitish; the flower purple, with some small yellow stamens, the fruit white, like a Cherry. In Temucasensis, &c. in New Spain.

Nature & Virtue. The root bitter and sharp, and hot almost in the third degree: Half an ounce of its bark, bruised, and drunk in water, purgeth all Humours; is good in Dropsies, Fevers, and Difficulty of Breathing.

This seems plainly to be the Spinachia frutescens America. Munting, and a species of Solanum, as Columna rightly notes; and of the kinds above (as we judge).

Amacóztic

Pomifera saxatilis, Mexican fructu caliculato polyspermos; Amacoztic [or] papyro lutea, [or] Tepeamatl, Sycamoro saxatili, Mexican Recchi. There are two species of this; the first is a large tree, with leaves as large as Ivy—leaves almost of the form of an heart, purplish and fat; the bark pale-green on the inside, yellow on the other; out of the stems, which are like them of the Fig-tree, and pliable like them of Sycamore, grows the flower like small Figs, purple, and well furnished with small seeds. Columna has further noted from the dry'd flowers of this, that it has a purplish fruit in a green calix at the bottom, where it is purplish, being at the top red, which cut open lengthwise, five flowers appear in good order, of a blueish colour; the second has the same name and virtue, having bright and smooth twiggs; they grow in rocky mountains of Chietla.

Nature & virtue. A decoction of the root is good to moisten the tongue of the feverish, to ease pains of the breast, & purgeth choler and phlegm both ways, if three ounces of it be put to three pound of water, and boiled to half; its milk cureth ulcers of the lips, and other inveterate sores.

Ahoacaquáhuitl

Ahuaca quahuitl, Mex. [or] Arbor querciformis butyraceo fructu, Recchi. The tree like the Oak, with odoriferous leaves like the Citron-leaves but greener, rougher, and larger; flower small, whitish; fruit, of the form and bigness of an early Fig, black without, green within, moist and fat like butter, of a grateful taste; the kernel whitish, inclining to red, being solid, hard, neat, oblong, a little larger than a Dove's egg, cleaving into 2 parts like that of an Almond, and bitter like the bitter Almonds; e.g. in New Spain.

Nature & virtue. The leaves hot and dry in the 2nd degree fitly us'd in Potions; the Apples hot, wonderfully provoke to Venery, and increase seed; the kernels have an oil press'd out of them, like that of bitter Almonds in savour, colour, and faculty; which helps Dysenteries, Tetters, and marks in the skin, and prevents the cleaving of the hair.

Tzopilotltzontecómatl

Tzopilotl Ximenis, De Laet. the large tree with long and narrow leaves and somewhat large, long fruit, which includes some small, bitter stones, and are of a musky scent, and bitter Almond-like taste, which they leave behind them when they are rotten. There is pressed from them an oily and softning liquor; which also seems to have the faculty of the Oil of bitter Almonds. An Tzopilotlzonte Comatl, seu Capite aureo, Recchi? the tree large, with long, narrow leaves, fruit large, oblong; including smooth bitter kernels. In New Spain.

Nature & virtue. The Oil press'd out of the flower lenifies and clears the skin: The kernels hot almost the 3rd degree, are good for the Breast: The oily liquor thereof is emollient, operates like the Oil of bitter Almonds, discusses Tumours, and helps Coughs; taken into the Nostrils, it purgeth the Head.

Tletlatia

Tetlatiam, [or] Arbor urens Nieremberg, Recchi. This seems also (as Recchi notes) to be the same [as Arbor Indica Pomifera venenata, already said to be the same as "another," whose juice the barbarians use to poison their arrows]; for it agrees in its venomous quality; and its milk so burns, that it makes the hair to fall off by the least touch; and such as work the wood, have their hands and face inflamed and swell'd thereby; but this tree is said to be large, the fruit green (perhaps whilst unripe) of the form and bigness of Unedo. In Tepotzlandt.

Nature & virtue. The bark is cold and dry; a Decoction thereof disperseth pains of the joints.

Illamatzapotli

Yllamatzapotli Recchi. This, as Terrentius notes, seems to be a tree with an ash-colour'd bark, and fruit like a Pine-cone, scaly, 3 fingers and an half long, 2 and an half broad, no ways agreeing with out Pine-cone (when[ce] very likely it may agree with some of these).

Erasmus Darwin

Manzanilla

Hippomane. With the milky juice of this tree the Indians poison their arrows; the dew-drops which fall from it are so caustic as to blister the skin, and produce dangerous ulcers; whence many have found their death by sleeping under its shade.

Afternote: John Ray

The second volume of John Ray's monumental botanical catalog, *Historia plantarum* (London, 1686; 2d ed., 1688) contained an appendix devoted entirely to Hernández. The first part of this appendix is a summary of the first four books of the Rome edition—almost like an annotated table of contents—which gets progressively less detailed as Ray goes through it. The second part is an alphabetical list of all the remaining plants, all the herbs, from the Rome edition. In both parts Ray's notes indicate identifications, some very terse botanical description, and occasionally a medicinal application. Ray's catalog proper also included a few of the plants described by Hernández, drawn from the Rome edition, de Laet, and Nieremberg.

Cocoz xochipatli

Medicine with yellow flowers, Buphthalmum luterum, leaves like bugloss, roots like peony. Glutinous root and stops fluxes.

Cozoyatic

Herb like palm. From root is Pori cap. Low leaves like palm, oblong purple flowers in form of calyxes. The ground root instilled in the nostrils induces sneezing at once; as the Indian doctors called Titici say, this gives an indication whether the sick patient will die or not. The other is a herb that predicts life and death according to Monardes.

Coen (*Coentic*)

Exotic bean with tuberous roots, serrate leaves, nodular pods, lentiform seed, edible.

Cohayelli (*Chichica hoazton*)

Eryngium or (if Terrentius is right) more likely Dipsacus Americanus. Hot and bitter, good against cold.

SPAIN, 1790

OPERA:
THE MADRID EDITION

The *Opera* of Hernández, edited by Casimiro Gómez Ortega from copies he made of the manuscripts that survive today in the Biblioteca Nacional and the Ministerio de Hacienda, was published in Madrid in 1790. The five projected volumes were intended to include descriptions of animals and minerals as well as plants, but only the first three volumes appeared. Gómez Ortega retained the order of the manuscripts, thus returning Hernández's texts to something like the organization he had envisaged more than two hundred years earlier. Gómez Ortega's edition, including his introduction, was translated into Spanish and published as *Historia de las plantas de la Nueva España* (Mexico City: Instituto de Biología, 1942–46). The modern edition of Hernández's descriptions of plants, volumes 2 and 3 of the *Obras completas,* is a Spanish translation of the Latin text of the Madrid edition.

Acocotli, or Herb with a Hollow Stem

(1.25)

The acocotli is a tall herb with a hollow stem, from which it takes its name, long serrated leaves rather like the lovage, but divided in parts by irregular inlets, and flowers and seeds like the canna ferula. The root smells like carrot but is much more sharp and fragrant; it is hot and dry in the third degree, somewhat astringent and bracing. It is, according to conjecture, a type of lovage unknown yet in our world. Its properties are the same as our own lovage, such as the virtue of relieving pains from a cold cause. The Indians use the hollow stems to extract sap from cavities in the trunk of the maguey, and they distill wine in them. They say it cures abrasions. It grows in warm or temperate regions such as Cuernavaca and Tetzcoco, where some call it xalacocotli.

Acocotli of Tepecuacuilco

(1.26)

The acocotli of Tepecuacuilco has a ramified, fibrous root, a round, hollow stem divided at intervals by nodes, almost one cubit long and extremely thin. It has oblong leaves, repeatedly divided at the edge, bland, in appearance like the lovage, and red flowers. This plant seems to be a species of lovage, although the leaves are tasteless, glutinous, and cold and moist in temperament. Ground and powdered like flour, they cure chronic ulcers and swollen legs when applied like a poultice, and mouth ulcers when washed with its juice. It grows in Tepecuacuilco, from where it takes its familiar name, in warm, flat places, near running water.

Tonalxíhuitl

(1.68)

The tonalxíhuitl has a fibrous root like the radish, somewhat purple stems, leaves like the willow, an oblong yellow flower, and seed in elongated capsules. The root is quite sweet, glutinous and refreshing in nature, and moist in temperament. A handful of leaves dissolved in water and either taken or rubbed on the body is said to reduce fevers, and ease fatigue, as well as the pains that come from the French disease, and tumors that invade the legs or the head as a result of a poor constitution. Whether taken or applied, it is also supposed to be a cure for asthma, mumps, diarrhea, burns, and ulcers both internal and external; it mitigates heat in the kidneys and relieves sunburn. It grows in temperate areas like Mexico, or slightly colder ones like Amaquemeca, in all kinds of places. It sprouts with the first rains and flowers with the last, which is why it is called axochíatl, or water flower. It also grows in Xilotépec, where it is known as quequexquicpatli, on account of its piercing property.

Altichipinca

(1.88)

The altichipinca is a small herb, not tall, thin and soft, with hairlike roots, and leaves like the mulberry or pimento, with longitudinal veins, but softer and more pointed. It lacks any discernible taste or aroma, and it is cold and moist. It is administered in doses of one ounce with natural water or water of bugloss, as a treatment for afflictions of the heart that cause the patient to feel great heat. It reduces the heat, gets rid of weakness of spirit, and dissipates fear and anxiety. It grows in the warm region of Pahuatlan in humid places surrounded by rocks.

Axochíatl

(1.91)

This has a root and leaves like an onion or narcissus, of which it seems to be a species; flowers and stems of omixóchitl that sprout upright. It has a certain viscosity with bitterness, and some heat. It is said to alleviate swellings in the feet and groin, to dissolve tumors, and to cure corrosive ulcers. Half an ounce of the powdered root taken with water prevents dysentery. Its sap, mixed in equal parts with human urine and instilled in the nose, stops bleeding. It grows in the country in Mexico.

Round Atlinan

(1.95)

The rounded atlinan, which others call apatli or remedy that grows next to water, has hairlike roots, rounded, hollow, reddish stems that grow four cubits high. The leaves look like those of sage, but are larger and rougher, like bugloss. Each shoot bears yellow flowers tinged with red, oblong, and like little baskets, from which grows a little capsule in the shape of an egg filled with thin, reddish seeds. The root and leaves are ground into a powder that is then dusted on putrid ulcers to cure them. It is astringent and dry, so that it controls diarrhea, dysentery, and other fluxes, especially those arising from a hot cause. It grows in warm areas, such as Hoaxtepec, in barren and wild places.

Apatli of Mayanalan

(1.96)

The apatli of Mayanalan has ash-gray, cylindrical stalks two cubits long, small oblong leaves, and long, slender pods filled with lengthy black seeds that have white filaments attached. It has a bitter taste and a hot and dry temperament. Made into flour and ground to powder, the leaves cure sores, warm what has suffered cooling, and fortify what is weak and slack. It grows in the lands of the Mayanalanese, from which it takes its epithet.

Xánatl, or Water Adobe

(1.97)

The xánatl is a shrub about four or five cubits high; from its fibrous root grow stalks filled with soft pith, nodular, twisted, and similar to those of a fig tree; leaves like a black mulberry's, although smaller, sparse and streaked through with many ribs; and flowers of hoauhtli. The decoction of the leaves soothes the pains of women in childbirth and aids their weakness. It grows in the hot climate of Papalotícpac, in moist and watery places, from which it takes its name. There are also other plants that have taken their denomination from water; but as they seem to belong to the ferns, they are put aside to be described in that place.

Ahoacaquáhuitl or Tree like the Oak and That Gives Fruit

(1.103)

This is a tree[1] with leaves like the cedar but greener, wider and rougher. The flowers are small and white, tinged with yellow. The fruit is shaped like an egg but in some places it is much larger or about the size of a caprifig—wild fig. It is black on the outside and green inside. The inside is fatty like butter and tastes like sweet nuts. The leaves are aromatic and are hot and dry in the second degree, and are commonly used for external medicinal cleansing. Its fruit is also hot, agreeable to the taste and of some nutritional value. It is fatty and moist and greatly excites the sexual appetite and augments semen. It has white seeds, somewhat reddish, which are solid, heavy, shiny and divided into two parts and like almonds, oblong and a little larger than pigeon eggs. These seeds have the taste of bitter almonds, and produce, when they are pressed, an oil similar to that of almonds not only in aroma but also in the taste and with respect to other properties. The oil cures itching and scars and is also good for those suffering from dysentery, for which it offers some astringency; and it keeps hair from breaking. The tree has leaves year round and grows spontaneously anywhere. It is also cultivated, even though it grows better and reaches its best development in warm places and in the plains.

Acaxaxan or Marsh Plant, Tender Plant That, If Squeezed between the Fingers, Crumbles

(1.106)

The acaxaxan, also called tochnacaztli or rabbit's ear, because of the shape of the leaves, is an herb that grows near

rivers and lakes. Its long root has fibers near the nodes, a stem like a stick of cane or of cinnamon, also with knots and internodular spaces, and leaves that look like those of the pondweed, of which it seems to be a variety, which become red toward the tip, and a small, scarlet-colored flower. It grows in mild or slightly warm regions, like Mexico, near marshy and watery places. Two varieties of this plant can be found, very similar in form and properties. Both are cool and moist in nature, bring fevers down, cure scabies and dysentery, help in cases of depression, dissipate irrational fears, and invigorate those lacking spirit.

Acacóyotl 2

(1.129)

The second acacóyotl, also called acoyo or acóyotl, has a fibrous root, thick stems five cubits long, large, almost heart-shaped leaves, and a flower like a large pimento. It is hot and dry in the third degree, very fragrant and pleasant tasting, with a flavor of caucalis and cinnamon, or anise. The tender shoots, which are like fennel, are edible, and are usually prepared with sugar. Although it seems to be entirely like anise in all its virtues, except that it is a little more astringent, the Indians, who recognize some virtue in all their herbs, say only that it binds the stomach and eases stomach inflammation and pain. Perhaps this is a species of the acueyo, of which we shall speak in its place, or possibly it is the same herb, different only because of the conditions in which it grows. It grows in the warm climate of Pahuatlan, next to streams.

Chayotli, or Plant That Bears Fruit like Burrs

(2.18)

This is a voluble, climbing plant that grows in cultivated places and gardens. It bears a thorny fruit the form and size of a very large testicle, with white pulp surrounding a stone like an acorn, almond, or bean. The stems are long and thin with many tendrils; spaced-out leaves, angular and, up to a point, like those of the vine or squash. The fruit is eaten cooked, and a lot of it is sold in the markets; the interior

1. Avocado tree.

stone tastes rather like cooked acorns, with a tang of the sea, like grilled oysters, although it also seems like sweet potatoes or chestnuts. It is not bad as food, and is quite pleasant, but as far as I know it has no other use. It grows in mild or warm climates, such as Cuernavaca.

Chiantzotzolto, or Herb Resembling the Chiantzotzolli

(2.64)

The chiantzotzolto—which some people call tecamactlactlatzin, or "medicine that makes a sound in the mouth"; and others quauhtilizpatli because it excites the sexual appetite; and others mecapatli—is an herb with a fibrous root, from which grow many stalks two spans long with leaves at approximately four-inch intervals: oblong, small, bunched together, intermingled with medium-sized, oblong, white blossoms with purple [in them] and many yellow filaments that grow in all directions. It has an astringent, sweet nature; and thus the leaves, when they have been crushed and taken with some astringent drink, stop up abdominal flux. The root, which is a little acrid, when it has been crushed and taken in a dose of two drams, provokes vomiting; it also cures swellings and sores, and its decoction alleviates the French disease. It grows in flat, hot places in Yacapichtla.

Apárequa or Warm Herb

(2.85)

Apárequa is a kind of nettle with large leaves, serrate and round, of which there appears to be another species with much smaller stems, scarcely four spans, and very much smaller leaves. They stimulate numb or half-dead flesh, or those who have pain without inflammation in any part of the body, with very good results. Both species are also highly regarded by the natives to treat fractures and the pain they cause, to which the ground, hot leaves are applied in the form of a plaster. It grows in cold and damp regions, such as Pátzquaro in the province of Michoacán.

Ocopiaztli 2

(3.49)

The second ocopiaztli, which also is called hoitzcolotli, or scorpion's tail, is a spiny herb with a rounded, fibrous root,

from which sprout leaves with very long and narrow thorns and long, cylindrical, smooth stalks, at whose ends are stuck on spiny little heads similar to the teasel's, covered with purplish small blossoms. The root is similar to that of the caraway, in [having] a certain sweet taste and in its scent, and its nature is hot and dry in the second degree. The liquid in which it has been steeped for some time is usually administered by Indian doctors to those recovering from fever; with the result that, when all the humors that caused [the fever] have been evacuated through urine or through sweat, the patient is rid of it completely. In like manner it benefits those who suffer from illnesses in the joints; and it is usually employed in other, similar cases with great usefulness. It grows in Tenayuca, in wooded hills and moist places.

Xochiocotzoquáhuitl or Liquidambar Tree of the Indies

(3.57)

This is a large tree with serrate leaves like the larch, divided into three points and two hollows, pale on one side and darker on the other, and it has burrlike fruit. It is hot and dry in nature, and has a pleasant fragrance. A cut in the bark, which is red and green releases a sap that the Creoles call liquidambar of the Indies, and the Mexicans call xochiocótzotl, very similar to storax in aroma. The sap is hot in the third degree. Mixed with tobacco it strengthens the head, stomach, and heart, it induces sleep and eases headaches from a cold cause. On its own it stops humors, eases pains, and cures rashes caused by punctured skin. An oil can be obtained from this tree, either spontaneously or by making incisions in it, just as good as the sap described above, both in fragrance and in medicinal use. Both get rid of flatulence, resolve tumors, aid digestion, improve tonicity in the stomach, alleviate affections of the uterus and other similar things, either alone or mixed with other medicines. Some people prepare a kind of perfume by boiling the stems in water, but it is inferior and less effective for the purposes I have spoken of. It grows in warm, wooded places, and sometimes also in milder ones, such as Hoeyacocotla, Quauhchinanco and Xicotépec.

Tlachichinoapatláhoac, or Burned Broad-Leafed Herb

(3.66)

The tlachichinoapatláhoac, which other people call texixiuhuitli, or (as it were) "herb of the rocks," has a thick and fibrous root, sweet and of a moderate temperament, or slightly cold and dry; from which grow stalks a cubit in length, with leaves like a cedar's or the greater heliotrope's, of which it seems to be a variety, and on the ends of the branches blossoms resembling those of that same heliotrope. They say that it cures sores, gets rid of toothaches, scabs over mouth ulcers, shrinks swellings, eases fevers, and cures the itch and alopecia. Especially when mixed with salt and soot, it alleviates dysenteries and purges those who suffer from acute fever, when it is taken in a half-ounce dose with sediments of xocóatl. It grows in Ocpayocan, Yauhtépec, Tlachmalácac, Apaztla, Teloloapa, and other equally hot regions.

Apoyomatli or Phatzisiranda

(3.96)

The apoyomatli is a type of pithy reed, nodular, a cubit and a half long. It has long roots, thin and villous, but with rounded, knotlike tubercles, and a small, narrow flower. It is fragrant, bitter, warm and dry in the third degree, almost reaching the fourth, somewhat astringent, and has a resinous taste. Crushed and taken, it eases pain in the skin; applied to the bowels it prevents diarrhea; it strengthens the stomach, brain, and heart, excites the sexual appetite and is good for the uterus. It grows in Tacámbaro and in Tepecuacuilco, next to streams and moist places. It seems to belong to the species of cypress. Some people call the roots of this herb the beads of Saint Helen.

Ecapatli

(3.128)

When the leaves are washed and placed on the stomach it helps infants who vomit their milk. When it is applied as an ointment, it relieves headaches and chills of fever. It is also good for surfeit and leprosy.

Ancoas or Male Ginger

(3.200)

This has rougher and thicker leaves than common ginger, but the same shape, also a bigger and thicker root, and a sharper taste with a certain bitterness. The natives use it, pounded and sprinkled with walnut oil and applied, to treat stomach and belly illnesses with a cold cause. It is also used for septic wounds, in the form of a wick soaked in the same oil and introduced. They say that the male has stronger medicinal powers than the female, from which the natives of the Philippine islands also make certain wines of which we will speak later. They take four parts of the juice of the female ginger, one of the male, two of cane sugar, a little tanglat root (which we will discuss in its place),[2] some basil or other aromatic herbs that come to hand, fifty grains of common pepper, two parts cinnamon and a quenice[3] of rice. They form all this into a mass and make it into cakes that they set out in the shade to dry four or five days, then expose them for a while to sunlight, and finally keep them in a smoky place for subsequent use; old ones are considered better. They then take a medimno[4] of rice, some millet, or if they have none, they substitute the seed called borona, and boil it in enough water until all the liquid has evaporated. Next they put it out in the open to cool, mix it with three quarters of a cake, ground, which the natives call tapai, keep it in a partially covered barrel, leaving an empty space of four inches, and they leave it there with the mouth uncovered until it solidifies; then they cover it with leaves of plantain and camotli and leave it for three days, after which they fill the empty space with mud of ashes, cover that with the same leaves, and keep it that way up to a year and a half, although after as little as a week it can be used, and can be taken willingly, this being how to drink it: remove the ashes from the top, cover the mouth of the barrel tightly with leaves, fill the empty space with water, and sucking on the end of a tube, drink your fill. As the wine is drunk it can be replaced

---

2. Unidentified.
3. 1.1 liters.

4. 52.5 liters.

by water until it is entirely diluted. One hundred Indians often gather together to drink the contents of one barrel, and they come away completely sober, which is surprising, but it is because they almost always fill the barrel with water six times and drink it all the same day it is opened, without keeping it any longer. They say that this type of drink is excellent and healthful, that it is superior to all the wines of those islands, with the exception of ours.

Second Anónima of Michoacán

(3.214)

This is a herb with ramified roots, which grows many narrow, cylindrical stems, with leaves spaced out and opposed, rounded and of medium size, and in the top branches yellow flowers, round, medium sized, and usually in groups of three. I know nothing of its properties yet.

Chuprei, or Charápeti 2

(4.6)

The chuprei is a shrub with a thick and long root, white and red on the outside and on the inside white and yellow with purple in it, whence comes the name; from it many slender branches grow: long and of a dark green ⟨color⟩ that tends toward blue, cylindrical, plain, and full of leaves like a citron's but bigger and yellow, and star-shaped flowers. It lacks noticeable flavor or scent, and is of a dry and astringent nature. The indigenous peoples consider this plant very valuable and hide its properties with great secrecy; but with diligence and care, we were able to wrest them out of them. They aver that it outdoes and surpasses the rest of the Michoacanese plants in easily calming the ills that the French disease creates, and in curing complaints of the nerves, scabies, and other pernicious and unruly illnesses that do not yield to lighter remedies. For this reason the root is boiled in the quantity of one ounce in two gallons of water, until reduced by a third; and the decoction is taken in a dose of half an ounce daily, ⟨the patient⟩ sticking to the same diet as is customarily prescribed to those who are taking the decoction of guaiacum. The same decoction, when it is taken and rubbed on as an ointment, cures the swel-

lings, the sores, and the rest of the symptoms that proceed from the French disease. It reduces swellings of the face and the arms, stops dysenteries, excites the appetite, and fattens up emaciated persons. It grows in the hot, watery, moist places of Michoacán.

Coconut Tree

(4.16)

This tree, which the Indians commonly call maron, and which Strabo (as some say) calls palm, and which bears a fruit that the Mexicans call coyolli, the Portuguese coco because of certain "eyes" resembling those of the cercopithecus, and which the Persians and Arabs call narel, is a tall tree, the size and shape of a palm, among whose species it should undoubtedly be classified, with spongy, light, and ferulaceous wood, and round or slightly square fruit the size of a human head, which slowly ripens in one to three months and sometimes weighs the tree down with seven or eight clusters weighing 160 pounds. Almost all the parts of this plant are very suitable for human use. The wood is fuel for bonfires and hearths glow with it; in several countries ships and their decks, rudders, and masts are made from it, as are roofs for houses. There are two main species of these palms, one good for its fruit, the other for the liquor that is extracted from it; the sap that exudes from the shoots and soft racemes, tied at the tip and cut, is collected in glass tubes and other containers and takes the place of wine. The first day it is sweet, then in the next three or four days it is unpleasant, and after that it is entirely useless, but always smells bad and produces gross humors and wind; it is moderately moist and hot, smoother than our wine, and causes fewer headaches if no other intoxicating substance—such as mangrove, of which we will speak in its proper place—is added to the glasses in which it is collected. They say that this kind of wine is wonderfully good for consumptives, and that it is equally effective for urinary and kidney trouble, that it is effective in the Philippine islands, among the natives or among us, for those who suffer from these illnesses, for they clean these parts out with this drink and they break down and expel stones. They say, furthermore, that it does harm to those suffering from obstructions, mainly if they are splenetic or dropsical. If this wine is exposed to the sun or kept in such a place for eight or ten days, it turns into a very strong vinegar, but less dry than ours, and put to the fire it immediately loses all its acidity, so it is mixed with foods when they have already cooled down. It keeps a long time, but if it is mixed with water it loses its potency very quickly and goes off. From this wine, heated and reduced, honey and sugar are made, pleasant enough that many people, mainly the natives, prefer them to real honey and sugar, which are also plentiful. The sugar's temperament is hot and moist, it tastes pleasant, and keeps well without rotting; it clears the skin, relieves catarrh, strengthens the stomach and brain, and aids digestion. The stone is covered by two layers; the outer one is bristly, like woven threads of hemp or burlap, edible at first in the species of sweet palms, with a flavor like the leaves of the artichoke plant, but sweeter and more astringent, very effective for stopping diarrhea, curing indigestion and toning up the stomach. This outer rind is used to make fuses for burning powder in warring armies, very strong cords and ships' ropes that do not deteriorate in the sea air, and the fiber is especially useful for filling the joints between planks, because it swells as it gets damp and so covers the gaps better and more effectively stops water getting in. The inner rind that covers the stone is shiny, harder, and black in color; beautiful vases are made from this, decorated with gold and silver, and it is reported that very healthy drinks can be made from it and that (for I know only its virtues) they alleviate paralysis and strengthen the nerves. Inside is the pulp or marrow, intense white, edible and with a flavor rather like sweet almonds. Chopped and crushed, the pulp yields, without any need for heating it, a milk that is very useful for killing worms, principally in children and youths if an eight-ounce dose is taken with salt in the mornings. It is added to certain dishes, such as rice, or the so-called blancmange, and others of that sort. Like the pulp, it provides a coarse food and is difficult to digest; it increases phlegmatic humors in people who already have plenty of them, without doing any immediate harm, so much so that those with robust constitutions who are accustomed to such food suf-

fer no ill effects at all; its only effect is greatly to excite the sexual appetite, as is corroborated by the experience of the inhabitants of the islands known as the Ladrones,[5] where it is the staple food. It is smashed and cut in chunks, then taken thus to places that do not produce it, and it replaces chestnuts, which are kept for later use. From the grated pulp, boiled in a sufficient quantity of water and stirred a lot, an oil is obtained that can be eaten straight away if it is freshly made, and is very good for medicinal purposes. It is sweet, liquid, transparent, and tastes like the oil of sweet almonds; in nature it is hot and moist, and taken in the quantity of six or eight ounces, with the addition of water in which tamarind has been dissolved, gently purges the stomach and the intestines, and mainly expels atrabilious and phlegmatic humors even though the pulp is said to bind the stomach; but it must be fresh when it is consumed. It eases pains, principally those that come from cold causes, and admirably heals wounds, since it slows the blood, cleans and washes out pus, relieves the pain and hastens scarring more effectively than the oil known as Aparicio.[6] Smeared on the skin, it smoothes and cleanses, and serves so many other purposes that it would be difficult to list them all. From those pieces mentioned above a good oil can be extracted for lamps as well as for preparing rice, and is very effective in relaxing strained nerves, relieving chronic pains in the joints, and killing worms. Each nut contains, besides, a white liquid like whey or milk, in a quantity of about three pounds, good for quenching the thirst, reducing fevers, moderating heat, curing and washing the eyes, and cleaning women's skin. This water refreshes and moistens, corrects the blood, purges the stomach, cleans the urinary tract, eases pains, cures inflamed eyes, eats away fleshy growths, soothes the skin, and has a most pleasant taste, above all for those suffering from heat and thirst, to whom it never does any harm although they may be bathed in sweat and no matter how much of it they drink, nor even if they take it the following day on an empty stomach. It is very nourishing and wonderful against bilious fevers; it can be taken the same day as another remedy has been ingested, although it does produce wind and should be avoided by any patient with

---

5. Unidentified.

6. A vulnerary unguent created by Aparicio de Zubio in the sixteenth century.

looseness of the bowel or diarrhea. The shoots or heads of these palms are eaten, though with some detriment to the tree, and are very pleasant; neither are the leaves entirely useless, since they can be used instead of a colander to filter the palm wine and they are sometimes used to sole shoes. They grow all over the place in the east Indies, and now in the west Indies as well, mainly in maritime and sandy places. The nuts go to seed and transplant themselves when they have taken root, and so they grow and bear fruit in a very short time, especially if they are carefully cultivated and planted in a warm climate. It is better to start them in winter in ashes or manure, and water in the summer. They grow much taller next to buildings, as they seem to benefit from dust and mud. I think it will be understood from all that I have said that there is no one species of these palms. But there is another in New Spain on the coast of the southern sea, with much smaller fruit, no bigger than we show in the illustration, although, in my view, it has the same properties. There are also in the Philippines, according to reliable witnesses, dwarf palms that scarcely sprout before they give fruit. There are others called bahey, whose fruit they brought to us and which we give in a picture, and those that are called sacsac.

Jícama

(4.29)

Jícama is a voluble plant with a thick root that almost always tends to a round, white shape, agreeable as a food and of a very refreshing temperament; from which sprout slender, cylindrical branches, long and spread about the ground, which have at long intervals clusters of three leaves arranged like a cross and as if cut in a circle through the middle, and medium-sized pods filled with seeds like lentils. The roots are used, which usually are served at the end of a meal and furnish a welcome food to those persons who suffer from heat: refreshing, albeit apt to produce flatulence, and not at all bad if they are hung up beforehand in a well-ventilated place and are left there to wilt. They quench thirst, combat heat and dryness of the tongue, provide a food very appro-

priate for those persons who have a fever, and refresh, moisten, and nourish the body. It grows everywhere, but especially in gardens or similar cultivated places. I have heard it said that these roots at times have been transported to Spain, preserved with sugar or covered with sand, and that they have arrived without decomposing. The Mexicans call it cátzotl, which is "root that abounds in juice."

Quauhcamotli, or Yucca

(4.32)

This is a shrub of ten palms in height and three or four fingers in width, surrounded by some semicircles like knots alternating on both sides. The bark is tawny-colored and the wood white, the pith soft, and the roots like the asphodel's or the sweet potato's—from which it takes its name—but thick, a palm in length, white on the inside, tender, ten or twelve in number, and encased in a black bark unlike any other plant that I have seen. The end of the stalk is red, as are the peduncles and the veins; the leaves are green, tending to purple, and sprout near the end of the stalk, at intervals of a palm's length, seven on each peduncle. The roots of this plant are eaten roasted, and are very similar in flavor to the sweet potato. There is another, poisonous, type, similar in shape to the previous one; but from which, after the juice first has been extracted, they make a healthful and tasty bread called cazabi[7] and xauhxauh on the island of Haiti, which is where it is principally used. We already have told how many kinds of bread are made from this plant, and how it is propagated and cultivated, in the little book that we dedicated to Haitian plants when I was there.[8]

Teucopalli, or Divine Copalli

(4.52)

The teucopalli is an herb with a fibrous root, from which is produced a hollow, nodular, white stalk similar to the giant fennel's; leaves like the acocotli's, or Indies lovage's; at the ends of the stalks a hirsute fruit like the flytrap's, but smaller; and downy blossoms. It has a hot nature, with the result

7. Cassava.

8. No such book is known to survive today.

that, when the root has been reduced to powder and mixed with nanahuapatli and yohualanense, it usually cures the little swellings that come from the French disease. It grows in hot regions.

Tlacochíchic of Ocopetlayuca

(4.93)

This is an herb with a ramified root, from which grow round, purple stalks three cubits in length; serrated leaves resembling those of the sage plant, but a little less broad, whitish underneath and green on top; and at the ends of the stalks white blossoms that break apart into thistledown. They say that the juice from one ounce of the root, taken with water, evacuates phlegmatic humors by means of the lower channel. It is hot and has an acrid, bitter flavor. The people of Pánuco say that it cures the itch and pain in the belly, and that it reduces spleen.

Temécatl 2

(5.85)

A single one of its blossoms would suffice to identify this herb, which grows in all places, for they are red and entirely similar to butterflies' wings. Mixed with the grease of the worms called axín—of which we will speak when we deal with animals—they are said to be an admirable cure for ills from a cold cause.

Purging Temécatl

(5.88)

This has a root resembling the radish's, but more slender, from which grow slender, flexible stalks that creep upon the earth; and upon them sparse, tricuspid, medium-sized leaves; round, medium-sized, yellow blossoms near the leaves' bases, and all along the stalks' length; and capsules filled with seed, villous and whitish on their undersides. When taken in a half-ounce dose with water, the roots evacuate bile and phlegmatic humors by means of ⟨both⟩ the upper and the lower channels. It grows in Acolman, in any place.

Zazacatzin

(5.176)

The zazacatzin has a fibrous root, purple stems, leaves like the pomegranate but much larger, and round fruit larger than a chickpea. The skin of the root, ground and taken in a dose of two drams with water, loosens the belly gently and without harm. It grows at high altitudes where there are no trees in cold areas, such as the pueblo of Tlilyuquitepec in Tlaxcala, where the Indians hold this herb in great esteem, because they believe that they live free of all illnesses thanks to the abundance of this plant.

Zozoyátic, or Plant like a Palm

(6.24)

This has a root and leaves like the leek or the palm, from which it takes its name. On its stem it has long purple flowers in calyxes. The root, crushed and applied to the nose, provokes sneezing instantly and clears away mucus, so that the Indian doctors called Titici use it to predict which of their patients will die and which will recover. A dram of the same thing is said to provoke urine and cure dysentery. Mixed with meat it kills mice, and washing the head with its decoction will kill lice. This is the famous plant that is sprinkled over honey, to exterminate all the insects that walk through the house, especially when they are so invasive and harmful in summer; they are attracted by the sweetness. It is bitter, and hot and dry in the fourth degree. Pills are made from the root and applied to the rectum; the root is good for the chest, purges phlegmatic humors and revives those suffering from an excess of them. In Michoacán they call it xahuique. It grows everywhere.

Wheat of Michoacán

(6.47)

I saw in Michoacán the wheat familiar from our country, but so luxuriant that each ear was three or four times as large. I thought it not unworthy of inclusion in this history. The European type grows here, but none knows it uses.

Tlalcacáhoatl or Small Cacáhoatl

(6.89)

To this herb, whose fruit the Haitians call manies, the Mexicans give the name tlalcacáhoatl[9] because they are similar to those that are called the second type of tlalcacáhoatl. This similarity is especially seen in the roots. These are similar to pine nuts not only in shape but also in the taste, which is like almonds. These are also prepared with sugar and excite the sexual appetite. They are pleasing because of their sweet and appetizing taste. If they are eaten in excess, they produce headaches. They grow in the lands of Cuernavaca even though they were previously found only on the island of Haiti.

Cozticpatli of Acatlan 2

(6.186)

This is a small herb like pond cilantro, with fiberlike roots, yellow within, thin stems with leaves rather like cilantro, and small, villous, delicate flowers. The root is sweet, with a little bitterness, and of subtle parts. A decoction of the roots, taken, provokes urine and eases heat and pain in the kidneys. Taken with water in a dose of half an ounce, the roots prevent fluxes of the belly in children; their juice is good for the eyes. It grows next to streams and in other watery places, mainly in lower Mixteca. It seems to belong to the species of cocóztic.

Curungariqua

(7.9)

The plant known as curungariqua has a thin, long, fibrous root, from which grow thin cylindrical stems about a span and a half long, full of leaves like the cinquefoil, rather long and narrow. At the tip grow little blue flowers that produce round capsules full of seeds. It grows in temperate and humid places in Uruapa, in the province of Michoacán. The root is bitter, hot and dry. It cures cough, asthma, and also diseases of the chest caused by cold or gross and viscous humors. Powder from the flowers mixed with sugar or

honey and made into a syrup, taken every morning in the quantity of two spoonfuls, sharpens the vision, and from this good effect it gets its name.

Cuixtapazolli or Sparrowhawk's Nest

(7.91)

This is a small tree with a whitish stem, smooth, obtuse leaves like oregano, without veins almost, and devoid, so they say, of either fruit or flowers. The leaves, if rubbed, get rid of feverish heat. It grows in the warm hills of Texaxahuaco, and is cold and moist in nature.

Zayulpatli of Oaxaca 2

(7.108)

This has a root an inch thick with a thick skin, serrate leaves in groups of five, like angelica or wild parsnip, to which species I think it belongs, because the white and yellow flowers are similarly arranged in umbels; the seed is round, succulent, fragrant, and slightly sharp. The root, which is hot and dry in the second degree, first tastes like carrot, but the aftertaste is bitter and piquant. Crushed and applied to the belly, it is said to prevent diarrhea, and when eaten, to get rid of a cough and alleviate hoarseness. It grows in flat, mild places and in the mountain passes of Oaxaca and Itzoacan, where it is called cacapúltic, and also in Michoacán, where they call it caniume.

Ixocuilpatli of Yacapichtla

(10.14)

This has fibrous roots, many delicate, narrow, whitish and slightly purple stems, leaves like crowned rosemary, and at the tip of the stems, flowers that separate into woolly threads. The root tastes at first like a legume, but then becomes sharp, is piquant in the throat and seems to be hot in the third degree. It cures the eyes by removing everything that impedes vision, which is how it gets its name. It grows in the warm hills of Yacapichtla.

---

9. Peanut.

Teizquixóchitl, or Izquixóchitl of the Rocks

(10.165)

This is a small herb with branched roots, tawny-colored on the outside and white on the inside, from which grow tender, cylindrical, purple, woody stalks with leaves like a flax plant's, and at their ends blossoms like a chamomile's but with a white fringe and yellow center that sometimes tends to purple. The root is cold and astringent. It is administered in any appropriate quantity to hemoptystical persons[10] with great benefit. It grows among rocks or in craggy places, and it is not completely different from the so-called lesser belis of Spain. The root is preserved for use throughout the year.

Iztapaltlácotl

(11.10)

This iztapaltlácotl, which some call chachayactli, others quauheloxóchitl, and others hoexotzin, is a large tree with leguminous leaves and broad pods full of flattened seeds. Mixed with bark of tzápotl it cures sores; its own bark is prescribed for those suffering from fever, to reduce heat, for which the decoction is also taken. It grows in warm or mild areas, such as Mexico, Yyauhtepec, and the like.

Peyotl from Zacatecas, or the Soft or Lanuginous Root

(15.25)

This plant has a root of medium size that sprouts neither stems nor leaves out from the earth, but only one bud adheres to it. For this reason it is difficult to depict in an appropriate manner. They say that there is a male plant and a female plant. It tastes sweet and is moderately hot. It is used in the following manner: it is pounded and applied and is said to cure pains of the joints. Marvelous things concerning this plant are recounted (if one is to believe what is widely held about this plant) and what they say is that those who eat it can have presentiments about what will happen and they are able to foretell future events. For example, if they are going to be attacked the next day by their enemies, or if they should expect to have happy times in the future. They also can tell who stole a particular object or utensil and other similar things that the Chichimeca try to find out by using this drug. In addition, when they want to know where to find this root, which is buried in the earth, they find out by eating another. It grows in hot and moist places.

Pitahaya of Tepéxic

(15.74)

This has a round root in the shape of a pig's kidney. The striated stems have spines at intervals. They are thin and round and it is on them that the tunas and flowers grow. They belong to the tunas species. The root, which is succulent, is sandy and has no notable aroma. They say that it can cure swelling of the belly and dropsy, but I do not see how this can happen unless it has some other special property.

Tlaelpatli or Medicine for Dysentery

(19.22)

This is an herb with a long root an inch thick, from which grow many narrow stems, almost a span long, covered with round leaves like veronica, serrate, small, and with fruit like the long pepper, but an inch thick. It grows next to rivers in warm places in lower Mixteca. The root is cold, dry, and very astringent; crushed and taken in a dose of half an ounce, it controls dysentery and all the excess flow that requires astringency; it also cures sores.

Xicalquáhuitl or Gourd Tree

(20.24)

This is a large tree with tricuspid leaves, colorless on the underside and with sharply pointed berries: hence its name. Half an ounce of the bark, ground and introduced, is very effective against dysentery. It grows in Cuernavaca.

---

10. I.e., persons coughing up blood.

Acaxílotl

(21.4)

This is an herb with a root in the shape of a radish but covered with a dry and arundinaceous nodular membrane quite like sugarcane. The point where the leaves grow is similar to the plantain but much larger. The root is eaten, either raw or cooked in place of bread, and makes a pleasant food, juicy and not at all bad. It grows in Pánuco.

Cachoz

(21.73)

This shrub is found in the woods of Peru, according to the testimony of reliable informants. It has round, thin and dark green leaves, and fruit that looks like the crab apple, edible and full of tiny seeds, gray, smooth and pleasant to taste, which are said to be diuretic, prevent stones from forming in the bladder, and generally expel any urinary obstruction. If this is a plant that we have described and had painted in New Spain, I cannot say, because I have never seen it: the Peruvians into whose hands my books come can decide and let me know.

Granadilla

(22.35)

They say that this[11] grows in the land of the Peruvians and that it is voluble and like ivy, that its flower is similar to a white rose, and that in its leaves one can see the figures and symbols of the instruments of the Passion of Christ. Its fruit is similar to that of the pomegranate in shape, color and size—from which the Spanish took its name[12]—but without a crown. When it is dry, you can hear the seed rattle, which is similar to that of the pear. The fruit has beautiful markings, is white inside, and has no aroma. When ripe, it is full of a somewhat acidic liquid. The Spanish and Indians break it open and suck out the juice as one would suck out an egg. It tastes good and comforts the stomach, and gives no sensation of heaviness.

---

11. Granadilla: passionflower.

12. Pomegranate is *granada* in Spanish.

AN EPISTLE TO ARIAS MONTANO

Hernández composed his poem to Benito Arias Montano probably in 1580, at about the time Recchi was appointed to produce his selection from Hernández's *Natural History*. The poem was not published until Gómez Ortega included it, as the preface to the *Opera*. The text survives today as Hac. MS 931, fols. 235v–237v. The English text of *An Epistle to Arias Montano* was first published by Rafael Chabrán and Simon Varey in *Huntington Library Quarterly* 55 (1992): 621–34.

An Epistle to Arias Montano

To the most learned and distinguished Arias Montano

Montano, do not scorn your old colleague, who has
already docked at Jerez,[1] who first saw
you in the land of Romulus and who has come, over
the years, to recognize in you
a rare miracle of nature, honor of your people,
5   and ornament of our time. I have come here now to
see you once more,

long after that retirement in which the nine Sisters
taught you, Montano, and filled your mind with the
causes of things,
with different languages, and with the light of
inspiration,
inside the igniferous rocks and walls dedicated
10   to Philip—the king's delight and blessed seat.[2]
You went from there, determined to shape the Bible in
four languages,
an immense and illustrious work, and one of enormous labor;
you went of your own accord to live among the peaceful Belgians and, leaving your country,

---

1. The Latin formula used here, "Astae ripis," gives the fluvial port of Jerez shores, literally.

2. Quite why the rocks are "igniferous" we cannot say (volcanic, perhaps?); but the allusion to the enclosed place seems to be to the Escorial, where Arias Montano was installed on March 1, 1577,

before being sent to Lisbon in January 1578. Reluctantly obeying a royal summons, Arias Montano had returned to Madrid on September 8, 1579. He probably stayed in or near Madrid, without necessarily having much to do with the Escorial, until he resigned the chaplaincy in 1584, after which he retired to Andalucía.

you trod the frozen lands as you traveled toward the
Arctic;[3]

15 while I, searching for the secrets of nature in distant
regions,

sailed—not slowly—to the west Indies,

pledged to obey the clement mandate of Philip,

ruler of the west, who lays claim to the lacerated
earth,[4]

who institutes holy laws and renovates decaying ones,

20 who destroys the unjust and the hostile in the name
of Christ.

Thus after numerous adventures, after holding on
to my cargo,

which I treated with care as I traveled by land and by
sea,

I have been driven by so many misfortunes. Bring me
back

and protect me in your bosom: then you will be called

25 the resourceful guardian and loyal patron of an exile.

There are those who snap at my heels and spread the
poison

of envy, who try to damn my innocuous labors,

which they will not see, or—if they read them—even
understand:

they do not deserve to know what the earth conceals,
yet the mass of good people

30 have to hear the venomous outpourings from their
wretched mouths.[5]

It would only be justice if you drove these people
away, sent them to hell

with your genuine candor, your wisdom and knowledge,

and with you gravitas, your faith, and your demon-
strable moral strength.[6]

Virtue does not rush to deprive itself of a patron,

35 any more than wild boars like to wallow in clean
spring waters.

The time will come soon when we will be able to
shake hands

and you may hear and receive my thanks in person.

Then, as if I were gazing at the sanctuaries of the
Muses,

exulting immensely, I will say not a word, O Montano,

40 concerning our private affairs, so that by my silence
you may know

how indebted to you are these writings of mine, and
how much

gratitude I owe you, and what glory awaits our efforts.

In all important matters, if one takes a great stride

toward the loftiest heights, the effort

45 brings honor to the endeavor—and still curses the
ears

of those detractors by exposing them to a fatal
disease that destroys them at the core.

I have forgotten how I bore such great burdens for
seven long years

(I languished, because I was already an old man without the ardent blood of my youth)[7]

having twice crossed the ocean, and experienced
remote lands

50 and foreign climates, having to eat food everywhere

that took a long time to get used to, and drinking
impure water.

I pass over the intense heat, and the extreme cold,

barely tolerable in any way by the frail or sick,

not to mention the forested hills and impassable
mountains,

55 rivers, swamps, vast lakes, and expansive lagoons.

I will not talk about the perverse Indian guides,

nor will I speak of all their fraudulence, or terrible
lies,

which caught me off guard more than once; how they
played tricks on me,

which I took care to avoid with all the tact at my
disposal;

60 and how often did I get the properties and even the
names of plants wrong

because I depended on false information from an
interpreter:

thus when I had to treat wounds, in some instances all
I had to rely on was my own

medical knowledge and the help of Christ.

I cannot begin to count the mistakes of the artists,
who

---

3. The rhetorical contrast is between Arias Montano footslogging
(*calcas*) across Europe and Hernández swimming (*adnamus*) the
Atlantic.

4. Why the earth should be "lacerated" (*lacerum*) is not clear.

5. No one knows who these detractors were, or if they existed outside Hernández's anxieties. The dual fears of being misunderstood

and being attacked by detractors become something of a leitmotif
in Hernández's letters, above.

6. This is the first of four instances of glaring pleonasms in the
poem noted by Herrera (*OC* 4.26). The others are at lines 37, 42,
and 74.

7. Hernández was about fifty-five when he went to Mexico.

65 were to illustrate my work, and yet were the greatest
        part of my care,
    so that nothing, from the point of view of a fat
        thumb,[8] would be different
    from what was being copied, but rather all would be
        as it was in reality.
        And the delays of the officials, who, time after
            time, when I needed to hurry,
    interfered with my enterprises and frustrated my
        efforts!
70 What do I say? Why did it fall to me to test the medi-
        cinal plants on myself,
    And at the same time put my life at great risk?
    Or those diseases, which caused me such excessive
        fatigue,
    with which I am still afflicted, and which will affect
        me for the rest of my life—
    how many more years will that be?
75 And the hostile encounters, and the monstrous crea-
        tures swimming in the lakes,
    which have stomachs vast enough that they can swal-
        low men whole?
    Oh, why talk of hunger and thirst? or of the thou-
        sands of nasty insects
    everywhere that lacerated my tender skin with their
        bloodsucking stings?
    The sullen guides and the inept servants?
80 The ingenuity of the Indians in the wild, who could
        not be persuaded to reveal
    a single secret of nature, and who were so insincere?
    I leave these things, I say again, and add that what we
        did
    we did only with the grace of Christ and the patron-
        age of his saints,
    as I traveled through the regions of New Spain.
85 Thus I wrote twenty books on plants, and some oth-
        ers too,
    at the same time (besides those that present minerals
    and whole species of animals to human eyes);

Spain cultivates not one of these plants in her fields,
    so I was searching for western ones
90 and, all at once, stalks, roots, and shimmering flow-
        ers of many colors;[9]
    I took into account the fruits, the leaves, and any of
        the names
    of the species as they vary from region to region,
    their medicinal powers, the native soil, the method of
        cultivation, and their taste,
    or the sap that drops from a cut in the bark of a tree:
        which
95 diseases can be cured by it, what is the limit of
        heat,[10]
    what color it is, and whatever substance grows
        beneath the bark;
    briefly, I noted whatever would be relevant to human
        health,
    or whatever else this natural narration of things
        would demand,
    in language as appropriate as I could manage, and
        with due brevity.[11]
100 Indeed, I gave twenty living plants, many seeds,
    and innumerable medicines, to the viceroy to send to
        Philip Augustus[12]
    so that they could be carried with the utmost care
        back to Spain where
    they will adorn the gardens and hillsides;[13]
    and guided throughout New Spain by the brightest
        star in the sky,
105 cities, and settlements, mountains, and rivers. It is a
        very
    desirable thing for our people, that there may be in
        the known world
    lands filled with such riches, called by so many
        names.
    I wrote down a method for identifying Indian plants
    as well as ours;[14] together with any way in which a
        plant may have
110 the power to cure any western disease,

8. Hernández seems to mean that the artists, or draftsmen, would normally estimate the scale of an object by measuring it against their outstretched thumb.

9. The emphasis is on the botanist's need to examine all parts of a plant, i.e., not to examine roots alone, or flowers alone.

10. Humoral heat.

11. Brevity might seem a surprising quality to claim for such a prolific work as Hernández, but see comments in his letters to the king, above.

12. In the translation of Pliny and in Letter 3 [November/December 1571], Hernández likens himself to a new Aristotle and correspondingly likens Philip II to Augustus.

13. Although Hernández is certainly not specific here, he may have had in mind the gardens at Seville.

14. A reference to one of his lost works.

and to differentiate the indigenous from those we
    brought from our mountains by sea
on the long voyage to these lands.
And I added, on the basis of solid proof
and my personal experiments, which medicines are
    rejected by the body,[15]
115 which are better than the ones already known to us,
    and which are worse:
the rest I am silent about, which, if God permits, you
    will see
and emend, when I have come joyfully to your house,
and you give me the benefit of your genius and your
    muse,[16]
and indulge a sweet passion, free of cares.
120   Therefore, if these writings of mine are to
    earn the approbation of another man and cause others
      to consult them,
who can be trusted to give the work all the care and

    scrutiny it requires?
And what if you cannot find, anywhere, people who
    can support
such labor on their own shoulders, and willingly?
125 Oh, who can be judge, censor, and expert,
    who knows nothing of plants wherever they come
      from?[17]
And then, who will see neither my books nor my hard
    work?[18]
And when will I find that my great achievements
    do not lack their detractors, motivated by envy or
      some other vile urge?
130 Will thunderbolts be hurled into humble valleys?[19]
    Therefore, most illustrious sir, read
through my books, and if they prove not unworthy of
    honor,
embrace the ideas just like those of a dear brother
and thus favoring me, embrace me for eternity.

---

15. *Succos,* which we translate here as "medicines," appears to mean the fluids derived from plants (i.e., by crushing, extraction, or mixing with other liquids).

16. Arias Montano's poetic muse was alive and well: his *Monumenta humanae salutis,* a collection of religious poems, had been published in 1571 by Plantin, who also published Arias Montano's *Poemata* in 1589 (though work on the printing seems to have begun in 1587). See *Correspondance de Christophe Plantin,* ed. Max Rooses and J. Denucé, 9 vols. in 8 (Antwerp, Ghent, and The Hague 1883–1918), vol. 8–9 (1918), 193–95.

17. Presumably an allusion to Nardo Antonio Recchi, whose medical expertise Hernández did not hold in high esteem.

18. Knowing that there were no plans for publication of his monumental work, Hernández feared that his writings would never see the light of day.

19. A nice allusion to Horace, *Odes* II, x, 11–12 ("feriuntque summos / fulgura montes"). Herrera (*OC* 6.26) notes allusions to Horace at: line 79 (*Epistles,* I, xix, 19); line 119 (*Odes,* II, vii, 28); and line 129 (*Epistles,* II, ii, 207).

APPENDIX

EXTRACT FROM WILLIAM SALMON, BOTANOLOGIA. THE ENGLISH HERBAL: OR, HISTORY OF PLANTS

(LONDON, 1710)

I. The Qualities of Medicaments are five-fold, according 1. To their Temperaments. 2. As they are Alteratives. 3. As they are Appropriate. 4. As they Diminish something. 5. As they Add or Restore something; all which Qualities we come now to explicate in order.

II. The Temperaments of Medicaments are five-fold, considered. 1. As they are perfectly Temperate, *viz.* neither Hot nor Cold, Dry nor Moist. 2. As they are Hot. 3. As they are Cold. 4. As they are Dry. 5. As they are Moist. In the four last of which, there are said to be 4 Degrees, receding from their principle, *ver. gr.* An Herb which is Hot, may be hot in the first, second, third, or fourth Degree of heat. Again, from the four prime Qualities, these also proceed, *viz.* that a Medicament, 1. as it is Hot, may be hot and dry, or hot and moist. 2. As it is Cold, also cold and dry, or cold and moist; and these likewise in all the four Degrees of Temperature.

III. Temperate Medicaments are such which work no change at all, in respect of heat, coldness, dryness, or moisture.

And these may be Temperate in some respect. 1. As being neither hot nor cold, and yet may be moist or dry. 2. As being neither moist nor dry, and yet may be hot or cold. Their Use is, where there are no apparent Excesses of the four other Qualities; to preserve the Body Temperate, conserve Strength, and restore decayed Nature.

IV. Hot Medicaments (and so also Cold) are considered in respect of our Bodies, and not of themselves: For those Simples are called Hot, which heat our Bodies.

Their Uses are, 1. To make the offending Humour thin, to be expell'd by Sweat, or thro' the Pores. 2. To help Concoction. 3. To warm and comfort the *Viscera*. 4. And by outward application, to discuss Tumours. 5. Or to raise Blisters, make Cauteries, &c. according to the degrees of Heat.

V. Cold Medicaments are such, as cool our Bodies being over-heat, by any adventitious or accidental Causes.

Their Uses are, 1. To cool the Parts or Bowels. 2. To condense Vapours. 3. To thicken Humours. 4. To abate the heat of Fevers. 5. To refresh the Spirits almost suffocated. 6. Allay Inflammations. 7. Repress Sweating. 8. Ease violent Pains.

VI. Drying Medicaments, are such as make dry the Parts overflowing with moisture.

They are used, 1. To stop Fluxes. 2. To comfort and strengthen Nature. 3. To consume a superfluity of Humours. 4. To fortify the Bowels. 5. To restore in Consumptions, where great fluxes of the Bowels have been.

VII.   Moist Medicaments, are such as are opposed to drying, which moisten, loosen, are lenitive, and make slippery.
They are used, 1. To moisten an over dry and constipated Habit of Body. 2. To ease Coughing. 3. To help the roughness of the Wind-pipe. 4. To loosen the Belly. 5. To relax Parts contracted or hardened.

VIII.   Things hot in the first Degree, gently warm the Body being over cooled, and outwardly open the Pores. Hot in the second Degree as much exceed the first, as the first exceed Temperature, and these cut tough Humours, open Obstructions, and the Pores also outwardly. Hot in the third Degree, more powerfully heat, and are able (if much used) to inflame the Body, and cause Fevers, provoke Sweat exceedingly, and resist the malignity of the Plague or Pestilence, and more powerfully also cut tough Humours. Hot in the fourth Degree, burn the Body, if outwardly applied, raise Blisters, corrode the Skin.

IX.   Things cold in the first Degree, qualify the heat of the Stomach, and refresh the Spirit. Cold in the second Degree, are chiefly of use to abate Inflammations. Cold in the third Degree, are Repercussive, and drive back the Matter, repress Sweat, and keep the Spirits from Fainting. Cold in the fourth Degree, stupify the Senses, ease violent Pains, and are used in extream Watchings.

X.   Things dry in the first Degree, Strengthen. In the second Degree, Bind. In the third Degree, stop Fluxes, and restore in Consumptions. In the fourth Degree, stop Catarrhs, and all Fluxes of Blood and Humours; are highly Stiptick, and dry up a super-abundancy of moisture.

XI.   Things moist in the first Degree, are opposed to drying in the same Degree: They moisten the Body, and Parts dryed. In the second degree, they Lenify, loosen the Belly, and make slippery. In the third degree, they smooth the roughness of the Wind-pipe. In the fourth degree, they cure a constipation of the Bowels.

XII.   Thus Medicines alter according to their Temperature: Whose active Qualities are Heat and Cold; and by them Diseases are said to be eradicated. The Passive are dryness and moisture, and they are subservient to Nature.

Doses: *Pouders,* if temperate, or hot, or cold in the first degree, may be given from one Dram to two Drams; in the second and third degrees, from half a Dram, to a Dram, or more; In the fourth degree, from half a Scruple to half a Dram.

GLOSSARY

Although we translate virtually everything except most names into English, some terms either have specialized meanings that resist exact translation into English or are unfamiliar to Anglophone readers in any form. In a few cases (*protomédico,* for example) we use a Spanish term and its English translation indifferently. We generally render the Latin vocabulary of Hernández's botanical and medical descriptions as closely as possible, thus avoiding, as he often did, a large number of technical or specialized terms. Seasoned historians of medicine will not need information about the Galenic theory of humors, but other readers may be puzzled by the repeated appearance, in descriptions of the medicinal properties of plants, of expressions such as "it is hot and dry in the fourth degree, and somewhat glutinous." This is no place to discuss humoral medicine, but we have included as an appendix a concise explanation in English of what such terms mean. Unorthodox as it may be, our source for this explanation is a text written by a hack English herbalist, William Salmon, and published in 1710. We also employ terms that are standard in botanical description: some, such as "elongate" and "serrate" are too obvious to require glossing, but others, which may be unfamiliar to the general reader, are included in the list below.

America, American   The Americas, particularly Spanish America; not the United States.

Audiencia   Strictly speaking, an appellate court, but commonly used to indicate a local governing body in the colonial administrative structure.

Bloody flux   Any flow of blood, but especially that accompanying diarrhea or dysentery.

Calyx   The outermost part of the floral leaves, usually consisting of the sepals and usually green.

Capsule   Dry, dehiscent fruit.

Corymb   An inflorescence in which the stems grow from different levels but reach about the same height, making the flower cluster flat on top.

Dehiscent   Opening to shed its fruit.

Discuss   To dissolve, particularly in expressions such as "it discusses tumors," favored by some seventeenth-century English translators. In our own translations we use the term "resolve."

Don   The honorific title that, in certain circumstances, means *esquire* or *sir* but otherwise cannot be rendered in normal English ("el rey don Felipe" would be King Sir Philip) and is therefore omitted silently. The same applies to the Latin "Dominus" (usually abbreviated to D.), which we omit.

Entire   Usually referring to the leaves of a plant: with an even margin.

Hispid   Of parts of a plant: covered with bristles or stiff hairs.

Mexico City and other place names   Hernández refers to Mexico when he means Mexico City, and to Tenochtitlan on the rare occasions when he is writing about the city at about the time of the Spanish conquest, or earlier. We generally use the form "Mexico City" for clarity. For other place names that have variant spellings we usually follow the recommendations of Ricardo J. Salvador (and others, possibly) found in <http://www.public.iastate.edu/~rjsalvad/scmfaq/PLACENAM>.

Mexico/New Spain   From the early sixteenth century, the Spanish referred to New Spain to indicate territories that came under the jurisdiction of the audiencia of Mexico, territories that correspond, more or less, to the modern country of Mexico. When referring to the territories, we use "New Spain" in appropriate historical contexts and "Mexico" otherwise. Until independence (1821), when "Mexico" was adopted as the name of the whole country, Mexico was just one part of the viceroyalty of New Spain. Hernández speaks of "Mexicans," without always being careful to specify exactly whom he meant.

Náhuatl   Náhuatl is the language spoken by a large group of peoples who, in Hernández's time, inhabited the central Valley of Mexico and points southeast, as far as Guatemala. It is an Uto-Aztecan language, whose speakers included the Azteca.

Names of plants   We give the Náhuatl names of plants in headings as they are generally spelled today. A large part of *OC*, vol. 7, is devoted to competing identifications.

Node, [nodular]   The place on a stem from which a leaf grows.

Opposite   Growing symmetrically on opposite sides of a stem.

Pilose   Of parts of a plant, hairy.

Protomedicato   An official board of overseers of the medical profession in general. The regulatory concept was taken from Spain to the Americas but not put into practice according to the Spanish model until 1646.

Protomédico   Chief medical officer. Generally used in this volume to refer to the *protomédico general de las Indias,* or chief medical officer in the Spanish colonies—the position that Hernández held throughout his time in New Spain.

Pueblo   A village or a small town, especially a country town.

Raceme   An inflorescence with flowers on stalks of about equal length, distributed along an elongated stem.

Scarious   Extremely thin; nearly transparent.

Terms   Menstruation; the common expression "to provoke the terms" meant "to induce menstruation."

Umbel   An inflorescence in which several pedicels all come from one center.

Units of measurement   The principal units of volume and weight are the real, dram, obolus, and scruple; of length, the span, vara, cuarta, and cubit. The weight of one real, a coin, appears to have been equal to 1 dram. It is likely, but not entirely certain, that Hernández was using the Attic standard for the dram, which was equivalent to about 0.15 ounce (4.3 grams), or the apothecaries' dram of 20 grains (about 0.13 ounce or 3.9 grams). An obolus weighed one-sixth of a dram, as Hernández himself explained (*QL* 1.1.9). An apothecaries' scruple was 2 oboli, or one-third of a dram. An ounce was the same as it is today, but the apothecaries' pound was 12 ounces. A span (*palmus*) would usually mean the width of a man's outstretched hand from the thumb to the little finger—about 9 inches. A vara measured 32 inches, and a cuarta 8 inches. A cubit, subject of heated debate for several centuries, was more or less generally agreed to be the distance from the point of the elbow to the tip of the middle finger—a measure that, of course, varies, from about 19 to 23 inches.

INDEX

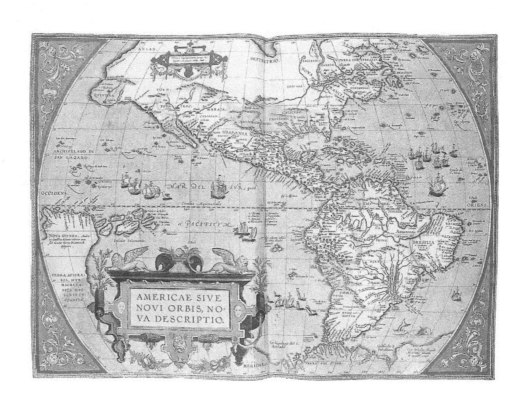

CPSIA information can be obtained
at www.ICGtesting.com
Printed in the USA
BVHW010934140922
646998BV00004B/138

9 780804 739634